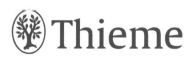

Venous Interventional Radiology

Laura K. Findeiss, MD, FSIR, FAHA
Professor of Radiology and Surgery
Emory University School of Medicine
Chief of Service
Department of Radiology
Grady Health System
Atlanta, Georgia

298 illustrations

Thieme
New York • Stuttgart • Delhi • Rio de Janeiro

Library of Congress Cataloging-in-Publication Data

Names: Findeiss, Laura K., editor.

Title: Venous interventional radiology / [edited by] Laura K. Findeiss.

Description: New York : Thieme, [2020] | Includes bibliographical references and index. | Summary: "The diagnosis and interventional management of venous disorders is a truly core area in radiology, representing a significant percentage of the caseload of an interventional radiologist-up to 75% in some institutions. Covering common disorders such as venous ulceration and varicose veins (affecting half of adults over the age of 50) as well as such serious disorders such as thromboembolic disease, this book will present the state of the art in minimally invasive diagnosis and management of these disorders. Highly practical and authoritative, this book will open with sections on epidemiology, anatomy, and the basics of venous access and then will cover the wide range of these disorders, with practical guidelines and case examples"– Provided by publisher.

Identifiers: LCCN 2020001751 (print) | LCCN 2020001752 (ebook) | ISBN 9781626232730 (hardcover) | ISBN 9781626232747 (ebook)

Subjects: MESH: Vascular Diseases–diagnostic imaging | Veins–pathology | Vascular Diseases–therapy | Radiology, Interventional–methods | Radiography, Interventional–methods

Classification: LCC RD598.67 (print) | LCC RD598.67 (ebook) | NLM WG 600 | DDC 616.1/307572–dc23

LC record available at https://lccn.loc.gov/2020001751

LC ebook record available at https://lccn.loc.gov/2020001752

© 2020 Thieme Medical Publishers, Inc.

Thieme Publishers New York
333 Seventh Avenue, New York, NY 10001 USA
+1 800 782 3488, customerservice@thieme.com

Thieme Publishers Stuttgart
Rüdigerstrasse 14, 70469 Stuttgart, Germany
+49 [0]711 8931 421, customerservice@thieme.de

Thieme Publishers Delhi
A-12, Second Floor, Sector-2, Noida-201301
Uttar Pradesh, India
+91 120 45 566 00, customerservice@thieme.in

Thieme Publishers Rio de Janeiro, Thieme Publicações Ltda.
Edifício Rodolpho de Paoli, 25º andar
Av. Nilo Peçanha, 50 – Sala 2508
Rio de Janeiro 20020-906 Brasil
+55 21 3172-2297 / +55 21 3172-1896
www.thiemerevinter.com.br

Cover design: Keith Palumbo and Konzeption
Typesetting by Thomson Digital, India

Printed in USA by King Printing Company, Inc.   5 4 3 2 1

ISBN 978-1-62623-273-0

Also available as an e-book:
eISBN 978-1-62623-274-7

Important note: Medicine is an ever-changing science undergoing continual development. Research and clinical experience are continually expanding our knowledge, in particular our knowledge of proper treatment and drug therapy. Insofar as this book mentions any dosage or application, readers may rest assured that the authors, editors, and publishers have made every effort to ensure that such references are in accordance with **the state of knowledge at the time of production of the book.**

Nevertheless, this does not involve, imply, or express any guarantee or responsibility on the part of the publishers in respect to any dosage instructions and forms of applications stated in the book. **Every user is requested to examine carefully** the manufacturers' leaflets accompanying each drug and to check, if necessary in consultation with a physician or specialist, whether the dosage schedules mentioned therein or the contraindications stated by the manufacturers differ from the statements made in the present book. Such examination is particularly important with drugs that are either rarely used or have been newly released on the market. Every dosage schedule or every form of application used is entirely at the user's own risk and responsibility. The authors and publishers request every user to report to the publishers any discrepancies or inaccuracies noticed. If errors in this work are found after publication, errata will be posted at www.thieme.com on the product description page.

Some of the product names, patents, and registered designs referred to in this book are in fact registered trademarks or proprietary names even though specific reference to this fact is not always made in the text. Therefore, the appearance of a name without designation as proprietary is not to be construed as a representation by the publisher that it is in the public domain.

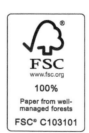

FSC
www.fsc.org
100%
Paper from well-managed forests
FSC® C103101

To my parents, who always encouraged me to keep going and let me believe that anything was possible.

And to my husband, Chuck Ray, who has shown me that everything is possible.

- Laura K. Findeiss

Contents

Preface

Venous Interventional Radiology was conceived as a comprehensive textbook of image guided intervention in the venous system and is intended to cover a broad range of disease states. It is well recognized that venous disorders are, in many ways, the mainstay of interventional radiology practice and are squarely within the purview of the interventional radiologist. However, there are few textbooks that comprehensively address the broad scope of venous interventional radiology practice beyond lower extremity venous insufficiency.

A foundation of this volume is an emphasis on the importance of the clinical management of patients with venous disorders, extending beyond the act of performing image-guided interventions. Using a standardized chapter format and a case-based approach, this text aims to address the nuances of decision-making in clinical encounters, and describes workup, non-interventional management, image guided interventions, and post-procedure care. This richly illustrated textbook begins with an in-depth discussion of anatomy and physiology, followed by a comprehensive review of thrombosis. These chapters are foundational, and the understanding of these topics is critical to excellence in the care of patients with venous disorders. Moving on to a broad range of topics, from chronic thrombosis and acute thromboembolism to portal venous disease and venous anomalies, the remainder of the text is designed to provide a practical guidance in treating patients with venous disorders and may be read in its entirety, or may serve as a reference in preparing for an individual patient encounter. The authors, recruited from both academics and private practice, are experts with extensive experience in venous disorders or venous interventions, and I am grateful for their generosity in participating in this endeavor.

Venous interventional radiology is a rapidly evolving field, and I anticipate that we will continue to increase our understanding of the optimal management of patients with the disorders described in this text. As this volume goes to press, the devices available for intervention in venous occlusive disease are rapidly increasing in number, such that the options described herein can in no way be considered exhaustive. Such is the nature of our dynamic specialty. It is my goal that the expert clinical guidance provided by the authors will serve as a foundation for outstanding patient care as this area of practice continues to develop.

Laura K. Findeiss, MD, FSIR, FAHA

Acknowledgments

I would like to express my deepest gratitude to all of the contributing authors for being willing to take this endeavor on in spite of their many other responsibilities. Their excellent contributions have allowed for the vision of this book to materialize. I also deeply appreciate their patience in getting to the finish line with me.

Contributors

Christopher R. Bailey, MD
Russell H. Morgan Department of Radiology and
  Radiological Science
Johns Hopkins Hospital
Baltimore, Maryland

Maria del Pilar Bayona-Milano, MD
Assistant Professor of Interventional Radiology
Mallinckrodt Institute of Radiology
Washington University
St. Louis, Missouri

Kyle Cooper, MD
Department of Radiology
Loma Linda University
Loma Linda, California

Mary Costantino, MD
Interventional Radiologist
Legacy Good Samaritan Medical Center
Medical Director
CIC-Portland
Portland, Oregon

Nitish Dhingra
Candidate, Bachelor of Health Sciences
McMaster University
Hamilton, Ontario, Canada

Hanadi M. Farrukh, MD
Assistant Professor of Medicine
Department of Internal Medicine
University of Utah
Salt Lake City, Utah

Hector Ferral, MD
Senior Clinician Educator
NorthShore University Health System
Evanston, Illinois

Laura K. Findeiss, MD, FSIR, FAHA
Professor of Radiology and Surgery
Emory University School of Medicine
Chief of Radiology
Grady Health System
Atlanta, Georgia

Kathleen Hamrick, MD
Interventional Radiology Fellow
Department of Radiology
Northwestern University
Evanston, Illinois

Todd Hoffman, MD
Quantum Imaging and Therapeutic Associates
Lewisberry, Pennsylvania

Matthew S. Johnson, MD
Indiana Radiology Partners
Department of Radiology
Indiana University
Bloomington, Indiana

Minhaj S. Khaja, MD, MBA
Department of Radiology
University of Virginia
Charlottesville, Virginia

Robert L. King, MD
Assistant Professor of Clinical Radiology
University of Illinois College of Medicine-Peoria
OSF St. Francis Medical Center
Peoria, Illinois

Bill S. Majdalany, MD
Division of Interventional Radiology
Department of Radiology
Emory University School of Medicine
Atlanta, Georgia

Gordon McLennan, MD
Department of Diagnostic Radiology
Cleveland Clinic
Cleveland, Ohio

Douglas A. Murrey, MD
Inland Imaging
Spokane, Washington

Kieran Murphy, MB, FRCPC, FSIR
Professor of Interventional Neuroradiology
University of Toronto
Toronto Western Hospital
Toronto, Ontario, Canada

Matthew T. Rondina, MD
Professor of Internal Medicine and Pathology
University of Utah Health Sciences Center
George E. Wahlen VAMC
Salt Lake City, Utah

Scott R. Shuldiner, BS
Medical Student
Johns Hopkins University School of Medicine
Baltimore, Maryland

Akhilesh K. Sista, MD, FSIR, FAHA
Associate Professor
New York University School of Medicine
Division of Vascular and Interventional Radiology
New York, New York

Deepak Sudheendra, MD, FSIR, RPVI
Assistant Professor
Clinical Radiology and Surgery
Hospital of the University of Pennsylvania
Philadelphia, Pennsylvania

Clifford R. Weiss, MD, FSIR
Associate Professor
Department of Interventional Radiology
Russell H. Morgan Department of Radiology and
  Radiological Science
Johns Hopkins Hospital
Baltimore, Maryland

Ronald S. Winokur, MD, FSIR, RPVI
Associate Professor of Radiology
Director of Venous Interventions
Thomas Jefferson University Hospital
Division of Vascular and Interventional Radiology
Philadelphia, Pennsylvania

1 Venous Anatomy and Physiology and Epidemiology of Venous Disorders

Kathleen Hamrick and Laura K. Findeiss

Summary

Venous anatomy and physiology, and the epidemiology of venous disorders are critical aspects of the knowledge base of any interventional radiologist caring for patients with venous disease. Venous disorders are a substantial component of interventional radiology clinical practices, with interventional radiologists performing a variety of procedures in multiple venous territories. This chapter provides a detailed overview of venous anatomy and embryology as a basis for understanding collateral pathways, which are described in detail. There is also a discussion of venous physiology, as well as an overview of the epidemiology of various venous disorders cared for by the interventional radiologist.

Keywords: collateral, venous, vein, embryology, intima, adventitia, media

1.1 Introduction

Venous anatomy and physiology have been topics of great interest for centuries. As minimally invasive image-guided procedures have become increasingly common and complex, a thorough understanding of venous anatomy and physiology is essential for interventional radiologists to ensure effective treatment and management of venous disease.

The venous system is an extensive network of vessels with the primary function of returning blood to the heart for reoxygenation and recirculation. Veins are equally important and complex as their arterial counterparts, but are distinct from both anatomic and physiologic perspectives. The manifestations and treatment of venous pathology are also different from those relevant to arterial disorders. Veins are more than blood return conduits; they are dynamic structures responsive to many anatomic and physiologic changes. Veins play essential roles in hemodynamics and contain approximately 60 to 80% of the blood volume at any given time.[1,2,3]

Histologically, vein walls are composed of three layers: the intima, media, and adventitia. The intima is uniformly comprised of a single layer of endothelial cells. Underlying the intima is the internal elastic lamina, a thin layer of connective tissue, present predominantly in larger veins. The internal elastic lamina may be incomplete or absent in small- to medium-sized veins. The media is a layer of smooth muscle cells that varies in thickness based on location and function. Interspersed within the media are connective tissue substances such as collagen and elastin. The adventitia is the outer layer comprised of loose connective tissue, the vasa vasorum, and nerve fibers.[2,4]

While these layers are similar to the anatomic layers of arteries, the relative composition of each layer differs. Arteries are typically thick-walled vessels due to a more abundant media layer. The arterial media contains many more smooth muscle cells and elastic fibers, allowing the large elastic arteries

and medium muscular arteries to accommodate higher blood pressures and pulsatile flow from the heart. Veins have a thinner media layer, decreasing wall thickness, and increasing vessel diameter. Therefore, veins at each anatomic location have a much larger capacitance than their companion arteries, and hold the majority of the blood volume in the vascular system. Regional composition of veins also varies based on vessel size and function. Valves are structures unique to veins and are essential in normal venous physiology. Valves are connective tissue infoldings of the intimal layer covered on both sides by endothelium. The primary functions of valves are the prevention of reflux and retrograde blood flow. Valves are predominantly found in larger veins and lower extremity veins.[2,4]

1.2 Embryology

Embryologic development of the venous system occurs in multiple stages. By the third week of gestation, biochemical signals induce differentiation of progenitor cells such as hemangioblasts and angioblasts. During stage 1, the undifferentiated stage, primitive channels of endothelial cells form a capillary network. The retiform stage, stage 2, is marked by the formation of large plexiform structures. The maturation stage, stage 3, consists of larger primitive vascular channels that begin differentiating into arteries and veins.[3,4] Differentiation was historically thought to be driven by differences in blood flow. However, specific molecular markers also have important roles in vascular differentiation.[5] For example, the attachment of vascular endothelial growth factor (VEGF) to angioblasts determines whether the angioblast will differentiate into an artery or a vein. VEGF binds to the VEGFR2-NP-1 complex in arterial development, while VEGF binds only to VEGFR2 for venous development.[6]

By the fourth week of gestation, venous networks begin to form. The cardinal system drains the body of the embryo. The vitelline (omphalomesenteric) system drains the yolk sac as well as the primitive gastrointestinal tract, and later becomes the hepatic portal venous system. The umbilical venous system carries oxygenated blood from the placenta to the embryo.[6]

The venous system of the trunk begins as paired symmetric structures. As the embryo develops, the left-sided venous structures regress and the right-sided vessels persist to form the major systemic drainage pathways. In the systemic circulation, the bilateral anterior and posterior cardinal veins drain the cranial and caudal structures of the embryo, respectively. The primitive veins of the neck and thorax develop via the anterior cardinal network, which eventually mature and drain into the superior vena cava (SVC). Cranial and facial structures drain into the proximal anterior cardinal veins. Venous plexuses of the bilateral upper limbs fuse to form the subclavian veins and then drain into the anterior cardinal veins. By week 8, an anastomosis forms between the left and right anterior cardinal veins, channeling blood to the right. The conduit becomes the left brachiocephalic vein. Cranial to this anastomosis, the anterior cardinal veins become the internal jugular veins. The anterior and posterior cardinal veins join and become the right and left common cardinal veins. These drain into a common channel, the sinus venosus, which returns blood to the primitive heart. The distal portion of the left anterior cardinal vein regresses. The left common cardinal vein becomes the coronary sinus. As the system matures, the SVC forms at the confluence of the right and left brachiocephalic veins.

Successive venous networks form during embryonic development of the caudal circulation. The paired posterior cardinal veins form an iliac anastomosis in what will become the pelvis. The caudal portions of the veins form the common, external, and internal iliac veins, as well as the medial sacral vein. The cranial portion of the right posterior cardinal vein becomes the arch of the azygous.[4] The subcardinal veins form during the fourth week of gestation and coincide with the development of the mesonephros. The subcardinal venous network arises from the anastomosis of the internal veins of the Wolffian body and the posterior cardinal veins and replaces the posterior cardinal system. The subcardinal sinus becomes the left renal vein. The right subcardinal vein forms the right gonadal vein and portions of the pararenal vena cava. By the seventh week, the supracardinal system develops. The supracardinal system is located dorsally and runs parallel to the sympathetic chain. The bilateral supracardinal veins form anastomoses with one another and with the subcardinal veins on the right. The right supracardinal vein becomes the azygous vein and the left supracardinal becomes the hemiazygous vein.[6]

The inferior vena cava (IVC) forms in segments arising from different embryologic networks. The hepatic segment of the IVC is formed by hepatic sinusoids. The right subcardinal vein forms the prerenal and pararenal IVC, accounting for the relatively anterior positioning of the IVC at this level.[4] The renal segment of the IVC forms from the subcardinal and supracardinal anastomosis. The caudal postrenal segment of the IVC originates from the right supracardinal vein. Due to the posterior development of supracardinal network, the distal IVC and common iliac veins are posterior to the distal aorta and common iliac arteries.[4,7]

Vascular development of the limbs begins with a capillary network arising from arterial structures. As blood drains through the capillary network, blood collects in a marginal sinus within the limb bud. Early on, blood drains through a small superficial network back to the heart. As the limb develops, deep venous structures begin to form parallel to major arteries, and blood is shunted into the deeper veins.[6]

Development of the portal venous system occurs separately through the vitelline or omphalomesenteric system. The vitelline vein transports blood from the yolk sac to the heart. During development, a vascular network from the vitelline vein forms around the primitive duodenum. As the liver primordium proliferates, the vitelline vein fragments and forms the hepatic sinusoids. Cranial to the liver, the vitelline vein drains into the sinus venosus. As the left side of the sinus regresses, the right vitelline vein forms an anastomosis and becomes the suprahepatic segment of the IVC. Caudal to the liver, the anastomotic network surrounding the duodenum becomes a single trunk and eventually develops into the main portal vein. Portions of the remaining right vitelline vein become the superior

mesenteric vein, and the distal left vitelline vein becomes the splenic vein. The proximal right and left vitelline veins become the right and left hepatic veins.[8,9]

The umbilical veins transport oxygenated blood from the placenta. The left umbilical vein persists during development and communicates with the IVC via the ductus venosus. By 12 weeks of gestation, the ductus venosus is developed and carries oxygenated placental blood directly to the heart and bypasses the hepatic circulation. Following birth, the ductus venosus atrophies and closes to form the ligamentum teres.[6,8]

1.3 Anatomy and Variants

1.3.1 Upper Extremity and Thoracic Veins

Veins of the upper extremities develop in both superficial and deep networks. Perforating veins connect the superficial and deep veins.[10] Cardiac function plays a major role in venous return from the upper extremities. Unlike in the lower extremities, the upper extremities do not rely heavily on valves for effective venous return.[4] The major deep veins include the radial, ulnar, brachial, and axillary veins. Deep veins course with the major arteries of the same name. The cephalic and basilic veins are the main superficial conduits. The median cubital vein connects the cephalic and basilic veins. The cephalic vein receives tributaries from the dorsal venous plexus on the radial side of the hand and continues on the ventral radial forearm. The cephalic vein courses over the lateral arm, traverses the clavipectoral fascia, and drains into the axillary vein. The basilic vein receives tributaries from the ulnar side of the dorsal venous plexus, courses up the ulnar forearm, and enters the deep fascia in the mid arm before continuing as the axillary vein.[10]

The axillary vein begins anatomically at the inferior border of the teres major and drains centrally into the subclavian vein, which begins at the border of the first rib.[4,10] The subclavian vein and internal jugular vein join to form the brachiocephalic vein at the medial border of the anterior scalene muscle. The left brachiocephalic vein traverses the chest to join the right brachiocephalic vein at the SVC. The axillary vein receives many tributaries from the chest and neck, and these serve as the basis for collateral pathways in cases of obstruction. The pectoral branch of the thoracoacromial trunk, the lateral thoracic vein, and thoracodorsal vein all drain into the axillary vein. Posterior intercostal veins freely communicate with the anterior intercostal veins and the lateral and internal thoracic veins. The vertebral, internal thoracic, inferior thyroid, and left superior intercostal vein all drain into the brachiocephalic vein.[4] The internal jugular vein receives tributaries from the superior and middle thyroid veins. The external jugular vein communicates with the internal jugular and receives drainage from the transverse cervical, suprascapular, and anterior jugular veins.[11]

A duplicated SVC is the most common SVC variant, occurring in approximately 0.3% of the general population.[12] Incidence is higher in individuals with congenital heart disease.[12] Duplication results from persistence of the caudal portion of the left anterior cardinal vein. An isolated left-sided SVC occurs when the caudal portion of the left anterior cardinal vein persists and

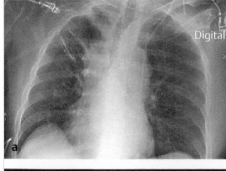
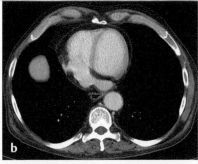
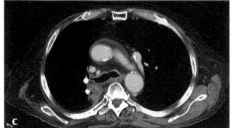
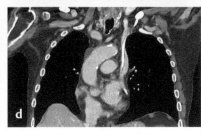

Fig. 1.1 Left-sided SVC. **(a)** Chest radiograph demonstrating alteration of the left cardiomediastinal contour with the central venous catheter projected over the left chest. **(b)** Axial CT demonstrating left-sided SVC at confluence with coronary sinus at the leftward border of the right atrium, anterior to descending aorta. **(c)** Axial CT shows left-sided SVC at lateral border of aortic arch. **(d)** Coronal CT demonstrating left-sided SVC descending to the left of the main pulmonary artery and aortic arch.

the caudal portion of the right anterior cardinal vein regresses. The brachiocephalic vein still forms, connecting the right anterior cardinal vein to the left anterior cardinal vein. The left-sided SVC maintains drainage into the right atrium through the coronary sinus (▶ Fig. 1.1).[4]

1.3.2 Abdominopelvic Veins

The IVC is the major venous conduit of the abdomen and courses along the right side of the vertebral column before terminating in the right atrium. Major abdominal tributaries to the IVC include the hepatic veins, bilateral renal veins, and the lumbar veins. The IVC also receives venous blood return from the pelvis. The inguinal ligament is the inferior anatomic landmark at which pelvic veins begin. The external iliac vein courses through the pelvis, receiving drainage from the inferior epigastric, deep circumflex iliac, and pubic veins. The internal iliac veins receive extrapelvic tributaries including the superior and inferior gluteal, internal pudendal, and obturator veins.[4] Intrapelvic drainage to the internal iliac vein comes from multiple venous plexuses within the pelvis. The presacral plexus, visceral plexus, and pudendal plexus provide free flow between both sides of the pelvis. Major tributaries include rectal, vesicular, uterine, prostatic, and vaginal veins. The external and internal iliac veins join in the region of the sacroiliac joint to form the bilateral common iliac veins, which then join to form the IVC.[4,13]

Duplication of the IVC occurs in about 2 to 3% of the population and results when the left supracardinal vein fails to regress (▶ Fig. 1.2). An isolated left-sided IVC occurs in less than 0.5% of the population and results from persistence of the left supracardinal vein and regression of the right supracardinal vein.[3,7] The IVC ascends to the left of the aorta and crosses over to the right at the level of the renal arteries. The right adrenal and gonadal veins empty into the right renal vein, while the left adrenal and gonadal veins drain directly into the IVC. Renal vein anomalies also occur and can be clinically significant. A posterior or retroaortic left renal vein occurs in approximately 1 to 2% of the population (▶ Fig. 1.3). A circumaortic renal vein is more common, occurring in 1 to 9% of the population.[3,4,14]

1.3.3 Azygous System

The azygous, hemiazygous, and accessory hemiazygous veins form a paired paravertebral venous pathway. The azygous system is an important collateral pathway between the SVC and IVC, and can serve as a shunt in cases of obstruction. The azygous vein is variable in origin, but usually begins at the junction of the right ascending lumbar and subcostal veins. The azygous vein ascends posteriorly on the right side to the level of T4–T6, where it passes anterior to the right mainstem bronchus and joins the SVC. The hemiazygous vein originates at the L1–L2 level and ascends on the left side of the vertebral column. The hemiazygous vein crosses midline at approximately T8 and passes posterior to the aorta and esophagus, draining into the azygous vein. The accessory hemiazygous vein originates from the left brachiocephalic vein and descends on the left side of the vertebral column, draining into the azygous or hemiazygous at approximately T7. The superior intercostal vein, bilateral posterior intercostal veins, bronchial veins, and the vertebral venous plexus also drain directly into the azygous system.[12,15]

The azygous system can be variable and congenital variants are rarely symptomatic. Azygous continuation of the IVC (▶ Fig. 1.4) occurs in roughly 0.6% of the population.[14,15] The hepatic segment of the IVC is absent and the hepatic veins drain directly into the right atrium.[15] Azygous continuation is commonly associated with duplication of the IVC. Typically, the left IVC will terminate at the left renal vein and the right IVC will remain as the azygous vein, bypass the liver, and join the SVC.[15] Separate right and left azygous veins occur in 1 to 2% of individuals. A single midline azygous vein also occurs in approximately 1 to 2%.[12] Incomplete medial migration of the right posterior cardinal vein results in an azygous lobe of the right lung in 0.5 to 1% of the population (▶ Fig. 1.5).[15]

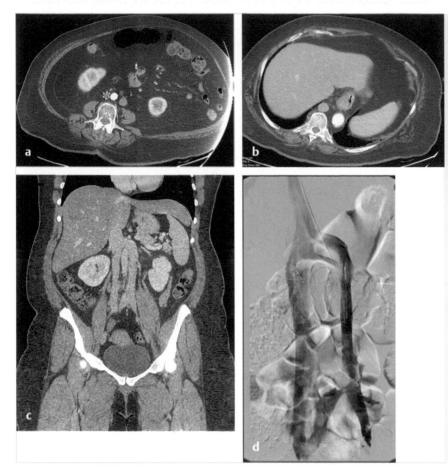

Fig. 1.2 Duplicated IVC. **(a)** Axial CT of the abdomen depicts a duplicated IVC, with IVC filter present in only the right-sided IVC lumen. **(b)** Axial CT of the abdomen showing the extrahepatic course of the duplicated IVC with azygos continuation. **(c)** Coronal CT of the abdomen demonstrates the IVC duplication with confluence at the renal veins and extrahepatic course. **(d)** Inferior vena cavogram of duplicated IVC with filters present in both lumens, demonstrating iliac venous configuration and confluence of IVC lumens at renal veins.

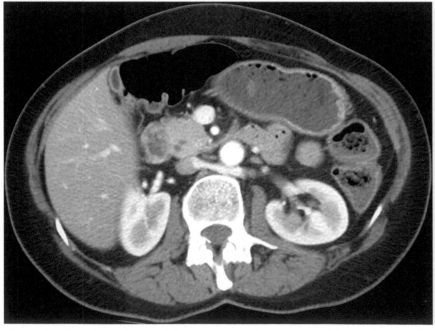

Fig. 1.3 Axial CT of the abdomen with contrast depicts a retroaortic left renal vein, with the left renal vein passing posterior to the aorta.

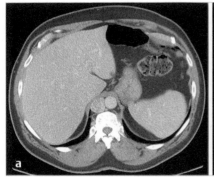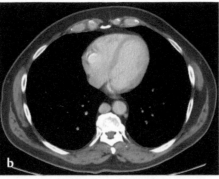

Fig. 1.4 Azygous continuation of the IVC. (a) Axial CT of the abdomen demonstrating IVC confluence located posterior to the diaphragm, with absent intrahepatic segment. (b) Axial CT of the chest shows azygous continuation of the IVC into the chest, with the enlarged azygous vein/IVC coursing parallel to the aorta and bypassing the right atrium.

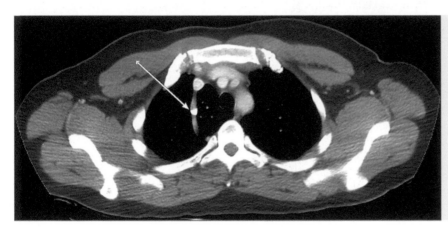

Fig. 1.5 Azygous fissure of the right lung, with the persistently lateral right posterior cardinal vein highlighted by the *white arrow*.

1.3.4 Lower Extremity Veins

Lower extremity veins, like upper extremity veins, are divided into superficial and deep networks. Perforating veins connect the superficial and deep systems. Intraluminal valves play an essential role in lower extremity venous return, helping to maintain unidirectional flow and regulate venous pressure as blood is returned to the heart.[13]

Superficial veins are located outside of the deep muscular fascia. The superficial veins of the lower extremity drain blood from the skin and subcutaneous tissues of the lower extremity. Superficial venous anatomy is highly variable. The dorsal and plantar venous networks comprise the superficial veins of the foot. The dorsal venous arch overlies the proximal metatarsal heads. The medial end of the arch becomes the medial marginal vein, which drains into the great saphenous vein. The lateral aspect becomes the lateral marginal vein, which drains into the small saphenous vein (SSV).[4,13]

The main conduit in the superficial system is the great saphenous vein (GSV), which is contained within the saphenous subcompartment and covered by a fascial layer. The saphenous fascia separates the GSV from the remainder of the superficial compartment.[4] The GSV ascends the medial aspect of the lower extremity, beginning anterior to the ankle and terminating at the fossa ovalis. Duplication of the GSV is a relatively common anatomic. Duplication below the knee is seen in approximately 25% of the population and duplication above the knee occurs in approximately 8%.[4] The SSV begins in the distal calf and ascends the calf laterally in the subcutaneous tissue. The SSV enters the deep fascia in the upper calf between the medial and lateral heads of the

gastrocnemius muscle. The SSV enters the popliteal fossa and drains into the popliteal vein. Often, a small cranial extension of the SSV ascends into the thigh.[3,4]

Deep veins are located within the fascial compartments and run parallel to the major arteries. The deep plantar venous arch receives drainage from the foot, becoming the plantar veins and eventually forming the paired posterior tibial veins.[4,13] The posterior tibial veins drain the deep and superficial posterior compartments in the calf and are located between the flexor digitorum longus and the tibialis posterior. Dorsally, the anterior tibial veins receive drainage from the dorsalis pedis veins. The anterior tibial veins drain the anterior compartment. The peroneal vein courses deep to the flexor hallucis longus muscle and communicates with both the anterior tibial and posterior tibial veins. The posterior tibial and peroneal veins form the tibioperoneal trunk. The anterior tibial vein and tibioperoneal trunk join to form the popliteal vein. The popliteal vein becomes the femoral vein in the adductor canal. The femoral vein and the profunda femoral veins join to become the common femoral vein. The common femoral vein courses medial to the artery and at the level of the inguinal ligament and becomes the external iliac vein.[4]

Perforating veins are the connection between the superficial and deep veins of the lower extremity. Like other lower extremity veins, perforating veins also contain valves, which ensure one-way flow from the superficial to the deep venous system.[13] While highly variable in location, there are several regions where perforating veins are predictably found. In the foot, a perforating vein is usually located between the first and second metatarsals connecting the dorsal venous arch to the pedal vein. Multiple perforating veins are present in the ankle, both medially and laterally. The medial calf perforating veins are the most widely studied, and can be divided into the posterior tibial and paratibial perforating veins.[4] The posterior tibial perforators are divided into lower, middle, and upper sections. The posterior tibial perforators connect the posterior accessory GSV to the posterior tibial veins, while the paratibial perforators drain the GSV.[4] Numerous other perforating veins occur superior to the knee, draining the superficial veins into the femoral vein.

1.3.5 Portal and Hepatic Venous System

The portal vein forms at the confluence of the splenic and superior mesenteric veins, posterior to the head of the pancreas and anterior to the IVC. The portal system receives blood from the mesenteric, splenic, gastroduodenal, pancreatic, and cystic veins. About 75 to 80% of the hepatic blood supply comes from the inflow from the portal system.[8] The main portal vein runs in the hepatoduodenal ligament with the common bile duct on the right and the hepatic artery on the left. The right portal vein divides into anterior and posterior segments in the right hepatic lobe. The left portal vein has a transverse segment supplying the caudate lobe and an umbilical segment that divides into superior and inferior branches. The hepatic veins and portal veins are major landmarks in the Couinaud functional segmental anatomy of the liver. The portal vein creates a horizontal plane, which divides the liver into superior and inferior portions. The major hepatic veins create vertical planes separating segments. The right hepatic vein divides the right lobe into anterior and posterior sections. The middle hepatic vein lies in the main lobar fissure and divides the liver into the right and left hepatic lobes. The left hepatic vein divides the left lobe into medial and lateral sections. The three vertical planes and one horizontal plane divide the liver into eight segments. The hepatic veins function to provide outflow from the liver into the systemic circulation. Intralobular veins coalesce from the hepatic sinusoids, eventually draining into the hepatic vein branches. The right hepatic vein drains the posterior and superior liver segments and commonly joins the IVC separately. The middle hepatic vein drains portions of the right hepatic lobe and medial portions of the left hepatic lobe. The left hepatic vein drains both lateral left hepatic lobe segments and the superior medial segment. The middle and left hepatic veins often form a common trunk before entering the IVC.[8]

1.4 Physiology

The venous system functions to return blood to the heart as well as provide cardiovascular homeostasis through changes in venous tone.[1] Venous return, the rate of blood flow toward the heart, is a complex process requiring a central pump, pressure gradients, peripheral muscle pumps, and one-way valves.[1,3] Veins, unlike arteries, are high-capacitance vessels able to accommodate highly variable blood volumes without significant changes in venous pressure.[3] The heart serves as the central pump, moving blood through both arteries and veins and creating dynamic pressure. Normal right atrial pressure ranges from 4 to 7 mm Hg and capillary bed pressures are approximately 12 to 18 mm Hg, and blood is returned to the heart along this gradient.[1,2]

Venous flow is highly dependent on hydrostatic pressure in the upright position. Hydrostatic pressure is the weight of the blood column below the right atrium, as determined by blood density and the acceleration of gravity. The effect of gravity increases by 0.77 mm Hg per cm of height below the right atrium and the effects of hydrostatic pressure must be overcome in order for blood to return from the dependent portions of the body.[1,2,3] The skeletal muscle pump and venous valves function to counteract hydrostatic pressure in the lower extremities. The calf muscle pump is the most widely studied and produces the most physiologic impact. Contraction of the gastrocnemius and soleus muscles forcefully advances blood back toward the heart, generating pressures of over 200 mm Hg with each contraction. This pressure is enough to eject 60% of the usual 100 to 150 mL blood contained within the veins of the calf.[1,3] Similar physiology is thought to occur in the plantar venous plexus, as well as the thigh; however, the effects on venous return are thought to be minimal in comparison to the calf.

Along with the muscle pump, valves play a critical role in lower extremity venous return. Deep veins in the lower extremity contain numerous valves, at increasingly frequent intervals moving proximal to distal. Deep veins of the calf have valves occurring in approximately 2-cm intervals.[4] A valve is almost always found at the junction of the femoral vein and profunda femoral vein. The proximal common femoral vein usually contains only one valve, and the common iliac vein and IVC contain no valves. Likewise, upper extremity veins contain fewer valves because the effects of gravity are significantly less.[4] The calf muscles also contain venous sinuses, thin-walled chambers able to hold a significant blood volume. Venous sinuses are frequently found within the soleus muscle, and contract with ambulation. Sinuses fill from superficial veins and subsequently drain into the deep posterior tibial veins. The sinuses are valveless, but the draining veins connecting the deep veins contain numerous valves, preventing backflow.[1,4]

Respiration also affects venous return by movement of the diaphragm and changes in intra-abdominal pressure. For blood to drain from the peripheral veins through the abdominal cavity, pressure in the IVC must exceed that of the abdominal cavity. Increase in intra-abdominal pressure, caused by descent of the diaphragm during inspiration, will cause a decrease in the pressure gradient and therefore slow or stop venous return. For blood return from the upper extremities, low intrathoracic pressure creates a pressure gradient favorable for venous return. Therefore, respiration has less effect on upper extremity venous return. In cases of congestive heart failure or pulmonary hypertension, central pressure is elevated and flow pattern depends on right heart function.[2]

In addition to blood return, veins play an important role in hemodynamic stability. Veins have both high capacitance and compliance, allowing the venous system to accommodate as much as a 20 to 30% increase in volume if needed.[1] Changes in vasomotor tone, distention, and recoil of the vein wall allow for these changes in volume. The venous wall is collapsible and varies in shape depending on volume and pressure. When volume is low, the vein walls are coapted and have an ellipsoid shape. Relatively large volume shifts can occur with little pressure change. As volume increases, veins distend to a circular shape, at which point pressure begins to increase more

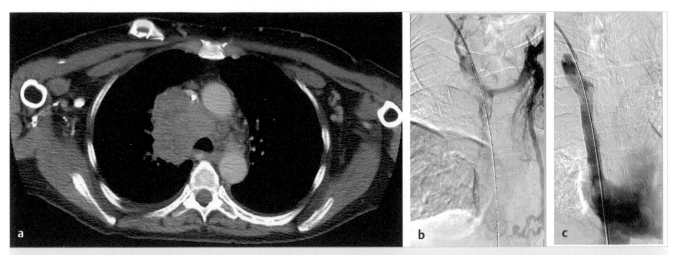

Fig. 1.6 Malignant SVC compression. **(a)** Axial CT of the chest demonstrates anterior displacement and compression of the SVC, caused by mediastinal mass. **(b)** Right brachiocephalic venography demonstrates near-occlusive obstruction of the SVC, with retrograde flow in the left brachiocephalic vein and opacification of a large left internal mammary vein and adjacent collateral venous structures. **(c)** Following deployment of a stent in the SVC, collateral flow through the left internal mammary vein has resolved, with elimination of retrograde flow in the left brachiocephalic vein.

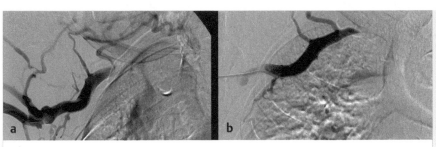

Fig. 1.7 Right subclavian venous stenosis secondary to central venous catheter. **(a)** Right upper extremity fistulogram for high venous pressures during dialysis demonstrates diversion of blood flow into cervical and chest wall collaterals with reduced blood flow into the SVC. **(b)** Selective right subclavian venography illustrates tapering stenosis of the central right subclavian vein, compatible with stenosis secondary to central venous catheter placement.

significantly per unit volume. The transmural pressure is the difference between intraluminal pressure distending the vein and the external pressures collapsing the vein. An increase in transmural pressure from 0 to 15 mm Hg corresponds to a 250% increase in volume.[2]

Smooth muscle activity in the wall of both arteries and veins is mediated by the sympathetic nervous system. Venous innervation is greatest in the splanchnic and cutaneous venous system, where smooth muscle is most prevalent. The splanchnic circulation usually accounts for approximately 25% of the total blood volume.[1] Stimulation of the sympathetic nervous system results in acute changes in splanchnic blood volume. Arterial receptors such as the carotid sinus can also cause changes in venous capacitance. For example, when blood pressure is low, catecholamine release causes increased venous smooth muscle tone and increase in venous return to the heart.[1,2]

1.5 Collateral Pathways

Extensive collateralization in the venous system affords the ability to bypass obstruction in order to maintain venous return. An understanding of collateral pathways and changes in venous flow is essential in the treatment of venous disease. Collateral pathways are important when large vessels, such as the SVC and IVC, are occluded. Many well-documented collateral networks of the venous system have been described.

SVC and IVC obstructions occur secondary to a number of causes. Pulmonary or mediastinal malignancy is the most common cause of SVC obstruction (▶ Fig. 1.6).[16] Growth of primary or metastatic malignancy over time causes mass effect on the adjacent SVC and can eventually lead to occlusion. Thrombosis of the major thoracic and upper extremity veins is also a common cause of obstruction, often secondary to central venous catheters.[11,16] Subclavian or brachiocephalic venous obstruction may be secondary to hypertrophied valves in the setting of arteriovenous fistulas or grafts placed for dialysis access (▶ Fig. 1.7). Other well-documented causes of thoracic venous obstruction include mediastinal fibrosis, aortic aneurysm, retrosternal thyroid, sarcoidosis, and radiation fibrosis.[16]

Causes of IVC obstruction are similar to those of SVC obstruction. Thrombosis is one of the most common causes, which often extends to the IVC from lower extremity deep venous thrombosis (DVT).[17] Extrinsic compression from surrounding tumor, fibrosis, lymphadenopathy, and aneurysm also occurs. Iatrogenic obstruction from IVC filter placement is also reported. Rarely, intrinsic causes such as congenital membranes or primary caval tumors are the cause of obstruction.[11,16,17]

Extensive collateralization of the venous system already exists, and many of the collateral pathways intercommunicate. Superficially, there are numerous collaterals in the chest wall. Chest wall collateral flow often occurs in cases of axillary vein occlusion.[11] The pectoral branches of the thoracoacromial trunk, the lateral thoracic, and thoracodorsal veins drain into the axillary vein. The posterior intercostal veins drain into the azygous system, but also communicate with the lateral thoracic, anterior intercostal, and internal mammary veins (▶ Fig. 1.8). When axillary occlusion occurs, flow reverses in these branches and returns via the intercostal veins (▶ Fig. 1.9). More central occlusion involving the subclavian and brachiocephalic veins may divert flow through collateral pathways within the chest wall and the neck (▶ Fig. 1.10). Venographic studies have demonstrated collateralization with the vertebral veins in the posterior neck. In addition, contralateral collaterals develop between the right and left external jugular veins via the jugular venous arch.[11] Important communications also exist between the internal and external mammary veins and the superior and inferior epigastric veins. For example, in IVC or iliofemoral obstruction, blood can return from the external iliac veins to the inferior epigastric veins (▶ Fig. 1.11). The inferior epigastric veins anastomose with the superior epigastric veins in the abdominal wall.[17] The superior epigastric veins communicate with the internal and external mammary veins, and ultimately return to the SVC.

The azygous system is a well-developed venous network with numerous communications.[12] Central SVC and IVC obstruction often causes blood flow to divert through the azygous system. The ascending lumbar plexus is a very common collateral pathway seen in iliac vein, renal vein, and IVC obstruction (▶ Fig. 1.12). Deep venous connections also exist between the ascending lumbar plexus and the internal and external vertebral plexuses, which ultimately empty into the azygous system. The Batson venous plexus connects deep pelvic veins to the vertebral network and may be important in pelvic venous obstruction.[17] The vertebral veins also communicate with the internal mammary pathway in the chest wall. In some cases of abdominal venous obstruction, blood may also divert through the retroperitoneum via the periureteral plexus, which drains into the renal veins and IVC. Collateral drainage with the gonadal veins is also relatively common (▶ Fig. 1.13). Blood flow through these collateral paths usually depends on patency of the renal veins, which may be affected depending on the level of IVC obstruction.[9,17]

The systemic-to-pulmonary pathway is a less common collateral path. SVC obstruction can rarely result in systemic-to-pulmonary flow between the brachiocephalic veins and the superior pulmonary veins. Anatomic connections between the bronchial and pulmonary veins already exist because of bronchial venous plexuses. Bronchial veins are also connected to the azygous/hemiazygous system with one-way valves preventing backflow. When the SVC is obstructed, the systemic venous pressure is increased, causing valve incompetence and resulting in flow reversal through the preexisting collateral pathways (▶ Fig. 1.14). The presence of pulmonary collateral pathways is clinically important because it results in a right-to-left shunt, placing patients at increased risk for stroke or other complications.[16]

Numerous connections exist between the systemic and portal venous systems and may be of clinical importance in both systemic and portal venous pathology. Cavoportal collateral pathways direct blood from the systemic veins to the portal vein. Superficial cavoportal collaterals develop in both SVC and IVC obstruction and this collateralization relies on the connection between the superior and inferior epigastric veins with the internal mammary veins. Blood flow is directed into the portal vein via a recanalized umbilical vein. Alternatively, blood may divert from the internal mammary vein to the inferior phrenic vein. The inferior phrenic vein communicates with capsular veins of the liver, and these in turn drain into the portal system.

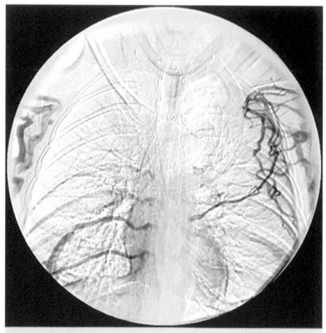

Fig. 1.9 Venogram of patient with bilateral axillary vein occlusion with opacification of bilateral intercostal veins.

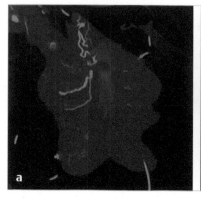
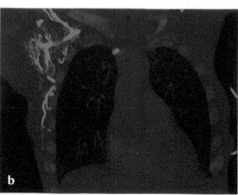

Fig. 1.8 Chest wall collaterals enlarge in the setting of brachiocephalic venous stenosis or occlusion. These include (a) internal mammary and intercostal veins and (b) lateral thoracic and thoracodorsal collaterals.

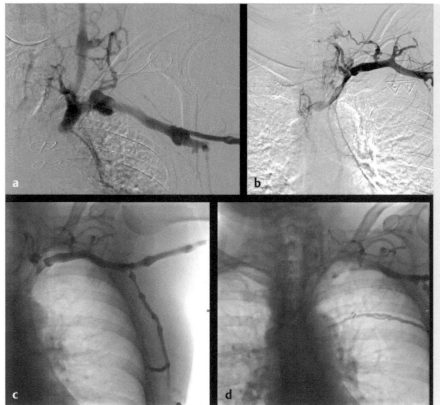

Fig. 1.10 Left upper extremity venogram demonstrating: **(a)** occlusion of the left subclavian vein with cervical collaterals; **(b)** brachiocephalic venous stenosis with cervical; **(c)** chest wall; **(d)** intercostal collaterals.

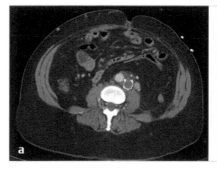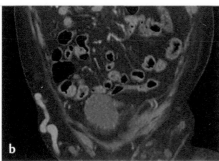

Fig. 1.11 Axial and coronal contrast-enhanced CT images showing **(a)** thrombosis of a left-sided IVC with caval filter and **(b)** inferior epigastric collateral veins.

SVC obstruction can also cause "downhill varices." The venous plexus surrounding the lower esophagus communicates with both the azygous system and the portal venous system. When the SVC is obstructed below the entry of the azygous vein, blood flow is directed toward the portal system. In IVC obstruction, blood can flow retrograde through the internal iliac veins to the hemorrhoidal plexus, through the mesenteric veins, and ultimately into the portal vein.[16,18]

Portosystemic collateral pathways develop in the setting of portal hypertension and divert blood from the elevated pressures in the portal veins to the systemic circulation. These collateral pathways are distinct from the cavoportal pathways described in systemic vein occlusion. While these pathways rely on similar anatomic communications, the difference is the direction of blood flow. In cavoportal pathways, the blood flow continues in the normal hepatopetal direction. Portosystemic collaterals demonstrate reversal of blood flow in the hepatofugal direction. Gastric (coronary) venous collaterals are common

in portal hypertension, seen in roughly 80% of patients with evidence of portal hypertension.[19] Esophageal and paraesophageal varices also occur frequently in portal hypertension. Esophageal varices are the most clinically relevant due to the risk of gastrointestinal bleeding. Esophageal varices are supplied by the anterior branch of the left gastric vein and are located within the lower esophageal mucosa. Paraesophageal varices are located outside the wall of the esophagus and are supplied by the posterior branch of the left gastric vein.[19] The paraesophageal varices connect the gastric veins with the azygous system and vertebral plexus. Perisplenic and gastric varices also develop. Gastric and esophageal varices often occur together and occur along the lesser or greater curvature of the stomach, draining into the azygous/hemiazygous system. Isolated gastric varices also occur, for example, in splenic vein occlusion. Splenorenal and gastrorenal shunts are spontaneous portosystemic shunts in which blood drains from dilated gastric or splenic veins into the left renal vein and IVC (▶ Fig. 1.15).

Rectal varices form between the superior rectal (hemorrhoidal) vein and the middle and inferior rectal (hemorrhoidal) veins. The superior rectal vein drains into the inferior mesenteric vein while the middle and inferior rectal veins join the internal iliac veins. In portal hypertension, varices develop and blood flow is directed toward the internal iliac veins.[20]

Abdominal wall varices (caput medusa) and paraumbilical varices develop on the abdominal wall. Paraumbilical varices occur in roughly 10 to 40% of patients with portal hypertension.[19] Collapsed paraumbilical veins, originating from the left portal vein, are present in the falciform ligament. These veins dilate in portal hypertension and are commonly referred to as recanalized umbilical veins. These veins communicate with the superior epigastric veins from the internal mammary vein, as well as the inferior epigastric and external iliac veins. Richly collateralized retroperitoneal and paravertebral veins may also become dilated. Omental and mesenteric varices are rare but also may occur.[19]

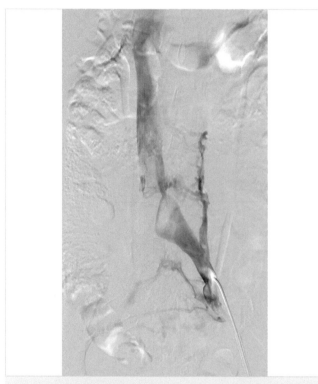

Fig. 1.12 Left external iliac venogram showing extrinsic compression and stenosis of the left common iliac vein with opacification of ascending lumbar collaterals.

1.6 Epidemiology of Venous Disorders

1.6.1 Thromboembolism

Venous thromboembolism (VTE), including DVT and pulmonary embolism (PE), contributes to significant disease burden in the United States and worldwide. VTE is the third leading cardiovascular disorder following myocardial infarction and stroke. Incidence of VTE reported in the literature is highly variable and dependent on population studies. A recent review of numerous population studies estimated average annual incidence of overall VTE among persons of European ancestry ranged from 104 to 183 per 100,000 person-years.[21] An estimated 900,000 total incident and recurrent VTE events occur in the United States annually.[22] Overall, incidence rates for VTE have been stable or increased, which may be partially due to improvement in diagnostic imaging studies.[21] A recent study by Bell et al quotes a lifetime risk of 8.1% of VTE after the age of 45 years based on data from the prospective cohort Cardiovascular Health Study (CHS) and the Atherosclerosis Risk in Communities (ARIC) study.[23]

Acute thromboembolic events are also a significant cause of mortality. PE is the third leading cause of cardiovascular-related death following myocardial infarction and stroke.[24] Fatality is higher in cases of PE than in cases of DVT alone.[22] One study

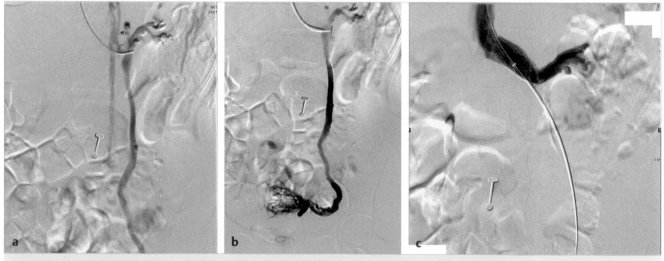

Fig. 1.13 **(a)** Venographic images demonstrating outflow obstruction of the left renal vein with resultant opacification of ascending lumbar and gonadal veins. **(b)** Delayed image from left renal venogram shows gonadal vein outflow via cross-pelvic collaterals. **(c)** Venogram following renal venous stent placement with a patent left renal vein and no collateral outflow.

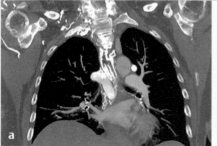
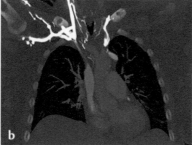
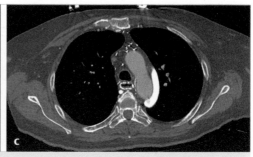

Fig. 1.14 SVC obstruction with **(a)** coronal CT image demonstrating dilated bronchial venous plexus, opacified via communication with **(b)** cervical venous collaterals with outflow **(c)** via azygous vein. Bronchial plexus collateralization is significant due to the potential for development of bronchial to pulmonary venous (right to left) shunting.

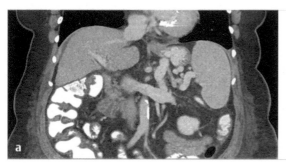
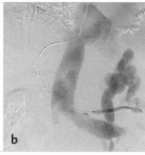

Fig. 1.15 (a) Coronal CT of the abdomen with contrast demonstrates large gastrorenal shunt, which opacifies on **(b)** images from a splenic venogram during a TIPS procedure.

reported 28-day case fatality rate of 9.4% after first-time DVT and 15.1% following first-time PE.[25,26] Overall, PE occurs in approximately 10% of cases of acute DVT, with an estimated incidence of first-time PE of 23 per 100,000 based on hospital discharge data.[26] All-cause mortality at 3 months associated with acute PE was 17% in the International Cooperative Pulmonary Embolism Registry, with 45% of deaths attributed to PE.[24,26] Studies show recurrence rates of approximately 7 to 10% within 1 year[26] and approximately 30% of patients develop recurrence within 10 years of a VTE event.[21,22] Recurrence rates are highest in the first 6 to 12 months following the incident event.

Well-documented chronic sequelae of thromboembolic disease include the postthrombotic syndrome (PTS). The PTS is a chronic condition characterized by pain and swelling in the affected limb. PTS may sometimes be accompanied by skin changes and ulceration. PTS develops in an estimated 20 to 50% of patient within 1 to 2 years of an acute DVT, with 5 to 10% classified as severe PTS.[27] PTS is not completely understood, but is thought to develop secondary to valvular damage and persistent venous obstruction after a thrombotic event. Valve incompetence and reflux lead to venous hypertension and stasis, similar to primary venous insufficiency. Inflammation may also be contributory to fibrosis and valvular incompetence.[27] Risk of developing PTS increases four- to sixfold with recurrent ipsilateral DVT.[27] Chronic postthrombotic pulmonary hypertension can also develop and lead to death from right ventricular failure.[24] Therefore, early thrombolysis and systemic anticoagulants may be helpful in the prevention of PTS. Cumulative rates of venous stasis following DVT in one study were 7.3 at 1 year and increased to 26.8% by 20 years.[28]

In addition to morbidity and mortality, VTE is associated with a significant health care cost burden. A 2016 study by Grosse et al analyzed the economic burden of VTE in the United States and estimated cost for incident VTE is approximately 7 to 10 billion dollars annually.[29] In patients who develop chronic complication such as PTS, annual cost per patient increases. One study found median total costs for patients who develop PTS to be $20,569. In matched controls with DVT without PTS, median total costs were $15,843.[30]

Cerebral venous thrombosis (CVT) is relatively rare in comparison to other forms of thrombosis, with an estimated annual incidence of 3 to 4 per 1 million. Incidence in children is slightly higher, occurring in about 7 per 1 million.[31] Diagnosis of CVT has increased in recent years, likely secondary to improvements in neuroimaging. Risk factors for development of CVT are similar to other forms of thrombosis. The most commonly cited causes include trauma, pregnancy, hormonal contraceptives, and either inherited or acquired hypercoagulable states. Infections such as otitis, mastoiditis, and meningitis have also been associated with CVT. The majority of patients affected are children and young adults, and approximately 75% of young adults with CVT are women.[31] Incidence is more equally distributed between genders in affected children and elderly patients. Thrombosis of the cerebral veins and dural sinuses can be a cause of stroke, accounting for approximately 0.5 to 1.0% of stroke.[32] Mortality rates from CVT has decreased over the years, now with acute mortality rates of approximately 5 to 10%.[33]

1.6.2 Venous Insufficiency

Chronic venous insufficiency (CVI) is a common medical condition with significant impact to patients and to health care. CVI encompasses a spectrum of disease manifestations including varicose veins, edema, skin changes, and ulceration. The underlying cause of venous insufficiency is venous hypertension. Studies suggest veins are unable to withstand increased pressures for a prolonged time. Longstanding hypertension leads to valve damage, remodeling, and inflammatory change. Insufficiency can result from both primary and secondary valvular incompetence. The exact mechanism of primary valvular incompetence is unknown. Some studies suggest varicose veins have decreased smooth muscle and elastin content.[34] Differences in the cellular makeup lead to a weak vessel wall, causing dilation. The valve leaflets are unable to coapt, resulting in reflux. Both reflux and obstruction may cause secondary venous insufficiency following venous thrombosis. Even when the occluded vein is recanalized, residual thrombus in the vessel may cause valve incompetence or entrapment. An estimated 80% of venous insufficiency is postthrombotic and only 20% is thought to be secondary to primary valvular incompetence.[3]

CVI affects roughly 5% of the adult population. Approximately 1% of patients suffer from skin ulceration and chronic wounds, the more severe consequences of CVI. In the United States, an estimated 2.5 million people have CVI, and 20% develop severe disease.[35] Prevalence and chronicity contribute to the economic impact of CVI. An estimated 1 to 3% of health care expenditure in developed countries relate to chronic venous disease. Wound care for venous ulcers costs an estimated $3 billion per year in the United States.[34,35] Patient disabilities related to ulcers lead to significant loss of work hours. An estimated 12.5% of patients with venous ulcers are consequently forced to retire early. CVI also contributes to decreased quality of life, social isolation, and limited physical function.[34]

Venous insufficiency can affect areas beyond the lower extremities. Pelvic congestion syndrome (PCS) is a condition often characterized by chronic pelvic pain, pelvic varicosities, and pelvic venous insufficiency. Pelvic varicosities arise in distinct areas such as the medial and posterior thigh, gluteal region, and vulvoperineum.[36,37] The pathophysiology of PCS is multifactorial and includes valvular insufficiency or congenital valvular absence, venous obstruction, and hormones.[36] Primary causes are nonobstructive, such as congenital valvular absence. Secondary insufficiency is the result of compression or obstruction, as seen in nutcracker syndrome (compression of the left renal vein by the superior mesenteric artery), retroaortic left renal vein, pregnancy, or May–Thurner syndrome (compression of the left iliac vein by the right iliac artery).[37] Unlike lower extremity veins, the pelvic venous plexus does not contain valves. However, valves are usually present at the ovarian vein terminus and serve to prevent reflux. Congenital absence of ovarian vein valves occurs in approximately 13 to 15% on the left side and 6% on the right.[38] When present, valves are incompetent in 41 to 43% on the left and 35 to 46% on the right. Incidence of PCS is likely underestimated secondary to underdiagnosis. One study of healthy female kidney donors demonstrated a 9.9% prevalence of ovarian varices on preoperative imaging studies, with 59% of those patients reporting pelvic pain in retrospective analysis.[39] A recent review quotes a prevalence of PCS in 10 to 30% of patients evaluated for chronic pelvic pain.[38]

1.6.3 Portal and Mesenteric Venous Disorders

Portal hypertension is defined as a hepatic venous pressure gradient greater than 5 mm Hg or direct portal venous pressure greater than 12 mm Hg. Normal portal venous pressure is between 5 and 10 mm Hg. Over time, portosystemic collateral pathways develop in response to elevated portal pressures. Portosystemic collaterals serve to decrease the pressure in the portal vein and shunt blood flow into the systemic circulation. Complications of portal hypertension usually manifest when the pressure gradient is greater than 10 mm Hg. Portosystemic collaterals begin to develop at watershed zones of portal and systemic drainage, and there is often recanalization of embryonic remnants such as the umbilical vein.[20]

Causes of portal hypertension can be divided into three categories: prehepatic (presinusoidal), intrahepatic (sinusoidal), and posthepatic (postsinusoidal). Portal vein, mesenteric, and splenic vein thromboses are common prehepatic causes of portal hypertension. Intrahepatic causes include cirrhosis, inflammation and infection, and congenital fibrosis. Classic posthepatic causes are the Budd–Chiari syndrome (BCS), as well as cardiac conditions such as congestive heart failure, tricuspid valve regurgitation, or constrictive pericarditis.

The incidence of prevalence of portal hypertension both in the United States and worldwide is not known. Underlying cirrhosis is a major cause of portal hypertension, and etiologies vary between the Eastern and Western hemispheres. Hepatitis C is a major cause of cirrhosis and portal hypertension worldwide. Alcoholic and viral cirrhosis are the leading causes of portal hypertension the Western countries. Nonalcoholic steatohepatitis is also becoming a major cause of cirrhosis in the United States. Esophageal varices are present in 60 to 70% of patients with decompensated cirrhosis.[40] Hepatic cirrhosis is the 12th leading cause of deaths in the United States yearly. In Eastern countries, Hepatitis B is endemic and is a major cause of portal hypertension. Overall, there is a 60% male predilection for chronic liver disease.[41] Certain causes such as thromboembolic disease and primary biliary cirrhosis have a female predilection.

Portal venous thrombosis (PVT) is a vascular disease of the liver that blocks portal vein inflow. Portal vein inflow accounts for roughly 75% of the blood supply to the hepatic parenchyma, and blocking portal flow has devastating consequence. Population studies estimate the prevalence of PVT is approximately 1%, with an incidence of approximately 4 per 1 million yearly.[42] PVT has been identified as a cause for roughly 30% of cases of portal hypertension in adults, and accounts for nearly 75% of cases of portal hypertension in children.[43] PVT occurs most commonly in patients with underlying cirrhosis. Prevalence increases with disease severity, occurring in less than 1% of patients with compensated cirrhosis, but increasing to 8 to 25% in end-stage cirrhosis.

Like other thrombotic conditions, inflammation, malignancy, trauma, and coagulopathy can play a role in the development of thrombosis in the portal and splanchnic vasculature. About 70% of cases are caused by a systemic factor, whereas about 30% have a local cause. Both inherited and acquired prothrombotic conditions are important systemic causes. In patients without a known tumor or cirrhosis, 30 to 40% of patients had an underlying myeloproliferative disorder.[43] Antiphospholipid syndrome was identified in 6 to 19% of patients. Other known hypercoagulable conditions such as factor V Leiden mutation, and protein C and protein S deficiency have also been cited. Local causes of PVT include inflammatory conditions such as pancreatitis, inflammatory bowel disease, or other gastrointestinal tract inflammation and infection. The leading local causes are cirrhosis and malignancy in the portal venous territory. Trauma and iatrogenic causes such as splenectomy, colectomy, and transjugular intrahepatic portosystemic shunts (TIPSs) can also play a role.[43]

PVT presents as both acute and chronic PVT, and the distinction is important for clinical management. Acute PVT can involve portions of the splenic or mesenteric veins, and severity of presentation depends on the extent of thrombus. Portal vein occlusion leads to hepatic hypoperfusion, which is overcome by increasing hepatic arterial inflow to the liver. When thrombus extends to the mesenteric venous arches, intestinal ischemia or infarct can occur secondary to venous hypertension. Collateral vessels form in chronic PVT to compensate for increased venous pressure. Large clot burden and occlusion of the main portal vein or major branches nearly always lead to portal hypertension if there is no recanalization.[43]

BCS is a group of disorders caused by impaired hepatic venous outflow, rather than primary parenchymal disorder. Obstruction can occur at the level of the large hepatic veins, the IVC, or the right atrium. Outflow obstruction causes increased pressure in the hepatic sinusoids and leads to hepatic congestion. Because of the increased sinusoidal pressure, hepatopetal portal flow is obstructed which results in portal hypertension and decreased perfusion. Portal venous inflow provides the majority of the hepatic blood supply, and as perfusion is decreased, hepatocyte ischemia and necrosis results. Over time, hepatocyte damage will evolve into hepatic fibrosis and cirrhosis. In chronic, progressive cases of BCS, collateral pathways develop to redirect drainage. If the increased sinusoidal pressure is not reversed, BCS will progress to liver failure.[44]

BCS is overall a rare condition, with an estimated incidence of 0.1 to 0.8 per 1 million per year. Prevalence is estimated at 1.4 to 2.4 per 1 million per year in the United States.[45] BCS demonstrates a female predilection and more frequently occurs in young adults. An underlying prothrombotic risk factor is identified in over 75% of patients.[44] Like PVT, underlying myeloproliferative disorders are frequently a cause, found in 40 to 50% of patients with primary BCS.[43] Rarely, malignant tumor invasion can also lead to BCS. In Asian populations, membranous intravascular obstructions have been described, both congenital and secondary.[44] Clinical presentation varies based on the acuity and extent of the obstruction, and the severity is dependent on the development of collateral circulation and the remaining venous outflow pathways.[45]

1.6.4 Venous Anomalies

Venous malformations are the most common vascular malformation, accounting for 44 to 64%. The Hamburg classification divides venous malformations into truncular or extratruncular. Forty percent of venous malformations occur on the extremities, 40% occur on the head and neck, and the remaining 20% occur on the trunk. Venous malformations are slow-flow lesions and are further characterized as focal or diffuse. Focal venous malformations are by far the most common (99%) and are only present in one tissue layer.[46] Focal lesions drain into normal adjacent veins via small communications. Diffuse venous malformations span multiple tissue layers and often connect to main venous branches. Diffuse lesions are much more likely to recur and are more difficult to treat. Venous malformations are benign and require treatment only for pain or disfigurement.

1.7 Importance to Interventional Radiology

Venous disorders are diverse, occurring in multiple anatomic territories and organ systems. Venous interventions have historically fallen within the scope of practice of interventional radiologists, as the full spectrum of percutaneous venous interventions has developed within the specialty as an outgrowth from historical invasive imaging of venous pathology.

The many manifestations of venous disease constitute a significant disease burden, and as venous pathologies are increasingly recognized and patients present for therapy, interventional radiologists are in a unique position to remain preeminent in treating the wide range of venous disorders. Doing so requires a thorough understanding of the complexities of the venous system in every anatomic territory. The successful practitioner will be comfortable with the pathophysiology of these disorders, the evaluation of the patient, the nonprocedural management of these diseases, and the full spectrum of therapeutic options. Many of these patients require longitudinal management, with intermittent therapeutic intervention needed, and successful long-term outcomes require lasting clinical relationships with patients.

There is a great opportunity for interventional radiologists to continue to impact outcomes in patients with venous disease, as many of the entities discussed in this volume present opportunities for improvement in treatment options. Interventional radiologists have led the way in innovating and optimizing therapies, and are well-suited to developing guidance regarding best practices in management of venous diseases by investigating the outstanding clinical questions.

References

[1] Padberg F. The physiology and hemodynamics of the normal venous circulation. In: Gloviczki P, ed. Handbook of Venous Disorders. 3rd ed. London: Hodder Arnold; 2009:25–35

[2] Pounds LL, Killewich LA. Venous physiology. In: Cronenwett JL, Johnston KW, eds. Rutherford's Vascular Surgery. Vol 1. 7th ed. Philadelphia, PA: Elsevier; 2010:151–162

[3] Meissner MH, Moneta G, Burnand K, et al. The hemodynamics and diagnosis of venous disease. J Vasc Surg. 2007; 46 Suppl S:4S–24S

[4] Gloviczki P, Mozes G. Development and anatomy of the venous system. In: Gloviczki P, ed. Handbook of Venous Disorders. 3rd ed. London: Hodder Arnold; 2009

[5] Swift MR, Weinstein BM. Arterial-venous specification during development. Circ Res. 2009; 104(5):576–588

[6] Guttmann GD, Endean E. Embryology. In: Cronenwett JL, Johnston KW, eds. Rutherford's Vascular Surgery. Vol 1. 7th ed. Philadelphia, PA: Elsevier; 2010:15–30

[7] Lundell C, Kadir S. Inferior vena cava and spinal veins. In: Kadir S, ed. Atlas of Normal and Variant Angiographic Anatomy. Philadelphia, PA: WB Saunders; 1991:187–190

[8] Lundell C, Kadir S. The portal venous system and hepatic veins. In: Kadir S, ed. Atlas of Normal and Variant Angiographic Anatomy. Philadelphia, PA: WB Saunders; 1991:365–369

[9] Valji K, ed. Vascular and Interventional Radiology. 2nd ed. Philadelphia, PA: Saunders; 2006

[10] Lundell C, Kadir S. Upper extremity veins. In: Kadir S, ed. Atlas of Normal and Variant Angiographic Anatomy. Philadelphia, PA: WB Saunders; 1991:177–179

[11] Richard HM, III, Selby JB, Jr, Gay SB, Tegtmeyer CJ. Normal venous anatomy and collateral pathways in upper extremity venous thrombosis. Radiographics. 1992; 12(3):527–534

[12] Lundell C, Kadir S. Superior vena cava and thoracic veins. In: Kadir S, ed. Atlas of Normal and Variant Angiographic Anatomy. Philadelphia, PA: WB Saunders; 1991:163–165

[13] Lundell C, Kadir S. Lower extremities and pelvis. In: Kadir S, ed. Atlas of Normal and Variant Angiographic Anatomy. Philadelphia, PA: WB Saunders; 1991:203–208

[14] Bass JE, Redwine MD, Kramer LA, Huynh PT, Harris JH, Jr. Spectrum of congenital anomalies of the inferior vena cava: cross-sectional imaging findings. Radiographics. 2000; 20(3):639–652

[15] Piciucchi S, Barone D, Sanna S, et al. The azygos vein pathway: an overview from anatomical variations to pathological changes. Insights Imaging. 2014; 5(5):619–628

[16] Kapur S, Paik E, Rezaei A, Vu DN. Where there is blood, there is a way: unusual collateral vessels in superior and inferior vena cava obstruction. Radiographics. 2010; 30(1):67–78

[17] Sonin AH, Mazer MJ, Powers TA. Obstruction of the inferior vena cava: a multiple-modality demonstration of causes, manifestations, and collateral pathways. Radiographics. 1992; 12(2):309–322

[18] Dahan H, Arrivé L, Monnier-Cholley L, Le Hir P, Zins M, Tubiana JM. Cavoportal collateral pathways in vena cava obstruction: imaging features. AJR Am J Roentgenol. 1998; 171(5):1405–1411

[19] Cho KC, Patel YD, Wachsberg RH, Seeff J. Varices in portal hypertension: evaluation with CT. Radiographics. 1995; 15(3):609–622

[20] Pillai AK, Andring B, Patel A, Trimmer C, Kalva SP. Portal hypertension: a review of portosystemic collateral pathways and endovascular interventions. Clin Radiol. 2015; 70(10):1047–1059

[21] Heit JA, Spencer FA, White RH. The epidemiology of venous thromboembolism. J Thromb Thrombolysis. 2016; 41(1):3–14

[22] Heit JA. The epidemiology of venous thromboembolism in the community. Arterioscler Thromb Vasc Biol. 2008; 28(3):370–372

[23] Bell EJ, Lutsey PL, Basu S, et al. Lifetime risk of venous thromboembolism in two cohort studies. Am J Med. 2016; 129(3):339.e19–339.e26

[24] Goldhaber SZ, Bounameaux H. Pulmonary embolism and deep vein thrombosis. Lancet. 2012; 379(9828):1835–1846

[25] Cushman M, Tsai AW, White RH, et al. Deep vein thrombosis and pulmonary embolism in two cohorts: the longitudinal investigation of thromboembolism etiology. Am J Med. 2004; 117(1):19–25

[26] White RH. The epidemiology of venous thromboembolism. Circulation. 2003; 107(23) Suppl 1:I4–I8

[27] Kahn SR, Galanaud JP, Vedantham S, Ginsberg JS. Guidance for the prevention and treatment of the post-thrombotic syndrome. J Thromb Thrombolysis. 2016; 41(1):144–153

[28] Kahn SR, Ginsberg JS. Relationship between deep venous thrombosis and the postthrombotic syndrome. Arch Intern Med. 2004; 164(1):17–26

[29] Grosse SD, Nelson RE, Nyarko KA, Richardson LC, Raskob GE. The economic burden of incident venous thromboembolism in the United States: a review of estimated attributable healthcare costs. Thromb Res. 2016; 137:3–10

[30] MacDougall DA, Feliu AL, Boccuzzi SJ, Lin J. Economic burden of deep-vein thrombosis, pulmonary embolism, and post-thrombotic syndrome. Am J Health Syst Pharm. 2006; 63(20) Suppl 6:S5–S15

[31] Stam J. Thrombosis of the cerebral veins and sinuses. N Engl J Med. 2005; 352(17):1791–1798

[32] Saposnik G, Barinagarrementeria F, Brown RD, Jr, et al. American Heart Association Stroke Council and the Council on Epidemiology and Prevention. Diagnosis and management of cerebral venous thrombosis: a statement for healthcare professionals from the American Heart Association/American Stroke Association. Stroke. 2011; 42(4):1158–1192

[33] Breteau G, Mounier-Vehier F, Godefroy O, et al. Cerebral venous thrombosis 3-year clinical outcome in 55 consecutive patients. J Neurol. 2003; 250(1):29–35

[34] Bergan JJ, Schmid-Schönbein GW, Smith PD, Nicolaides AN, Boisseau MR, Eklof B. Chronic venous disease. N Engl J Med. 2006; 355(5):488–498

[35] Eberhardt RT, Raffetto JD. Chronic venous insufficiency. Circulation. 2005; 111(18):2398–2409

[36] Durham JD, Machan L. Pelvic congestion syndrome. Semin Intervent Radiol. 2013; 30(4):372–380

[37] Richardson GD. Management of pelvic venous congestion syndrome. In: Gloviczki P, ed. Handbook of Venous Disorders. 3rd ed. London: Hodder Arnold; 2009:617–626

[38] Borghi C, Dell'Atti L. Pelvic congestion syndrome: the current state of the literature. Arch Gynecol Obstet. 2016; 293(2):291–301

[39] Belenky A, Bartal G, Atar E, Cohen M, Bachar GN. Ovarian varices in healthy female kidney donors: incidence, morbidity, and clinical outcome. AJR Am J Roentgenol. 2002; 179(3):625–627

[40] Garcia-Tsao G, Sanyal AJ, Grace ND, Carey W, Practice Guidelines Committee of the American Association for the Study of Liver Diseases, Practice Parameters Committee of the American College of Gastroenterology. Prevention and management of gastroesophageal varices and variceal hemorrhage in cirrhosis. Hepatology. 2007; 46(3):922–938

[41] Kim WR, Brown RS, Jr, Terrault NA, El-Serag H. Burden of liver disease in the United States: summary of a workshop. Hepatology. 2002; 36(1):227–242

[42] Qi X, Jia J, Ren W, et al. Scientific publications on portal vein thrombosis and Budd-Chiari syndrome: a global survey of the literature. J Gastrointestin Liver Dis. 2014; 23(1):65–71

[43] DeLeve LD, Valla D-C, Garcia-Tsao G, American Association for the Study Liver Diseases. Vascular disorders of the liver. Hepatology. 2009; 49(5):1729–1764

[44] Cura M, Haskal Z, Lopera J. Diagnostic and interventional radiology for Budd-Chiari syndrome. Radiographics. 2009; 29(3):669–681

[45] Sabol TP, Molina M, Wu GY. Thrombotic venous diseases of the liver. J Clin Transl Hepatol. 2015; 3(3):189–194

[46] Mulligan PR, Prajapati HJ, Martin LG, Patel TH. Vascular anomalies: classification, imaging characteristics and implications for interventional radiology treatment approaches. Br J Radiol. 2014; 87(1035):20130392

2 Venous Thromboembolism

Matthew T. Rondina and Hanadi Farrukh

Summary

Venous thromboembolism has been increasingly recognized as a significant contributor to patient morbidity and mortality, and there has been rapid growth in the application of interventional techniques to the management of venous thrombotic disorders. For the physician managing a patient with a venous thrombosis, an excellent understanding of the mechanisms of disease, thrombosis physiology, pathophysiology of clotting disorders, data to support the application of different pharmacologic interventions, and risks and benefits of different therapies is critical to success. This chapter provides a thorough overview of the science and pharmacologic management of thrombosis, as well as details of patient evaluation, epidemiology, and expected outcomes of intervention.

Keywords: venous thromboembolism, pulmonary embolism, deep vein thrombosis, diagnosis, anticoagulation, DOAC, Treatment, Warfarin, D-dimer, ultrasound

2.1 Introduction

Venous thromboembolism (VTE) is a major public health burden globally and, after myocardial infarction and stroke, the third most common cardiovascular disease. The causes of VTE are complex and multifactorial and include both inherited and acquired factors. As our population ages and develops VTE risk factors, the incidence and prevalence of VTE will continue to increase—as likely will its attendant complications, including postthrombotic syndrome (PTS) and pulmonary hypertension. Thus, for providers in all settings, an understanding of VTE is warranted.

Starting with a clinical vignette, this chapter will review the pathophysiology and epidemiology of VTE, including common provoking risk factors and inherited thrombophilias. The appropriate use of algorithms to diagnosis deep vein thrombosis (DVT) and pulmonary embolism (PE) will be reviewed, including a discussion on potentially more complex and challenging diagnostic issues—such as recurrent ipsilateral DVT and when computed tomography pulmonary angiography (CTPA) is contraindicated in patients suspected of having acute PE. With the advent of the direct oral anticoagulants (DOACs), therapeutic options for the treatment of VTE have broadened. Accordingly, we will discuss central issues in the management of VTE, including acute antithrombotic therapy, thrombolytics for massive PE, and the duration of anticoagulation for provoked and unprovoked events.

2.2 Clinical Vignette

2.2.1 Patient Presentation

A 46-year-old white female presented to clinic with a 2-week history of progressive exertional dyspnea that had worsened over the past 2 days. She also had the onset of right pleuritic chest pain 1 day earlier and two episodes of presyncope with palpitations and chills. She denied fevers, cough, or wheezing. She had tried an albuterol inhaler prescribed by a friend without benefit. She was a lifetime nonsmoker. Her past medical history was notable for gastroesophageal reflux disease, irritable bowel syndrome, and menorrhagia. Her past surgical history included a remote left oophorectomy for an ovarian cyst. Her current medications included lansoprazole, oral contraceptive pills (taken for the past 2 years), and dicyclomine.

2.2.2 Physical Exam

She was a pleasant obese white female in no acute respiratory distress, although she appeared mildly anxious. Her body mass index was $42\,kg/m^2$, blood pressure was 116/76 mm Hg, pulse was 91 beats per minute, respiratory rate was 16 breaths per minute, the temperature was 98.6 °F, and her room air oxygen saturation was 96%. Her cardiovascular exam noted a jugular venous pulsation of 5 cm H_2O, and there was a regular heart rate and rhythm without murmurs or gallops. Her lungs were clear to auscultation and her abdomen was soft, nontender, with normal bowel sounds and no masses or organomegaly. Her extremities were without edema, there was no calf tenderness to palpation, and distal pulses were intact.

2.2.3 Lab Evaluation

Complete blood count, prothrombin time and international normalized ratio (INR), partial thromboplastin time, and comprehensive metabolic panel were within normal range. The troponin-I was 0.03 ng/mL (normal: 0.0–0.03 ng/mL) and the D-dimer was elevated at 2.5 µg/mL (normal 0.0–0.04 µg/mL).

2.2.4 Noninvasive Testing

An electrocardiogram demonstrated normal sinus rhythm with a rate of 90 beats per minute and diffusely inverted T waves across precordial leads.

2.2.5 Imaging

A posteroanterior and lateral chest X-ray was normal. CTPA demonstrated bilateral filling defects involving both the right and left main pulmonary arteries and extending into the segmental and subsegmental arteries, with distention of the right ventricle suggestive of right heart strain. A transthoracic echocardiogram demonstrated normal left ventricular systolic function with an ejection fraction of 68%, normal right ventricular systolic function, and mildly elevated pulmonary artery systolic pressure.

2.2.6 Plan of Care

She was admitted to the hospital with a diagnosis of acute, submassive PE and was treated with antithrombotic therapy.

2.3 Pathophysiology and Epidemiology of Venous Thromboembolism

Venous thrombi are classically comprised largely of red blood cells, with some leukocytes and platelets, interwoven in a fibrin lattice (▶ Fig. 2.1a). The formation of venous thrombosis occurs commonly in settings where there is vessel wall injury or stasis (e.g., surgery, trauma, malignancy), systemic inflammation (e.g., lupus, sepsis), and/or a procoagulant state (e.g., inherited thrombophilia, antiphospholipid antibodies). Vessel wall injury exposes tissue factor and collagen, leading to activation of the coagulation cascade. Historically, the coagulation cascade has been divided into the intrinsic and extrinsic pathways (▶ Fig. 2.1b). More recently, a cell-based model of coagulation has been put forth, whereby activation of the coagulation cascade occurs on the cell surface in four overlapping steps: (1) initiation, (2) amplification, (3) propagation, and (4) termination. The primary event for initiation of this cascade is the interaction of activated factor VII (FVIIa) with exposed tissue factor, converting factor II (FII, also known as prothrombin) to thrombin (FIIa) and fibrinogen to fibrin.

The epidemiology of VTE—including PE and DVT of the leg, pelvis, and arm—has recently been reviewed.[1,2] VTE carries a major global disease burden with respect to incidence, morbidity, mortality, and cost.[3,4] After myocardial infarction and stroke, VTE is the third most common cardiovascular disease, with a lifetime risk after age 45 years of 8.1%.[5] The age-adjusted annual incidence of VTE has increased by 80% from 1985 to 2009 to 1.7/1,000/year. While DVT incidence has remained stable, PE incidence has progressively increased, possibly due to a combination of an aging population, improved diagnostic techniques, and/or poorly defined increases in VTE risk factors.[6]

VTE results in some 550,000 hospitalizations per year in the United States—350,000 for DVT and 200,000 for PE[7]—with at least 44,000 deaths per year. Moreover, this mortality rate is likely an underestimate as 10 to 25% of PE patients in the community may present with sudden death prior to diagnosis.[8] Other consequences of VTE include a VTE recurrence rate of 15% over 3 years and 30% over 5 to 10 years in the absence of anticoagulation[2,9] and a 6% rate of major bleeding over 3 years.[10] In addition, PTS (▶ Fig. 2.2) occurs in 20 to 50% of patients within 2 years of a first episode of proximal DVT.[11] Severe PTS symptoms and/or venous ulceration develop in 5 to 10% of patients.[12] There is also a 2.8% incidence of chronic thromboembolic pulmonary hypertension within 1.5 years of

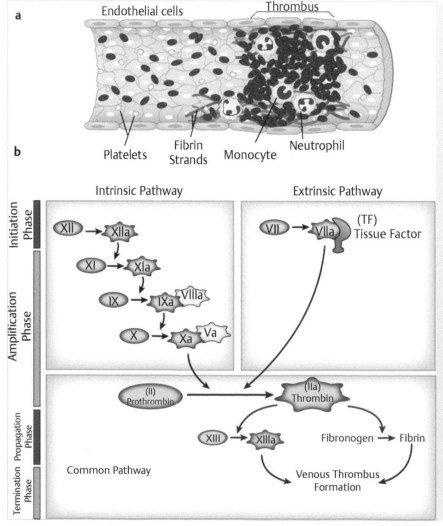

Fig. 2.1 (a) Venous thrombi are classically comprised largely of red blood cells, with some monocytes, neutrophils, and platelets, interwoven in a fibrin lattice. (b) The coagulation comprises the intrinsic and extrinsic pathways, whereas the cell-based model of coagulation occurs on the cell surface in four sequential phases: (1) initiation, (2) amplification, (3) propagation, and (4) termination. The intrinsic pathway begins with activation of factor XII, driving subsequent activation of factors XI, IX, and X. The primary event for initiation of the extrinsic pathway is the interaction between FVIIa and tissue factor (TF). Both the intrinsic and extrinsic pathways result in the conversion of prothrombin (FII) to thrombin (FIIa), in the common pathway. Thrombin then converts fibrinogen to fibrin and fibrin strands are cross-linked and stabilized by activated factor XIII (FXIIIa), leading to venous thrombus formation.

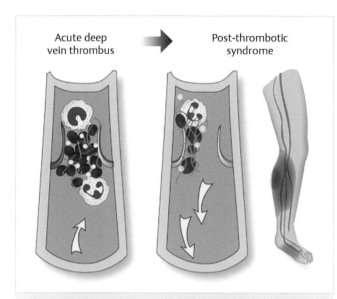

Fig. 2.2 Postthrombotic syndrome (PTS) is a complication of acute deep vein thrombosis. While still incompletely understood, the pathophysiology is thought to involve damage to the valves in the deep venous system with resulting venous insufficiency and inflammation. Patients with PTS have typical, often intermittent symptoms of leg erythema, cramping, heaviness, aching, and, in severe cases, ulceration.

Table 2.1 Risk factors for VTE

Inherited risk factors	Acquired risk factors	Temporary risk factors
Genetic thrombophilia	Age	Major surgery
• Major	Cancer	Acute medical
• Minor	Antiphospholipid	hospitalization
Family history of	antibodies	Major trauma
VTE	Obesity	Pregnancy
Male sex	Inflammatory	Puerperium
Ethnicity	diseases	Estrogen therapy
Tall height	• Inflammatory	Acute immobilization
Race	bowel disease	for ≥ 3–4 d
Blood group (ABO)	• Rheumatoid	Acute urinary or
	arthritis	respiratory infection
	• Systemic lupus	Acute neurologic illness
	Superficial phlebitis	with leg paresis
	Venous insufficiency	Cancer chemotherapy
	Hypertension	Central vein catheters
	Hyperlipidemia	or pacemakers
	Smoking	Minor trauma
	Metabolic syndrome	

an episode of PE.[13] The result is an estimated annual cost of VTE in the United States of $7 to 10 billion per year.[3]

2.3.1 Risk Factors for Venous Thromboembolism

VTE results from the complex, multiplicative interaction of inherited and/or acquired predisposing risk factors, often superimposed by the appearance of temporary clinical risk factors (▶ Table 2.1).[2,14,15] Recent cohort studies suggest that about 35% of first-episode VTE events are provoked by an identified temporary clinical risk factor, 20% are cancer-associated, and up to 45% are unprovoked (idiopathic).[10,16] The most common of the temporary clinical risk factors include surgical hospitalization within 3 months (24%), medical hospitalization within 3 months (22%), nursing home residence (14%), and central vein cannulation of the upper extremity (10%).[2,17] The incidence of VTE is strongly age-related, increasing three- to fivefold from patients aged 50 to 60 years to patients aged 70 to 80 years.[18] In adults aged 70 years and older, the annual VTE incidence is nearly 1%.[8,16,19] The incidence of VTE is also higher in blacks than whites, with Asian Americans and Native Americans at lowest risk, perhaps due in part to a variable prevalence of genetic thrombophilia.[20] Major (e.g., deficiencies of proteins C and S and antithrombin III) and minor (e.g., heterozygous factor V Leiden and prothrombin gene mutations) genetic thrombophilia increases the risk of a first VTE episode but minimally increase the risk of recurrent VTE.[21] For this reason, thrombophilia testing in VTE patients or their asymptomatic relatives rarely alters management decisions, may result in harm because of inaccurate interpretation and decision-making, and should be performed only in highly selected situations.[21]

Testing for acquired antiphospholipid antibody syndrome may be useful in some patients. Independent risk factors for a first episode of VTE among cancer patients include: cancer site (especially brain, pancreas, other gastrointestinal organs, lymphoma, and leukemia), advanced cancer stage (especially with liver metastases), chemotherapy, central vein cannulation, and hospitalization or nursing home placement.[22]

Independent risk factors for recurrent VTE include active cancer, unprovoked VTE, multiple VTE recurrences, male sex, increasing obesity, advancing age, antiphospholipid antibody syndrome, and persistently increased plasma D-dimer following cessation of anticoagulation.[2] PTS, even when severe, does not appear to be a risk factor for recurrent VTE.[23]

2.4 The Diagnosis of Venous Thromboembolism

The diagnosis of lower extremity DVT and PE is currently based on validated, Bayesian algorithms derived from outcome-management studies.[24,25,26] These studies prospectively enrolled consecutive patients with suspected VTE. All patients progressed through a particular diagnostic algorithm to confirm or exclude VTE with at least a 3-month follow-up when VTE was excluded. The pretest probability (PTP) of VTE was assessed using validated clinical decision rules to stratify VTE risk as low, moderate (intermediate), or high, or alternatively as unlikely or likely. Patients with low, moderate, or unlikely PTP were then tested for high-sensitivity D-dimer (HS-DD). A normal HS-DD in these patients safely excluded VTE without the need for diagnostic imaging in 20 to 30% of patients, with the likelihood of a new VTE diagnosis over the next 3 months being less than 2% (upper 95% confidence boundary less than 3%). Nevertheless, as discussed below, this is not a safe approach in cancer patients with suspected DVT.[24,27,28,29] A normal HS-DD was also not sufficient to safely exclude VTE in patients with high or likely PTP and should not be routinely ordered. These patients and those with elevated HS-DD generally should proceed to diagnostic imaging with compression ultrasound (CUS) for suspected DVT

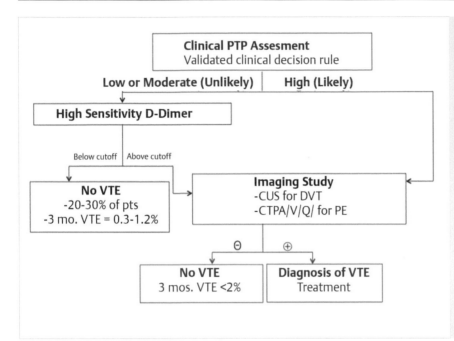

Fig. 2.3 Venous thromboembolism (VTE), either deep vein thrombosis (DVT) or pulmonary embolism (PE), is accurately ruled out in 20 to 30% of patients by the combination of low/moderate/unlikely pretest probability (PTP) and a normal high-sensitivity D-dimer without imaging. With high/likely PTP or elevated D-dimer, a normal imaging study with compression ultrasound (CUS) for suspected DVT or computed tomography pulmonary angiography (CTPA) for suspected PE accurately rules out VTE.

Table 2.2 10-point Wells score for suspected DVT

Item	Points
Active cancer	1
Paralysis, paresis, recent leg plaster immobilization	1
Bedridden ≥ 3 d or major surgery within 12 wk	1
Localized tenderness of deep venous system	1
Entire leg swollen	1
Calf swelling ≥ 3 cm vs. asymptomatic leg, 10 cm below tibial tuberosity	1
Pitting edema confined to symptomatic leg	1
Collateral, nonvaricose superficial veins	1
History of prior DVT	1
Alternative diagnosis as or more likely than DVT	−2

Note: Trichotomized scoring: low (≤ 0); moderate (1–2); high (≥ 3). Dichotomized scoring: unlikely (≤ 1); likely (≥ 2).

or to CTPA, or alternative pulmonary imaging, for suspected PE. After a negative imaging study in these patients, the 3-month VTE rate is generally less than 2% for both suspected DVT and PE (▶ Fig. 2.1).[24,27,28,29] Unfortunately, while these algorithms provide accurate and safe diagnosis of VTE, their actual utilization in clinical practice is suboptimal.[29] Omission or miscalculation of PTP assessment and/or omission of HS-DD testing has led to unnecessary imaging in many patients with consequent expense, radiation exposure, contrast nephropathy, contrast allergy, falsely positive or inconsequential incidental findings, and missed diagnoses with adverse patient outcomes. An algorithm for providers, based on these and other studies, is shown in ▶ Fig. 2.3.

2.4.1 The Diagnosis of Deep Vein Thrombosis

A large, individual patient meta-analysis found that the combination of a low/moderate/unlikely 10-point Wells score (▶ Table 2.2)

and a normal HS-DD safely rules out DVT (3-month VTE recurrence rate < 2%) in about one-third of outpatients with suspected first-episode DVT.[24] However, the Wells score combined with HS-DD approach does not appear to be sufficiently safe or efficient to be used in cancer patients,[24] hospitalized patients,[30] or possibly in patients with suspected recurrent ipsilateral DVT. These patients should proceed directly to CUS evaluation. The use of an age-adjusted HS-DD cut-off (age × 10 for patients age > 50 years) rather than ≥ 500 µg/L has not yet been sufficiently validated for use in clinical practice for patients with suspected DVT.[24]

CUS for DVT diagnosis may be applied only to proximal leg veins (termed limited CUS) or instead to both proximal and distal leg veins below the popliteal vein (termed whole-leg CUS). Direct comparisons of the two approaches demonstrate equivalent diagnostic accuracy.[31] Consistent with this, current guidelines[26,32] indicate that either approach may be used (▶ Fig. 2.4). However, a normal limited CUS study requires a repeat CUS study in 1 week in patients with moderate PTP and an elevated HS-DD and in patients with high or likely PTP, in order to detect progression of isolated distal DVT (IDDVT) into the popliteal vein. This progression occurs in 8 to 15% of patients and primarily in the first week.[33] While a single, whole-leg CUS by a skilled operator safely rules out DVT,[34,35] 40 to 50% of DVT events detected by whole-leg CUS are IDDVT. The clinical significance of IDDVT events and their need for anticoagulation remain controversial.[32,33] Recently, the prospective, multicenter PALLADIO study with 1,162 outpatients validated the safety and convenience of an algorithm combining limited CUS and whole-leg CUS to diagnose DVT. This approach eliminated the need for repeat CUS but also reduced the detection of clinically insignificant IDDVT.[36] With this diagnostic strategy (▶ Fig. 2.4), the 3-month VTE incidence in untreated patients was 0.87% (95% confidence interval [CI]: 0.44–1.70).

2.4.2 Diagnosis of Upper Extremity DVT

Upper extremity DVT (UEDVT) includes thrombosis in the brachial, axillary, subclavian, internal jugular, and brachiocephalic

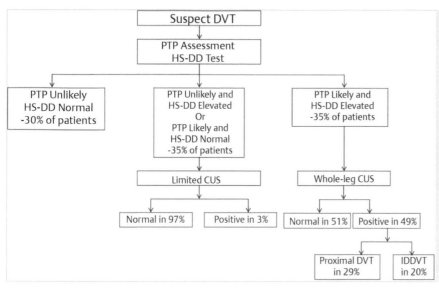

Fig. 2.4 The PALLADIO study algorithm to diagnose deep vein thrombosis (DVT). Depending on the results of the pretest probability (PTP) assessment and a high-sensitivity D-dimer (HS-DD), either no imaging at all, limited compression ultrasound (CUS) of the proximal leg veins, or whole-leg CUS of the proximal and distal leg veins may be used to accurately and efficiently diagnose DVT. However, in cancer patients, progress directly to CUS because of the more limited utility of PTP and HS-DD.

veins; the cephalic and basilic veins are considered distal, superficial veins.[37] UEDVT now constitutes about 10% of all DVT but up to 50% of DVT in hospitalized patients.[38,39,40] About 30% of cases of UEDVT may be classified as primary—that is, idiopathic or due to excessive upper extremity exercise or thoracic outlet vein compression.[41] Secondary UEDVT is associated with placement of central venous catheters or pacemakers and/or with cancer.[41] In some settings, central venous catheters may also increase the risk of lower extremity DVT, independent of causing UEDVT.[17] Complications from UEDVT are less frequent than with lower extremity DVT but PE (3–12%), PTS (7–46%), and recurrent VTE (2–9%) may still occur.[41,42] A high-quality, outcome-management study of 483 patients with suspected UEDVT has recently confirmed the safety of a normal single whole-arm CUS to exclude UEDVT.[43] In this study, the 3-month VTE rate was only 0.3% (95% CI: 0.05–1.68).[43] Another outcome-management study has found that an algorithm combining the Constans Clinical Decision Score, HS-DD, and whole-arm CUS safely ruled out UEDVT and did not require CUS imaging in 21% of patients, but further studies are necessary to confirm its safety.[44,45,46]

2.4.3 Diagnosis of Recurrent Ipsilateral DVT

The accurate diagnosis of recurrent ipsilateral DVT may be challenging.[29,47,48] For over 10 years, up to 40% of patients with prior DVT present with signs and/or symptoms of possible recurrence. About one-half of these patients will have DVT recurrence confirmed, about one-third will have an inconclusive evaluation, and the rest will have an acute exacerbation of PTS or other diagnoses.[29,48] Missing the diagnosis of recurrent DVT exposes the patient to the complications of untreated VTE. Nevertheless, conversely, making a falsely positive diagnosis may commit the patient to indefinite or life-long anticoagulation with its attendant risks of bleeding and other adverse effects. Unfortunately, a validated, safe algorithm incorporating PTP assessment, HS-DD, and CUS is not yet available. While the 10-point Wells score includes one point for prior VTE, its

reliability to safely exclude VTE when combined with a normal HS-DD has not been validated in a large outcome study.[24] The efficiency of this approach is also reduced as HS-DD may remain elevated in nearly 50% of VTE patients 3 months or longer after cessation of anticoagulation. Recommendations vary as to whether an unlikely PTP and normal HS-DD can[47] or cannot[29,48] be used to exclude recurrent ipsilateral DVT.

CUS results may be often inconclusive in these situations. A normal whole-leg CUS does rule out recurrent DVT. However, 1 year after a first DVT event, 40 to 50% of patients have persistent noncompressibility that cannot be definitively distinguished from acute thrombus. If a prior CUS study is available for comparison, new, noncompressible venous segments confirm the diagnosis of recurrent DVT. In settings where there may be residual vein thrombosis, whether a greater than 2- to 4-mm increase in the residual vein diameter of affected proximal leg veins confirms recurrent DVT, or its absence rules out recurrent DVT, is controversial. If the current CUS is nondiagnostic in comparison to a prior CUS, or if a prior CUS is unavailable, careful clinical judgment and consultation with a VTE specialist, where available, is recommended. ▶ Fig. 2.5 provides potential options for diagnosing recurrent ipsilateral DVT as suggested by several investigators.[29,47,48,49] A promising new diagnostic approach not yet validated by a large outcome-management study is magnetic resonance direct thrombus imaging. In a small study of 81 patients, this procedure differentiated acute recurrent from chronic residual thrombi with a sensitivity of 95% and specificity of 100% with good interobserver agreement.[50] A prospective outcome-management study is in progress. 18F-fluorodeoxyglucose positron emission tomography (^{18}F-FDG-PET) is also being investigated as a potential imaging tool to distinguish the acuity of DVT.[51,52,53]

2.4.4 The Diagnosis of Pulmonary Embolism

The underdiagnosis of PE has long been a concern, but recent studies suggest there may be increasing overdiagnosis of PE in community settings. CTPA utilization to diagnose PE has

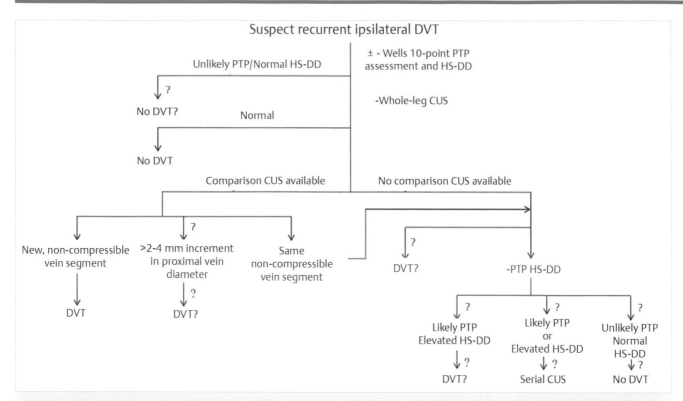

Fig. 2.5 In patients with suspected recurrent ipsilateral deep vein thrombosis (DVT), the utility of the Wells 10-point pretest probability (PTP) assessment and high-sensitivity D-dimer (HS-DD) is controversial; some clinicians instead progress directly to whole-leg compression ultrasound (CUS). If available, a comparison CUS can help make the diagnosis of recurrent DVT. If no comparison CUS is available, or if the same noncompressible vein segment is present in both CUS studies, a clear diagnosis may often be more difficult. Some clinicians would treat these patients as recurrent DVT, while others would consider PTP and HS-DD results as listed.

increased between 4- and 27-fold in recent years.[54] During this time, the age-adjusted incidence of PE increased by 80%, but PE mortality rates did not decrease.[55] These data may suggest that some detected PE either are clinically inconsequential because of small size and low recurrence risk, were asymptomatic incidental diagnosis, or were false-positive diagnoses.[55] Patients at very low risk for PE now undergo unnecessary diagnostic evaluation as indicated by the increasingly very low yield of PE diagnoses by CTPA, currently ranging from just 2.7 to 10% in U.S. emergency departments.[56,57] As many as 25% of currently detected PE may be false-positive diagnoses when the CTPA images undergo reinterpretation by a panel of subspecialty chest radiologists.[58] There may be multiple explanations for excessive use of CTPA and HS-DD to diagnose PE. These include clinician desire to rule out a potentially fatal diagnosis at any cost, clinician fear of litigation if a PE diagnosis is missed, patient expectations, the easy, immediate availability of CTPA, and clinician lack of knowledge about or simple failure to use evidence-based PE diagnostic algorithms.[25] A recent study found that only 45% of CTPA studies were ordered appropriately according to the results of PTP assessment and HS-DD measurement.[59] Over one-half of clinicians reported that they used formal PTP assessment tools in less than one-half of suspected PE cases.[60]

Several new approaches have been proposed to reduce excessive diagnostic testing for PE and consequent overdiagnosis and overtreatment, unnecessary radiation exposure and expense, and other potential complications of CTPA.[25,26] First, it may be useful to increase the utilization of evidence-based PTP

assessment and HS-DD by requiring these evaluations on CTPA order sheets and/or by incorporating the necessary clinical decision support into the electronic medical record. A systematic review of recent studies found that implementation of the Wells criteria for PE diagnosis increased the yield of CTPA by 33%.[56] A recent systematic review suggested that the modified and simplified Wells rules may be slightly more useful than the revised and simplified revised Geneva models in primary care settings.[61] ▶ Table 2.3 shows the simplified Wells rule and revised Geneva score. In contrast, a previous direct comparison of these rules in an outcome-management study found them equivalent, although the revised Geneva score has been validated only in outpatients.[62] Some investigators propose that clinician gestalt, especially by more experienced clinicians, is potentially equivalent to use of the formal PTP assessments.[63]

A second approach reduces unnecessary testing with HS-DD in patients with very low probability of PE by combining the Pulmonary Embolism Rule-Out Criteria (PERC) with the Wells or revised Geneva models. The PERC criteria are listed in ▶ Table 2.4.[64] A meta-analysis of 12 studies found that when the PERC criteria were applied to patients with low PTP assessment assessed by a validated clinical decision rule, and all 8 PERC criteria were met, the proportion of missed PEs was only 0.3%, eliminating the need for HS-DD testing in 22% of patients with suspected PE.[25,64] However, the PERC criteria may only be applied to patients with low PTP.[25]

A third approach to reduce unnecessary CTPA imaging is to use age-adjusted normal/abnormal cut-off levels for HS-DD in

Table 2.3 Clinical decision rules for PE

	Wells rule			Revised Geneva score		
Item	Original	Simplified	Item	Original	Simplified
Previous PE or DVT	1.5	1	Previous PE or DVT	3	1
Heart rate > 100/min	1.5	1	Heart rate 75–94/min	3	1
			Heart rate ≥ 95/min	5	2
Surgery or immobilization < 4 wk	1.5	1	Surgery or fracture ≤ 1 mo	2	1
Hemoptysis	1	1	Hemoptysis	2	1
Active malignancy	1	1	Active malignancy	2	1
Clinical signs of DVT	3	1	Unilateral lower limb pain	3	1
Alternative diagnosis less likely than PE	3	1	Pain on lower limb deep vein palpation *and* unilateral edema	4	1
			Age ≥ 65 y	1	1
Clinical probability			**clinical probability**		
Low	< 2		Low	0–3	
Intermediate	2–6		Intermediate	4–10	
High	> 6		High	≥ 11	
PE unlikely	≤ 4	≤ 1	PE unlikely	≤ 5	≤ 2
PE likely	> 4	> 1	PE likely	> 5	> 2

Table 2.4 The Pulmonary Embolism Rule-Out Criteria (PERC)

Age < 50 y

Initial heart rate < 100 beats/min

Initial room air oxygen saturation > 94%

No unilateral leg swelling

No hemoptysis

No surgery or trauma within 4 wk

No history of venous thromboembolism

No estrogen use

order to improve the specificity of the HS-DD test for PE. HS-DD levels increases progressively with age in the general population such that 90% of persons aged ≥ 80 years evaluated for suspected PE will have an HS-DD ≥ 500 ng/mL.[65] A meta-analysis[66] and a large prospective management trial[67] have evaluated the safety of using an age-adjusted, HS-DD cut-off level in patients aged > 50 years. In these studies, the HS-DD cut-off was the patient's age multiplied by 10 (in ng/mL), rather than the standard cut-off of 500 ng/mL, to help rule out PE. In patients aged over 50 years with a low, moderate, or unlikely PTP and a normal, age-adjusted HS-DD, the 3-month incidence of VTE was just 0.3% (95% CI: 0.1–1.7). Thus, in these studies, use of an age-adjusted HS-DD allowed PE to be ruled out without diagnostic imaging in an additional 12% of patients aged over 50 years and in 30% of patients aged ≥ 75 years.[67] Based on these studies, in 2015 the American College of Physicians recommended the diagnostic approach in ▶ Fig. 2.6.[25]

Most guidelines favor CTPA to confirm the diagnosis of PE in patients with an elevated HS-DD or high PTP in both outpatients and inpatients in the absence of contraindications.[25,26] An unresolved controversy is the clinical significance and management of isolated, small subsegmental pulmonary emboli (SSPE), which constitute up to 15% of all detected PE.[32,68,69] No prospec-

tive outcome-management studies are yet available to define optimal management of isolated SSPE, although such a trial is in progress in patients with SSPE who have normal bilateral CUS and no cancer (NCTO1455818). Some detected SSPE likely represent false-positive diagnoses, while others may carry no clinical significance.[32,55] Small retrospective studies have come to opposing conclusions as to whether treatment is indicated.[70,71] If bilateral CUS is normal, the 2016 Chest Expert Panel Report suggests that the decision to anticoagulate patients with SSPE (that has been confirmed by an experienced chest radiologist) depends on balancing the presence and strength of VTE recurrence risk factors, bleeding risk, baseline cardiopulmonary reserve, symptom severity, and patient preference (▶ Table 2.5).[32]

In the presence of relative contraindications to CTPA (e.g., renal insufficiency, severe contrast allergy, or a desire to limit radiation exposure, particularly in women under age 50 and in patients with prior CTPA or CT exposure), ventilation-perfusion lung scintigraphy combined with PTP assessment, HS-DD, and serial bilateral CUS can safely exclude and diagnose PE as well as CTPA, as demonstrated in outcome-management studies.[72,73] ▶ Fig. 2.7 shows the diagnostic algorithm from one of the studies.[72]

2.5 Acute Treatment of Venous Thromboembolism

The cornerstone of the acute treatment of VTE, once VTE has been diagnosed or is strongly clinically suspected, is the use of an antithrombotic agent with a rapid onset of action.[54,74] This helps prevent thrombus propagation or embolization. While traditionally accomplished through a parenteral antithrombotic agent, including intravenously or subcutaneously delivered unfractionated heparin (UFH), subcutaneous low-molecular-weight heparin (LMWH), or subcutaneous fondaparinux, in recent years the approval of the DOACs provides alternative

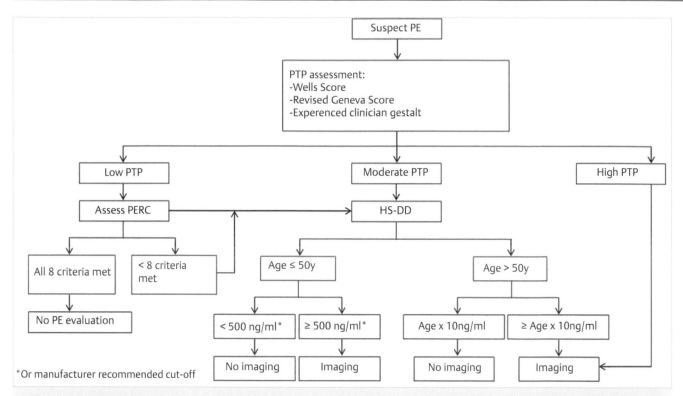

Fig. 2.6 The American College of Physicians algorithm for evaluation of suspected pulmonary embolism (PE) combines a low pretest probability (PTP) assessment with the Pulmonary Embolism Rule-Out Criteria (PERC) to decide on the need to test for high-sensitivity D-dimer (HS-DD). If less than eight PERC criteria are met, or if the PTP is moderate, an age-adjusted approach to the use of HS-DD is used. Patients with high PTP or an elevated age-adjusted HS-DD require an imaging study for PE.

Table 2.5 Contraindications to thrombolytic therapy: Chest Expert Panel, 2016

Major contraindications	Relative contraindications
Previous ICH	Recent nonintracranial bleeding
Ischemic stroke within 3 mo	Ischemic stroke > 3 mo previously
Active bleeding or bleeding diathesis	Anticoagulation (e.g., VKA, DOAC, etc.)
Recent brain or spinal surgery	Other recent surgery or invasive procedure
	Traumatic cardiopulmonary resuscitation
Structural intracranial disease	Systolic blood pressure > 180 mm Hg *or* diastolic blood pressure > 110 mm Hg
	Diabetic retinopathy
	Pericarditis or pericardial fluid
	Pregnancy
	Age > 75 y
	Low body weight (e.g., < 60 kg)
	Female gender
	Black race

Abbreviations: DOAC, direct oral anticoagulant; ICH, intracranial hemorrhage; VKA, vitamin K antagonist.

therapeutic tools for providers. The DOACs, discussed in more detail below, include rivaroxaban, dabigatran, apixaban, and edoxaban (▶ Table 2.6). As discussed below, in some instances the use of a DOAC for the acute treatment of VTE still requires lead-in therapy with a heparinoid, while other DOACs may be used as monotherapy without initial heparin therapy. While the use of UFH is declining for the acute treatment of VTE, particularly as more patients are treated in the outpatient setting, rather than being hospitalized, UFH remains a useful agent in patients with severe renal insufficiency or patients with a high bleeding risk where rapid anticoagulant reversal may be needed. Subcutaneous LMWH has more predictable pharmacology than UFH, allowing for outpatient VTE treatment with fixed, weight-based dosing. LMWH is also associated with fewer thrombotic complications, less major bleeding, and a mortality benefit when compared to UFH for VTE treatment.[75] In some patients, routine lab monitoring while LMWHs are being used may not be necessary.

The outpatient treatment of VTE is well established for appropriate patients with DVT without PE. Consistent with this, recent guidelines emphasize that patients with DVT alone may generally be treated as outpatients. Emerging data suggest that in carefully selected, low-risk patients with acute PE, outpatient therapy may also be safe and cost-effective,[32,76,77,78,79] although some uncertainties remain with regard to appropriate patient selection and treatment.

Often initiated concurrent with antithrombotic therapy, warfarin was the cornerstone of oral VTE treatment for nearly 60 years until the introduction of DOACs. Warfarin's narrow therapeutic window and numerous food and drug interactions necessitate routine INR monitoring for the duration of therapy. DOACs are a class of oral anticoagulants that more directly

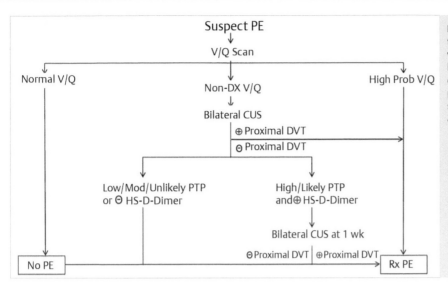

Fig. 2.7 If a contraindication to computed tomography pulmonary angiography is present, ventilation/perfusion (V/Q) scans combined with bilateral compression ultrasound (CUS) to diagnose coexisting deep vein thrombosis (DVT), pretest probability (PTP) assessment, and high-sensitivity (HS) D-dimer can be used to accurately and safely diagnose pulmonary embolism (PE).

Table 2.6 Comparisons of the direct oral anticoagulants (DOACs) for the treatment of VTE

	Apixaban (Eliquis)	Dabigatran (Pradaxa)	Edoxaban (Savaysa)	Rivaroxaban (Xarelto)
Mechanism of action	Factor Xa inhibitor	Direct thrombin inhibitor	Factor Xa inhibitor	Factor Xa inhibitor
Half-life $(t_{1/2})^a$	~12 h	~12–17 h	~10–14 h	~5–9 h
C_{max}^a	~3–4 h	~1 h	~1–2 h	~2–4 h
Renal excretion	~27%	~80%	~50%	~36%
Dosing regimen for acute VTE[b]	10 mg BID × 7 d 5 mg BID following day 7	150 mg BID	60 mg once daily	15 mg BID × 21 d 20 mg once daily following day 21
Parenteral anticoagulation lead-in	No	Yes	Yes	No
Dosing regimen for secondary VTE prevention[b]	2.5 mg BID ≥ 6 mo of treatment	150 mg BID	60 mg once daily	20 mg once daily
Specific FDA-approved antidote	No	Yes	No	No

Abbreviation: BID, twice daily (see package inserts for more details including information on dose adjustments in certain patients).
aPharmacokinetics may vary in some patients.
bFDA-approved dosing.

target specific coagulation factors. The DOACs currently FDA-approved for the treatment of VTE include dabigatran, rivaroxaban, apixaban, and edoxaban. Each of these agents has unique pharmacology and pharmacokinetics (▶ Table 2.4). In addition, indications and dosing of the DOACs vary. A comprehensive review of each of these DOACs is beyond the scope of this chapter and the reader is referred to each product's package insert and several recent reviews for more information.[54,74,80,81,82]

Dabigatran is a direct thrombin inhibitor that competitively binds to soluble and fibrin-bound thrombin, inhibiting the conversion of fibrinogen to fibrin and subsequent thrombus formation. Rivaroxaban, apixaban, and edoxaban are factor Xa inhibitors that selectively block the active site of factor Xa, inhibiting the coagulation cascade without the use of a cofactor (antithrombin). Additional appealing attributes of the DOACs include fewer drug interactions and more predictable pharmacology than warfarin, minimizing the need for routine lab monitoring and frequent dose adjustments.[83] Randomized clinical

VTE treatment trials have demonstrated the DOACs are noninferior to warfarin with respect to efficacy, and some agents may have superior safety profiles.[84,85,86,87,88,89] Some of these trials are discussed in more detail below.

The RE-COVER[88,89] and Hokusai VTE[85] studies compared warfarin to dabigatran and edoxaban, respectively. One design of these studies to highlight was the requirement of an initial course of heparin (UFH or LMWH) prior to DOAC initiation. In comparison, the EINSTEIN[86,87] and AMPLIFY[84] studies compared conventional therapy to rivaroxaban and apixaban as monotherapy without preceding heparin. These studies also established that the bleeding risk with apixaban, edoxaban, and rivaroxaban is lower compared to warfarin. Dabigatran has a similar bleeding risk profile to warfarin. Given the generally favorable bleeding profiles, the ability to forego parenteral anticoagulation with certain agents, and avoidance of routine lab monitoring, VTE treatment with DOACs provides some advantages for health care providers and carefully selected patients.

Unlike heparin and warfarin that can be reversed with protamine and vitamin K or plasma administration, respectively, DOAC reversal can be more challenging. Currently, the only FDA-approved reversal agent for any DOAC is idarucizumab: a monoclonal antibody fragment specific to dabigatran.[90] Specific reversal agents for factor Xa inhibitors (e.g., rivaroxaban, apixaban, and edoxaban) are in late-stage development.[91,92,93] Four-factor PCC (prothrombin complex concentrates), comprised of coagulation factors II, VII, IX, and X, has been evaluated in small studies and may be effective in correcting coagulation assay derangements following rivaroxaban administration.[94] Activated forms of PCC (aPCC) or recombinant FVIIa may be effective in reversing effects of dabigatran.[95] Unfortunately, observational data on novel oral anticoagulant–associated intracranial hemorrhage failed to demonstrate significant improvements in clinical outcomes among patients receiving PCC.[96] Until specific reversal agents for factor Xa inhibitors are approved, management of major or life-threatening bleeding remains supportive care with blood-product transfusion and mechanical intervention whenever possible (e.g., endoscopy, manual compression of compressible sites, intravascular embolization). With major or life-threatening bleeding associated with dabigatran use, idarucizumab administration should be considered.

Regardless of the antithrombotic agent and/or oral anticoagulant chosen, baseline assessment of bleeding risk, measurement of renal and hepatic function, platelet count, baseline coagulation measurements, and a thorough medication review are essential.[97] Patient and caregiver education is also paramount and may help inform decisions regarding the anticoagulant, intensity, and duration of therapy chosen. Patient preferences are especially important to ascertain in settings where there may be equipoise on anticoagulation initiation and/or duration (e.g., for a single, unprovoked distal DVT). Once anticoagulation is initiated, regular monitoring of renal function and other indicated laboratory tests, and medication compliance is important in older adults, given their increased bleeding risk.[97] In some settings, anticoagulation clinics, which historically managed patients on a vitamin K antagonist (VKA), now also follow patients on DOACs. Anticoagulation clinics may serve as key resources for patients and providers, helping ensure compliance, providing patient education, and assisting with periprocedural anticoagulation management. Patient-focused educational materials for anticoagulation are also recommended.[98,99]

2.5.1 Thrombolysis for Acute, Massive Pulmonary Embolism

Adverse outcomes in patients with PE vary, based in part on initial presentation and the presence or absence of sustained hypotension (e.g., systolic blood pressure < 90 mm Hg or requiring inotropic support; commonly termed "massive PE").[32,100] While published mortality rates vary, hypotension and/or cardiopulmonary arrest in patients with massive PE is associated with a significantly higher risk of short-term death than patients with submassive PE (e.g., systolic blood pressure > 90 mm Hg but with evidence of right heart strain or dysfunction) or patients with nonmassive PE (systolic blood pressure > 90 mm Hg and *no* evidence of right heart strain). For example, in-hospital mortality in patients enrolled in the Management Strategy and Prognosis of Pulmonary Embolism Registry (MAPPET) ranged from 8.1% (hemodynamically stable) to 25% (cardiogenic shock) to 65% (cardiopulmonary resuscitation).[100,101] Similarly, 90-day mortality rates in patients studied in the International Cooperative Pulmonary Embolism Registry (ICOPER) were 52.4% in PE patients with hypotension versus 14.7% in PE patients without hypotension upon initial presentation.[60,102] Given this high mortality, patients with confirmed massive PE and no contraindications (▶ Table 2.6) are often considered for fibrinolysis. While the fibrinolytic agent chosen, as well as dosing and route of administration, may vary, the use of fibrinolytics improves lung perfusion and reduces mortality in patients with massive PE.[100,103,104,105] These clinical benefits with fibrinolytics are offset by an increased risk of major bleeding (10% or greater in unselected patients) and intracranial hemorrhage (2 to 3%) compared to anticoagulation alone.[101,106,107,108] Recent meta-analyses suggest that in massive PE, the number needed to treat to prevent recurrent PE or death was 10, while the number needed to harm was 8.[109] As such, current guidelines recommend the administration of fibrinolytics in patients with massive PE who do not have a high bleeding risk.[32,100]

2.5.2 Duration of Anticoagulation for VTE

The optimal duration of anticoagulation is determined primarily by the risk of recurrent VTE but may be modified in some patients by the risk of major bleeding, effects on lifestyle, expense, and patient preference.[32,110] The minimum recommended duration of anticoagulation for VTE is 3 months. Randomized trials and their meta-analyses demonstrate that anticoagulation of VTE for less than 3 months increases the risk of recurrent VTE during the 6- to 12-month period following cessation of therapy.[110] Extending anticoagulation duration to 6 to 18 months after a first VTE event reduces VTE recurrence during the period of anticoagulation by 80 to 90%,[110,111] reduces the composite outcome of VTE recurrence and major bleeding by 78%,[112] and may reduce all-cause mortality and PE-related mortality by 53 and 68%, respectively.[113] However, extended duration anticoagulation beyond 3 months does not further reduce VTE recurrence rate once anticoagulation is discontinued.[32,112]

The primary determinant of recurrent proximal DVT or PE once anticoagulant therapy is stopped is whether the event was provoked by a transient surgical or nonsurgical risk factor (3 and 15% 5-year recurrence rates, respectively), or was unprovoked (30% 5-year recurrence rate), or occurred in the setting of active cancer (15% per year recurrence rate).[80,110] A second VTE event may increase the risk for a third VTE event by 50% above the recurrence rates listed above.[110] On the other hand, patients with IDDVT appear to have 50% lower recurrence rates than those listed above.[58] VTE recurrence rates above 5 to 8% at 1 year and above 15% at 5 years are generally considered as unacceptable and require careful consideration of extended duration anticoagulation.[80,110,114]

For patients with unprovoked proximal DVT or PE, finding risk factors or clinical decision rules that may help distinguish the 30% who will have a VTE recurrence over 5 years, from the 70% who will not, has been the aim of recent investigation. Several factors may strengthen borderline decisions to recommend extended anticoagulation. First, multiple studies demonstrate that the risk of recurrent VTE is twofold higher in men than women without reproductive risk factors.[115,116] Second, for patients whose initial presentation is PE, 70 to 80% of VTE recurrences are as PE rather than DVT.[117] PE recurrence may carry an 8 to 27% case fatality rate.[112,118] Third, patients with unprovoked VTE who have elevated D-dimer levels following cessation of anticoagulation have a higher VTE recurrence risk.[119] One recent management study found a low, 3% per year, VTE recurrence rate in patients with persistently normal HS-DD levels at 15, 30, 60, and 90 days following cessation of anticoagulation.[120] In contrast, another recent management study measured D-dimer 1 month after cessation of anticoagulation. Annual VTE recurrence rates in patients with normal D-dimer levels were 9.7% in men and 5.4% in women whose VTE was not associated with estrogen therapy, suggesting that only women with unprovoked VTE might benefit from D-dimer testing to help guide duration of anticoagulation.[121] However, current uncertainty about the type, timing, and cut-off levels for D-dimer and how D-dimer relates to patient gender may limit its use at this time to borderline decisions to stop or extend anticoagulation.[110] The predictive strength for recurrent VTE of either residual venous obstruction on CUS[122] or detection of antiphospholipid antibodies[123] remains uncertain. Nevertheless, these factors might be considered in patients where there is equipoise for extended anticoagulation. Although three clinical decision rules (Vienna Prediction Model, HERDOO-2, DASH score) that combine clinical and laboratory parameters to predict the likelihood of VTE recurrence have been proposed,[124,125,126] only the Vienna Prediction Model currently has an external validation study.[127] Some guidelines use the Vienna tool to provide patients an approximation of their VTE recurrence risk off anticoagulation.[26] Finally, in most cases, the presence or absence of hereditary thrombophilia disorders does not strongly predict VTE recurrence and current guidelines recommend against routine thrombophilia testing for both unprovoked and provoked VTE.[21,32]

The benefits of extended duration anticoagulation to reduce VTE recurrence must be balanced against the increased risk of major bleeding, particularly fatal bleeding. During the initial 3 months of treatment, the case fatality rates for major bleeding are much higher than those for recurrent VTE—11.3 versus 3.6%.[128] The gap between these case fatality rates may narrow during extended duration anticoagulation.[110] For this reason, the 2016 Chest Expert Panel Report recommends against extended anticoagulation for patients at high risk of bleeding (► Table 2.7).[32] Unfortunately, adequately validated bleeding risk assessment tools are not currently available to accurately quantify major bleeding risk during extended anticoagulation. The Chest Expert Panel Report recommends the use of a list of bleeding risk factors to stratify major bleeding risk: high, two or more risks; moderate, one risk; and low, 0 risks.[32] However, the recommendations for duration of anticoagulation for VTE listed in ► Table 2.8 are frequently not utilized in routine clinical practice. This may result in underuse of extended anticoagulation in 45% of patients with unprovoked VTE but also overuse in 58% of patients with transient risk factors who should be anticoagulated for only 3 months.

Table 2.7 Risk factors for bleeding with anticoagulation therapy

Age ≥ 65 (especially > 75 years old)
Frequent falls
Renal impairment with creatinine clearance < 50 mL/min
Hepatic failure
Cancer (especially metastatic)
Previous stroke
Recent bleeding
Labile INR
Alcohol abuse
Concurrent use of aspirin or NSAIDs
Diabetes
Anemia
Thrombocytopenia
Low risk= 0 risk factors
Moderate risk= 1 risk factor (absolute risk of bleeding 1.6% 0–3 mo; 0.8% > 3 mo)
High risk ≥ 2 risk factors (absolute risk of bleeding 3.2% 0–3 mo; 1.6% > 3 mo)

Abbreviations: INR, international normalized ratio; NSAIDs, nonsteroidal anti-inflammatory drugs.

2.6 Pearls of Wisdom

- The evaluation of suspected VTE should typically start with a PTP assessment, which can then guide appropriate use of laboratory testing (e.g., the HS-DD) and imaging (e.g., CUS, CTPA, etc.).
- DOACs for the acute treatment and secondary prevention of VTE provide alternatives to VKAs (e.g., warfarin). The decision on whether to use a DOAC or a VKA should take into consideration patient-specific factors, cost, and patient preference.
- The duration of oral anticoagulation (OAC) should be carefully tailored to patient risk factors, including both VTE recurrence and bleeding. Patient compliance, education, and preference should be considered in decisions regarding the duration of OAC.

2.7 Unanswered Questions

- Does systemic or catheter-directed thrombolysis improve net clinical benefit in patients with submassive PE or DVT?
- How can we more accurately determine a patient's risk of recurrent VTE in order to guide optimal duration of OAC?
- What is the role of measuring the HS-DD in determining an individual patient's risk of recurrent VTE?

2.8 Acknowledgments

We thank Ms. Diana Lim for her creativity and excellent figure preparation and Ms. Kendra Richardson for her editorial assistance. We also appreciate the critical review and helpful feedback from Dr. Barry Stults.

Table 2.8 Duration of anticoagulation for VTE: Chest Expert Panel, 2016

Indication	Estimated VTE recurrence rate		Proposed duration of anticoagulation
	1 y	5 y	
First proximal DVT/PE			
• Provoked by surgery	1%	3%	3 mo
First proximal DVT/PE			
• Provoked by nonsurgical transient risk factor	5%	15%	3 mo (or until resolution of the transient risk factor)
First isolated distal DVT			
• Provoked	0.5%	1.5%	3 mo
• Unprovoked	5%	15%	3 mo
First proximal DVT/PE			
• Unprovoked	10%	30%	
• Nonhigh bleeding risk			Extended (indefinite)
• High bleeding risk			3 mo
Second VTE			
• Unprovoked	15%	45%	
• Nonhigh bleeding risk			Extended (indefinite)
• High bleeding risk			3 mo
Active cancer VTE	15%/y		Extended (indefinite) until cancer inactive

2.9 Conflict of Interest

Dr. Rondina has received honoraria from Janssen Pharmaceuticals, Inc., for participation on a scientific advisory board. None of the other authors declare a relevant conflict of interest.

2.10 Author's Contributions

Conception and design of manuscript: M.T.R. and H.F.; drafting and critical revision of manuscript: M.T.R. and H.F.; and final approval of the manuscript version to be published: M.T.R. and H.F.

References

[1] Heit JA. Epidemiology of venous thromboembolism. Nat Rev Cardiol. 2015; 12(8):464–474
[2] Heit JA, Spencer FA, White RH. The epidemiology of venous thromboembolism. J Thromb Thrombolysis. 2016; 41(1):3–14
[3] Grosse SD, Nelson RE, Nyarko KA, Richardson LC, Raskob GE. The economic burden of incident venous thromboembolism in the United States: A review of estimated attributable healthcare costs. Thromb Res. 2016; 137:3–10
[4] ISTH Steering Committee for World Thrombosis Day. Thrombosis: a major contributor to global disease burden. Thromb Res. 2014; 134(5):931–938
[5] Bell EJ, Lutsey PL, Basu S, et al. Lifetime risk of venous thromboembolism in two cohort studies. Am J Med. 2016; 129(3):339.e19–339.e26
[6] Huang W, Goldberg RJ, Anderson FA, Kiefe CI, Spencer FA. Secular trends in occurrence of acute venous thromboembolism: the Worcester VTE study (1985–2009). Am J Med. 2014; 127(9):829–39.e5
[7] Li C, Hirsh J, Xie C, Johnston MA, Eikelboom JW. Reversal of the anti-platelet effects of aspirin and clopidogrel. J Thromb Haemost. 2012; 10(4):521–528
[8] Mozaffarian D, Benjamin EJ, Go AS, et al. American Heart Association Statistics Committee and Stroke Statistics Subcommittee. Heart disease and stroke statistics–2015 update: a report from the American Heart Association. Circulation. 2015; 131(4):e29–e322

[9] Huang W, Goldberg RJ, Anderson FA, Cohen AT, Spencer FA. Occurrence and predictors of recurrence after a first episode of acute venous thromboembolism: population-based Worcester Venous Thromboembolism Study. J Thromb Thrombolysis. 2016; 41(3):525–538
[10] Huang W, Goldberg RJ, Cohen AT, et al. Declining long-term risk of adverse events after first-time community-presenting venous thromboembolism: the population-based Worcester VTE study (1999 to 2009). Thromb Res. 2015; 135(6):1100–1106
[11] Vazquez SR, Freeman A, VanWoerkom RC, Rondina MT. Contemporary issues in the prevention and management of postthrombotic syndrome. Ann Pharmacother. 2009; 43(11):1824–1835
[12] Kahn SR, Galanaud JP, Vedantham S, Ginsberg JS. Guidance for the prevention and treatment of the post-thrombotic syndrome. J Thromb Thrombolysis. 2016; 41(1):144–153
[13] Klok FA, Dzikowska-Diduch O, Kostrubiec M, et al. Derivation of a clinical prediction score for chronic thromboembolic pulmonary hypertension after acute pulmonary embolism. J Thromb Haemost. 2016; 14(1):121–128
[14] Riva N, Donadini MP, Ageno W. Epidemiology and pathophysiology of venous thromboembolism: similarities with atherothrombosis and the role of inflammation. Thromb Haemost. 2015; 113(6):1176–1183
[15] Rosendaal FR. Venous thrombosis: a multicausal disease. Lancet. 1999; 353 (9159):1167–1173
[16] Martinez C, Cohen AT, Bamber L, Rietbrock S. Epidemiology of first and recurrent venous thromboembolism: a population-based cohort study in patients without active cancer. Thromb Haemost. 2014; 112(2):255–263
[17] Kaplan D, Casper TC, Elliott CG, et al. VTE incidence and risk factors in patients with severe sepsis and septic shock. Chest. 2015; 148(5):1224–1230
[18] Mohebali D, Kaplan D, Carlisle M, Supiano MA, Rondina MT. Alterations in platelet function during aging: clinical correlations with thromboinflammatory disease in older adults. J Am Geriatr Soc. 2014; 62(3):529–535
[19] Blix K, Brækkan SK, le Cessie S, Skjeldestad FE, Cannegieter SC, Hansen JB. The increased risk of venous thromboembolism by advancing age cannot be attributed to the higher incidence of cancer in the elderly: the Tromsø study. Eur J Epidemiol. 2014; 29(4):277–284
[20] Zakai NA, McClure LA, Judd SE, et al. Racial and regional differences in venous thromboembolism in the United States in 3 cohorts. Circulation. 2014; 129(14):1502–1509
[21] Stevens SM, Woller SC, Bauer KA, et al. Guidance for the evaluation and treatment of hereditary and acquired thrombophilia. J Thromb Thrombolysis. 2016; 41(1):154–164

[22] Ashrani AA, Gullerud RE, Petterson TM, Marks RS, Bailey KR, Heit JA. Risk factors for incident venous thromboembolism in active cancer patients: A population based case-control study. Thromb Res. 2016; 139:29–37

[23] Prandoni P, Noventa F, Lensing AW, Prins MH, Villalta S. Post-thrombotic syndrome and the risk of subsequent recurrent thromboembolism. Thromb Res. 2016; 141:91–92

[24] Geersing GJ, Zuithoff NP, Kearon C, et al. Exclusion of deep vein thrombosis using the Wells rule in clinically important subgroups: individual patient data meta-analysis. BMJ. 2014; 348:g1340

[25] Raja AS, Greenberg JO, Qaseem A, Denberg TD, Fitterman N, Schuur JD, Clinical Guidelines Committee of the American College of Physicians. Evaluation of patients with suspected acute pulmonary embolism: best practice advice from the Clinical Guidelines Committee of the American College of Physicians. Ann Intern Med. 2015; 163(9):701–711

[26] Streiff MB, Agnelli G, Connors JM, et al. Guidance for the treatment of deep vein thrombosis and pulmonary embolism. J Thromb Thrombolysis. 2016; 41(1):32–67

[27] Mos IC, Klok FA, Kroft LJ, DE Roos A, Dekkers OM, Huisman MV. Safety of ruling out acute pulmonary embolism by normal computed tomography pulmonary angiography in patients with an indication for computed tomography: systematic review and meta-analysis. J Thromb Haemost. 2009; 7(9):1491–1498

[28] Pasha SM, Klok FA, Snoep JD, et al. Safety of excluding acute pulmonary embolism based on an unlikely clinical probability by the Wells rule and normal D-dimer concentration: a meta-analysis. Thromb Res. 2010; 125(4):e123–e127

[29] van der Hulle T, Dronkers CE, Huisman MV, Klok FA. Current standings in diagnostic management of acute venous thromboembolism: still rough around the edges. Blood Rev. 2016; 30(1):21–26

[30] Silveira PC, Ip IK, Goldhaber SZ, Piazza G, Benson CB, Khorasani R. Performance of Wells score for deep vein thrombosis in the inpatient setting. JAMA Intern Med. 2015; 175(7):1112–1117

[31] Le Gal G, Righini M. Controversies in the diagnosis of venous thromboembolism. J Thromb Haemost. 2015; 13 Suppl 1:S259–S265

[32] Kearon C, Akl EA, Ornelas J, et al. Antithrombotic therapy for VTE disease: CHEST guideline and expert panel report. Chest. 2016; 149(2):315–352

[33] Palareti G. How I treat isolated distal deep vein thrombosis (IDDVT). Blood. 2014; 123(12):1802–1809

[34] Johnson SA, Stevens SM, Woller SC, et al. Risk of deep vein thrombosis following a single negative whole-leg compression ultrasound: a systematic review and meta-analysis. JAMA. 2010; 303(5):438–445

[35] Stevens SM, Woller SC, Graves KK, et al. Withholding anticoagulation following a single negative whole-leg ultrasound in patients at high pretest probability for deep vein thrombosis. Clin Appl Thromb Hemost. 2013; 19(1):79–85

[36] Ageno W, Camporese G, Riva N, et al. PALLADIO Study Investigators. Analysis of an algorithm incorporating limited and whole-leg assessment of the deep venous system in symptomatic outpatients with suspected deep-vein thrombosis (PALLADIO): a prospective, multicentre, cohort study. Lancet Haematol. 2015; 2(11):e474–e480

[37] Zwicker JI, Connolly G, Carrier M, Kamphuisen PW, Lee AY. Catheter-associated deep vein thrombosis of the upper extremity in cancer patients: guidance from the SSC of the ISTH. J Thromb Haemost. 2014; 12(5):796–800

[38] Bates SM, Jaeschke R, Stevens SM, et al. Diagnosis of DVT: Antithrombotic Therapy and Prevention of Thrombosis, 9th ed: American College of Chest Physicians Evidence-Based Clinical Practice Guidelines. Chest. 2012; 141 2 Suppl:e351S–418S

[39] Spencer FA, Emery C, Lessard D, Goldberg RJ, Worcester Venous Thromboembolism S, Worcester Venous Thromboembolism Study. Upper extremity deep vein thrombosis: a community-based perspective. Am J Med. 2007; 120(8):678–684

[40] Winters JP, Callas PW, Cushman M, Repp AB, Zakai NA. Central venous catheters and upper extremity deep vein thrombosis in medical inpatients: the Medical Inpatients and Thrombosis (MITH) study. J Thromb Haemost. 2015; 13(12):2155–2160

[41] Grant JD, Stevens SM, Woller SC, et al. Diagnosis and management of upper extremity deep-vein thrombosis in adults. Thromb Haemost. 2012; 108(6):1097–1108

[42] Bleker SM, van Es N, Kleinjan A, et al. Current management strategies and long-term clinical outcomes of upper extremity venous thrombosis. J Thromb Haemost. 2016; 14(5):973–981

[43] Sartori M, Migliaccio L, Favaretto E, et al. Whole-arm ultrasound to rule out suspected upper-extremity deep venous thrombosis in outpatients. JAMA Intern Med. 2015; 175(7):1226–1227

[44] Constans J, Salmi LR, Sevestre-Pietri MA, et al. A clinical prediction score for upper extremity deep venous thrombosis. Thromb haemost. 2008; 99(1):202–207

[45] Delluc A, Wells PS. Low failure rate reported of diagnosis algorithm for suspected upper extremity deep vein thrombosis. Evid Based Med. 2014; 19(5):189

[46] Kleinjan A, Di Nisio M, Beyer-Westendorf J, et al. Safety and feasibility of a diagnostic algorithm combining clinical probability, d-dimer testing, and ultrasonography for suspected upper extremity deep venous thrombosis: a prospective management study. Ann Intern Med. 2014; 160(7):451–457

[47] Ageno W, Squizzato A, Wells PS, Büller HR, Johnson G. The diagnosis of symptomatic recurrent pulmonary embolism and deep vein thrombosis: guidance from the SSC of the ISTH. J Thromb Haemost. 2013; 11(8):1597–1602

[48] Kyrle PA. How I treat recurrent deep-vein thrombosis. Blood. 2016; 127(6):696–702

[49] Tan M, Velthuis SI, Westerbeek RE, VAN Rooden CJ, VAN DER Meer FJ, Huisman MV. High percentage of non-diagnostic compression ultrasonography results and the diagnosis of ipsilateral recurrent proximal deep vein thrombosis. J Thromb Haemost. 2010; 8(4):848–850

[50] Tan M, Mol GC, van Rooden CJ, et al. Magnetic resonance direct thrombus imaging differentiates acute recurrent ipsilateral deep vein thrombosis from residual thrombosis. Blood. 2014; 124(4):623–627

[51] Hara T, Truelove J, Tawakol A, et al. 18F-fluorodeoxyglucose positron emission tomography/computed tomography enables the detection of recurrent same-site deep vein thrombosis by illuminating recently formed, neutrophil-rich thrombus. Circulation. 2014; 130(13):1044–1052

[52] Hess S, Madsen PH, Iversen ED, Frifelt JJ, Høilund-Carlsen PF, Alavi A. Efficacy of FDG PET/CT imaging for venous thromboembolic disorders: preliminary results from a prospective, observational pilot study. Clin Nucl Med. 2015; 40(1):e23–e26

[53] Rondina MT, Wanner N, Pendleton R, et al. The utility of 18F-FDG-PET/CT for the diagnosis of occult malignancy in patients with acute, unprovoked venous thromboembolism. Paper presented at: the Society of Vascular Medicine; 2011; Boston, MA

[54] Wells PS, Forgie MA, Rodger MA. Treatment of venous thromboembolism. JAMA. 2014; 311(7):717–728

[55] Wiener RS, Schwartz LM, Woloshin S. Time trends in pulmonary embolism in the United States: evidence of overdiagnosis. Arch Intern Med. 2011; 171(9):831–837

[56] Feng LB, Pines JM, Yusuf HR, Grosse SD. U.S. trends in computed tomography use and diagnoses in emergency department visits by patients with symptoms suggestive of pulmonary embolism, 2001–2009. Acad Emerg Med. 2013; 20(10):1033–1040

[57] Wang RC, Bent S, Weber E, Neilson J, Smith-Bindman R, Fahimi J. The impact of clinical decision rules on computed tomography use and yield for pulmonary embolism: a systematic review and meta-analysis. Ann Emerg Med. 2016; 67(6):693–701.e1

[58] Hutchinson BD, Navin P, Marom EM, Truong MT, Bruzzi JF. Overdiagnosis of pulmonary embolism by pulmonary CT angiography. AJR Am J Roentgenol. 2015; 205(2):271–277

[59] Adams DM, Stevens SM, Woller SC, et al. Adherence to PIOPED II investigators' recommendations for computed tomography pulmonary angiography. Am J Med. 2013; 126(1):36–42

[60] Runyon MS, Richman PB, Kline JA, Pulmonary Embolism Research Consortium Study Group. Emergency medicine practitioner knowledge and use of decision rules for the evaluation of patients with suspected pulmonary embolism: variations by practice setting and training level. Acad Emerg Med. 2007; 14(1):53–57

[61] Hendriksen JM, Geersing GJ, Lucassen WA, et al. Diagnostic prediction models for suspected pulmonary embolism: systematic review and independent external validation in primary care. BMJ. 2015; 351:h4438

[62] Douma RA, Mos IC, Erkens PM, et al. Prometheus Study Group. Performance of 4 clinical decision rules in the diagnostic management of acute pulmonary embolism: a prospective cohort study. Ann Intern Med. 2011; 154(11):709–718

[63] Penaloza A, Verschuren F, Meyer G, et al. Comparison of the unstructured clinician gestalt, the wells score, and the revised Geneva score to estimate pretest probability for suspected pulmonary embolism. Ann Emerg Med. 2013; 62(2):117–124.e2

[64] Singh B, Mommer SK, Erwin PJ, Mascarenhas SS, Parsaik AK. Pulmonary embolism rule-out criteria (PERC) in pulmonary embolism–revisited: a systematic review and meta-analysis. Emerg Med J. 2013; 30(9):701–706

[65] Righini M, Nendaz M, Le Gal G, Bounameaux H, Perrier A. Influence of age on the cost-effectiveness of diagnostic strategies for suspected pulmonary embolism. J Thromb Haemost. 2007; 5(9):1869–1877

[66] Schouten HJ, Geersing GJ, Koek HL, et al. Diagnostic accuracy of conventional or age adjusted D-dimer cut-off values in older patients with suspected venous thromboembolism: systematic review and meta-analysis. BMJ. 2013; 346:f2492

[67] Righini M, Van Es J, Den Exter PL, et al. Age-adjusted D-dimer cutoff levels to rule out pulmonary embolism: the ADJUST-PE study. JAMA. 2014; 311(11): 1117–1124

[68] Carrier M, Righini M, Wells PS, et al. Subsegmental pulmonary embolism diagnosed by computed tomography: incidence and clinical implications. A systematic review and meta-analysis of the management outcome studies. J Thromb Haemost. 2010; 8(8):1716–1722

[69] Ikesaka R, Carrier M. Clinical significance and management of subsegmental pulmonary embolism. J Thromb Thrombolysis. 2015; 39(3):311–314

[70] den Exter PL, van Es J, Klok FA, et al. Risk profile and clinical outcome of symptomatic subsegmental acute pulmonary embolism. Blood. 2013; 122(7):1144–1149, quiz 1329

[71] Goy J, Lee J, Levine O, Chaudhry S, Crowther M. Sub-segmental pulmonary embolism in three academic teaching hospitals: a review of management and outcomes. J Thromb Haemost. 2015; 13(2):214–218

[72] Anderson DR, Kahn SR, Rodger MA, et al. Computed tomographic pulmonary angiography vs ventilation-perfusion lung scanning in patients with suspected pulmonary embolism: a randomized controlled trial. JAMA. 2007; 298(23):2743–2753

[73] Salaun PY, Couturaud F, Le Duc-Pennec A, et al. Noninvasive diagnosis of pulmonary embolism. Chest. 2011; 139(6):1294–1298

[74] Hillis C, Crowther MA. Acute phase treatment of VTE: Anticoagulation, including non-vitamin K antagonist oral anticoagulants. Thromb Haemost. 2015; 113(6):1193–1202

[75] Erkens PM, Prins MH. Fixed dose subcutaneous low molecular weight heparins versus adjusted dose unfractionated heparin for venous thromboembolism. Cochrane Database Syst Rev. 2010(9):CD001100

[76] Beam DM, Kahler ZP, Kline JA. Immediate discharge and home treatment with rivaroxaban of low-risk venous thromboembolism diagnosed in two U.S. emergency departments: a one-year preplanned analysis. Acad Emerg Med. 2015; 22(7):788–795

[77] Kahler ZP, Beam DM, Kline JA. Cost of treating venous thromboembolism with heparin and warfarin versus home treatment with rivaroxaban. Acad Emerg Med. 2015; 22(7):796–802

[78] Piran S, Le Gal G, Wells PS, et al. Outpatient treatment of symptomatic pulmonary embolism: a systematic review and meta-analysis. Thromb Res. 2013; 132(5):515–519

[79] Zondag W, Mos IC, Creemers-Schild D, et al. Hestia Study Investigators. Outpatient treatment in patients with acute pulmonary embolism: the Hestia Study. J Thromb Haemost. 2011; 9(8):1500–1507

[80] Robertson L, Kesteven P, McCaslin JE. Oral direct thrombin inhibitors or oral factor Xa inhibitors for the treatment of deep vein thrombosis. Cochrane Database Syst Rev. 2015a; 6(6):CD010956

[81] Robertson L, Kesteven P, McCaslin JE. Oral direct thrombin inhibitors or oral factor Xa inhibitors for the treatment of pulmonary embolism. Cochrane Database Syst Rev. 2015b; 12(12):CD010957

[82] van Es N, Coppens M, Schulman S, Middeldorp S, Büller HR. Direct oral anticoagulants compared with vitamin K antagonists for acute venous thromboembolism: evidence from phase 3 trials. Blood. 2014; 124(12):1968–1975

[83] Eikelboom JW, Weitz JI. New anticoagulants. Circulation. 2010; 121(13):1523–1532

[84] Agnelli G, Buller HR, Cohen A, et al. AMPLIFY Investigators. Oral apixaban for the treatment of acute venous thromboembolism. N Engl J Med. 2013; 369(9):799–808

[85] Büller HR, Décousus H, Grosso MA, et al. Hokusai-VTE Investigators. Edoxaban versus warfarin for the treatment of symptomatic venous thromboembolism. N Engl J Med. 2013; 369(15):1406–1415

[86] Bauersachs R, Berkowitz SD, Brenner B, et al. EINSTEIN Investigators. Oral rivaroxaban for symptomatic venous thromboembolism. N Engl J Med. 2010; 363(26):2499–2510

[87] Büller HR, Prins MH, Lensin AW, et al. EINSTEIN-PE Investigators. Oral rivaroxaban for the treatment of symptomatic pulmonary embolism. N Engl J Med. 2012; 366(14):1287–1297

[88] Schulman S, Kakkar AK, Goldhaber SZ, et al. RE-COVER II Trial Investigators. Treatment of acute venous thromboembolism with dabigatran or warfarin and pooled analysis. Circulation. 2014; 129(7):764–772

[89] Schulman S, Kearon C, Kakkar AK, et al. RE-COVER Study Group. Dabigatran versus warfarin in the treatment of acute venous thromboembolism. N Engl J Med. 2009; 361(24):2342–2352

[90] Pollack CV, Jr, Reilly PA, Eikelboom J, et al. Idarucizumab for dabigatran reversal. N Engl J Med. 2015; 373(6):511–520

[91] Greinacher A, Thiele T, Selleng K. Reversal of anticoagulants: an overview of current developments. Thromb Haemost. 2015; 113(5):931–942

[92] Lu G, DeGuzman FR, Hollenbach SJ, et al. A specific antidote for reversal of anticoagulation by direct and indirect inhibitors of coagulation factor Xa. Nat Med. 2013; 19(4):446–451

[93] Siegal DM, Curnutte JT, Connolly SJ, et al. Andexanet alfa for the reversal of factor Xa inhibitor activity. N Engl J Med. 2015; 373(25):2413–2424

[94] Eerenberg ES, Kamphuisen PW, Sijpkens MK, Meijers JC, Buller HR, Levi M. Reversal of rivaroxaban and dabigatran by prothrombin complex concentrate: a randomized, placebo-controlled, crossover study in healthy subjects. Circulation. 2011; 124(14):1573–1579

[95] Marlu R, Hodaj E, Paris A, Albaladejo P, Cracowski JL, Pernod G. Effect of nonspecific reversal agents on anticoagulant activity of dabigatran and rivaroxaban: a randomised crossover ex vivo study in healthy volunteers. Thromb Haemost. 2012; 108(2):217–224

[96] Purrucker JC, Haas K, Rizos T, et al. Early clinical and radiological course, management, and outcome of intracerebral hemorrhage related to new oral anticoagulants. JAMA Neurol. 2016; 73(2):169–177

[97] Ho P, Brooy BL, Hayes L, Lim WK. Direct oral anticoagulants in frail older adults: a geriatric perspective. Semin Thromb Hemost. 2015; 41(4):389–394

[98] Vazquez S, Rondina MT. Direct oral anticoagulants (DOACs). Vasc Med. 2015; 20(6):575–577

[99] Wadhera RK, Russell CE, Piazza G. Cardiology patient page. Warfarin versus novel oral anticoagulants: how to choose? Circulation. 2014; 130(22):e191–e193

[100] Jaff MR, McMurtry MS, Archer SL, et al. American Heart Association Council on Cardiopulmonary, Critical Care, Perioperative and Resuscitation, American Heart Association Council on Peripheral Vascular Disease, American Heart Association Council on Arteriosclerosis, Thrombosis and Vascular Biology. Management of massive and submassive pulmonary embolism, iliofemoral deep vein thrombosis, and chronic thromboembolic pulmonary hypertension: a scientific statement from the American Heart Association. Circulation. 2011; 123(16):1788–1830

[101] Kasper W, Konstantinides S, Geibel A, et al. Management strategies and determinants of outcome in acute major pulmonary embolism: results of a multicenter registry. J Am Coll Cardiol. 1997; 30(5):1165–1171

[102] Kucher N, Rossi E, De Rosa M, Goldhaber SZ. Massive pulmonary embolism. Circulation. 2006; 113(4):577–582

[103] Dalla-Volta S, Palla A, Santolicandro A, et al. PAIMS 2: alteplase combined with heparin versus heparin in the treatment of acute pulmonary embolism. Plasminogen activator Italian multicenter study 2. J Am Coll Cardiol. 1992; 20(3):520–526

[104] Daniels LB, Parker JA, Patel SR, Grodstein F, Goldhaber SZ. Relation of duration of symptoms with response to thrombolytic therapy in pulmonary embolism. Am J Cardiol. 1997; 80(2):184–188

[105] Tibbutt DA, Davies JA, Anderson JA, et al. Comparison by controlled clinical trial of streptokinase and heparin in treatment of life-threatening pulmonay embolism. BMJ. 1974; 1(5904):343–347

[106] Goldhaber SZ, Visani L, De Rosa M. Acute pulmonary embolism: clinical outcomes in the International Cooperative Pulmonary Embolism Registry (ICOPER). Lancet. 1999; 353(9162):1386–1389

[107] Laporte S, Mismetti P, Décousus H, et al. RIETE Investigators. Clinical predictors for fatal pulmonary embolism in 15,520 patients with venous thromboembolism: findings from the Registro Informatizado de la Enfermedad TromboEmbolica venosa (RIETE) Registry. Circulation. 2008; 117(13):1711–1716

[108] Mostafa A, Briasoulis A, Telila T, Belgrave K, Grines C. Treatment of massive or submassive acute pulmonary embolism with catheter-directed thrombolysis. Am J Cardiol. 2016; 117(6):1014–1020

[109] Wan S, Quinlan DJ, Agnelli G, Eikelboom JW. Thrombolysis compared with heparin for the initial treatment of pulmonary embolism: a meta-analysis of the randomized controlled trials. Circulation. 2004; 110(6):744–749

[110] Kearon C, Akl EA. Duration of anticoagulant therapy for deep vein thrombosis and pulmonary embolism. Blood. 2014; 123(12):1794–1801

[111] Middeldorp S, Prins MH, Hutten BA. Duration of treatment with vitamin K antagonists in symptomatic venous thromboembolism. Cochrane Database Syst Rev. 2014; 8(8):CD001367

[112] Couturaud F, Sanchez O, Pernod G, et al. PADIS-PE Investigators. Six months vs extended oral anticoagulation after a first episode of pulmonary embolism: the PADIS-PE randomized clinical trial. JAMA. 2015; 314(1):31–40

[113] Bova C, Bianco A, Mascaro V, Nobile CG. Extended anticoagulation and mortality in venous thromboembolism. A meta-analysis of six randomized trials. Thromb Res. 2016; 139:22–28

[114] Kearon C, Iorio A, Palareti G, Subcommittee on Control of Anticoagulation of the SSC of the ISTH. Risk of recurrent venous thromboembolism after stopping treatment in cohort studies: recommendation for acceptable rates and standardized reporting. J Thromb Haemost. 2010; 8(10):2313–2315

[115] Roach RE, Lijfering WM, Rosendaal FR, Cannegieter SC, le Cessie S. Sex difference in risk of second but not of first venous thrombosis: paradox explained. Circulation. 2014; 129(1):51–56

[116] Roach RE, Lijfering WM, Tait RC, et al. Sex difference in the risk of recurrent venous thrombosis: a detailed analysis in four European cohorts. J Thromb Haemost. 2015; 13(10):1815–1822

[117] Baglin T, Douketis J, Tosetto A, et al. Does the clinical presentation and extent of venous thrombosis predict likelihood and type of recurrence? A patient-level meta-analysis. J Thromb Haemost. 2010; 8(11):2436–2442

[118] Mearns ES, Coleman CI, Patel D, et al. Index clinical manifestation of venous thromboembolism predicts early recurrence type and frequency: a meta-analysis of randomized controlled trials. J Thromb Haemost. 2015; 13(6):1043–1052

[119] Douketis J, Tosetto A, Marcucci M, et al. Patient-level meta-analysis: effect of measurement timing, threshold, and patient age on ability of D-dimer testing to assess recurrence risk after unprovoked venous thromboembolism. Ann Intern Med. 2010; 153(8):523–531

[120] Palareti G, Cosmi B, Legnani C, et al. DULCIS (D-dimer and ULtrasonography in Combination Italian Study) Investigators. D-dimer to guide the duration of anticoagulation in patients with venous thromboembolism: a management study. Blood. 2014; 124(2):196–203

[121] Kearon C, Spencer FA, O'Keeffe D, et al. D-dimer Optimal Duration Study Investigators. D-dimer testing to select patients with a first unprovoked venous thromboembolism who can stop anticoagulant therapy: a cohort study. Ann Intern Med. 2015; 162(1):27–34

[122] Donadini MP, Ageno W, Antonucci E, et al. Prognostic significance of residual venous obstruction in patients with treated unprovoked deep vein thrombosis: a patient-level meta-analysis. Thromb Haemost. 2014; 111(1):172–179

[123] Garcia D, Akl EA, Carr R, Kearon C. Antiphospholipid antibodies and the risk of recurrence after a first episode of venous thromboembolism: a systematic review. Blood. 2013; 122(5):817–824

[124] Eichinger S, Heinze G, Jandeck LM, Kyrle PA. Risk assessment of recurrence in patients with unprovoked deep vein thrombosis or pulmonary embolism: the Vienna prediction model. Circulation. 2010; 121(14):1630–1636

[125] Rodger MA, Kahn SR, Wells PS, et al. Identifying unprovoked thromboembolism patients at low risk for recurrence who can discontinue anticoagulant therapy. CMAJ. 2008; 179(5):417–426

[126] Tosetto A, Iorio A, Marcucci M, et al. Predicting disease recurrence in patients with previous unprovoked venous thromboembolism: a proposed prediction score (DASH). J Thromb Haemost. 2012; 10(6):1019–1025

[127] Marcucci M, Iorio A, Douketis JD, et al. Risk of recurrence after a first unprovoked venous thromboembolism: external validation of the Vienna Prediction Model with pooled individual patient data. J Thromb Haemost. 2015; 13(5):775–781

[128] Carrier M, Le Gal G, Wells PS, Rodger MA. Systematic review: case-fatality rates of recurrent venous thromboembolism and major bleeding events among patients treated for venous thromboembolism. Ann Intern Med. 2010; 152(9):578–589

3 Cerebral Venous Thrombosis

Nitish Dhingra and Kieran Murphy

Summary

While relatively uncommon, cerebral venous thrombosis is a potentially catastrophic condition. Management requires a multidisciplinary expert team and, in rare instances, intervention; the experienced interventional radiologist with expertise in intracranial catheter manipulation may have a role in facilitating rescue. This chapter provides a review of the management of these patients, and provides a case example in which off-label use of devices by an experienced operator led to recanalization with correction of neurologic deficits.

Keywords: stroke, cerebral edema, cerebral venous congestion, dural sinus

3.1 Introduction

Cerebral venous thrombosis (CVT), which includes the thrombosis of cerebral veins and major dural sinuses, is quite a rare disorder when looked at from a societal perspective. In fact, the annual incidence rate is estimated to be around three to four cases per million.[1,2] However, its several risk factors can make certain groups very susceptible, with the implications being rather severe. This chapter will provide a detailed overview of CVT, through analyzing its epidemiology and scope, its manifestation in patients, and the consequent appropriate evaluation and interpretation, as well as treatment options including some procedural tips.

3.2 Clinical Vignette

3.2.1 Patient Presentation

A 79-year-old woman presented with acute confusion and deteriorating levels of responsiveness.

Physical Exam

Physical examination was difficult, as the patient was not following commands.

Imaging

Unenhanced CT of the head demonstrated bilateral parasagittal edema (▸ Fig. 3.1). CT venography showed thrombosis of the midsuperior sagittal sinus.

Treatment Approach

The patient received intravenous heparinization and supportive care but continued to deteriorate over 24 hours. The decision was made to offer catheter-directed intervention.

Specifics of Consent

After a discussion of the risks and benefits, consent for recanalization of the superior sagittal sinus was obtained from the family. A 10 to 20% risk of periprocedural death was discussed, and the off-label use of technology was explicitly disclosed.

Details of Procedure

The procedure was performed under general anesthesia. First, right transfemoral arterial access was obtained for transarterial cerebral angiography, which demonstrated occlusion of the midsuperior sagittal sinus, with venous congestion and antegrade venous drainage proximal to the occlusion (▸ Fig. 3.2).

With ultrasound guidance, a retrograde left internal jugular (IJ) access was achieved, as this facilitates navigation of the jugular sigmoid tortuosity. The left IJ was chosen, as direction of flow was from the superior sagittal sinus to the left transverse sinus. A standard 6F vascular sheath was placed, with its tip positioned just into the jugular bulb. This did away with the need for guiding a catheter. Road map guidance was provided by angiography performed via an arterial catheter in the left carotid artery, capturing the road map at the venous phase of the injection. A catheter was advanced through the sheath and navigated to the level of occlusion. A 0.014-inch coronary Hi Torque Cross It wire (Abbott Vascular, Inc., Abbott Park, IL) was then delivered to the level of occlusion through a coronary 4 mm × 20 mm angioplasty balloon. The recanalization wire was used to puncture and cross the dense obstruction and the balloon was passed across the occlusion for venoplasty (▸ Fig. 3.3). Immediate recanalization was achieved and restoration of anatomic retrograde venous drainage established (▸ Fig. 3.4).

Follow-up

Serial CTs over the next few days showed that the venous congestion was improved. The patient's mentation and mobility improved and mobility was restored over the following few weeks.

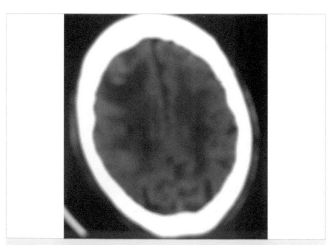

Fig. 3.1 Unenhanced CT demonstrated bilateral parasagittal edema.

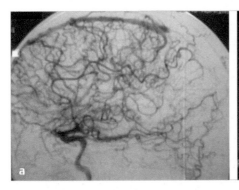

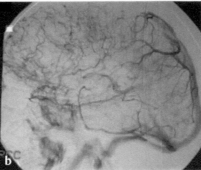

Fig. 3.2 (a) Early venous phase of cerebral angiography demonstrating occlusion of the midsuperior sagittal sinus with antegrade venous drainage anterior to the occlusion. (b) Late venous phase of cerebral angiography demonstrating venous congestion and late reconstitution of the posterior sagittal sinus and transverse sinuses.

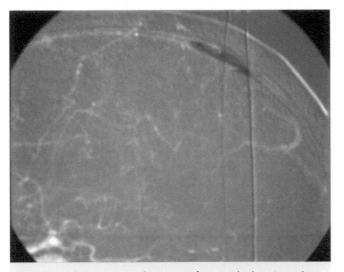

Fig. 3.3 Road map venous phase image from cerebral angiography demonstrating coronary angioplasty balloon passed from retrograde jugular venous approach through the transverse sinus to cross sagittal sinus occlusion. Balloon is inflated for focal venoplasty.

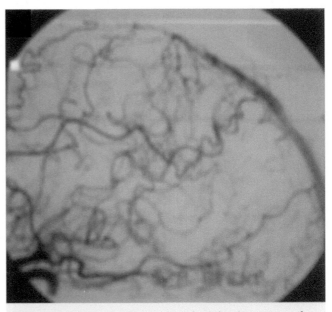

Fig. 3.4 Immediate recanalization was achieved and restoration of anatomic retrograde venous drainage established.

3.3 Epidemiology and Scope of Problem

While the annual occurrence of CVT is low, there are clear risk factors that increase the likelihood of specific groups of people developing this condition. The first major risk factor is a patient with a known prothrombotic state. In the International Study on Cerebral Vein and Dural Sinus Thrombosis (ISCVT), 22% of all CVT patients had an inherited prothrombotic state, while 34% were found after presentation to have a constellation of risk factors that resulted in a prothrombotic state.[1,3] A prothrombotic state, otherwise known as thrombophilia, may be understood as a tendency to develop clots inappropriately. This disorder can originate based off of genetic factors, acquired factors, or an interaction between the two. Moreover, women who are pregnant, in a post-partum state, or receiving oral contraceptives or other hormonal therapy are also at a higher risk of developing CVT.[4] CVT is also associated with cancer, nephrotic syndrome, localized infections such as otitis, mastoiditis, sinusitis, and meningitis along with systemic infectious disorders, as well as chronic inflammatory diseases like vasculitides and inflammatory bowel disease. Malignancy and hematologic conditions, like sickle cell disease, thrombocythemia, essential thrombocytosis, thrombotic thrombocytopenia purpura, polycythemia, leukemia, and anemia (including paroxysmal nocturnal hemoglobinuria) can also increase a patient's risk of developing CVT.[1,2,4] Head trauma, local injury to cerebral sinuses or veins, jugular venous cannulation, neurosurgical procedures, and uncommonly lumbar puncture are possible causes of CVT.[1,2] Finally, CVT has a higher frequency in patients under the age of 40.[1]

CVT manifests itself pathophysiologically through two major mechanisms. The first is through the increase of the cerebral venous pressure, which leads to decreased perfusion and, ultimately, ischemia, analogous to peripheral compartment syndromes. Moreover, parenchymal hemorrhage can occur secondary to elevated venous pressure.[1,2] A second mechanism leading to hemorrhage is decreased absorption of cerebrospinal fluid as a result of the obstructed cerebral sinuses, causing elevated intracranial pressure, which perpetuates the cycle of increased capillary pressure.[4] Distribution of hemorrhage can be posterior temporal if thrombosis is in the transverse sinus, or frontoparietal if the clot is in the superior sagittal sinus.

Table 3.1 MRI of acute, subacute, and chronic cerebral venous thrombosis

	Acute	Subacute	Chronic
MRI characteristics	On T1-weighted images, CVT appears isointense to brain tissue; on T2-weighed images, CVT appears hypointense.[1,10]	In both T1- and T2- weighted images, thrombus appears hyperintense.[1]	Thrombus can be heterogeneous with variable intensity compared to surrounding brain tissue; thrombus may be directly visualized in cerebral veins and dural sinuses and appear as a hypointense area on T2-weighted images.[1]

Mortality from CVT is significant. A meta-analysis of 1,190 patents with this condition showed that there was a 5.6% mean 30-day mortality rate.[5] Transtentorial herniation, often as a result of large venous hemorrhage, was shown to be the primary cause of death during the acute phase of CVT.[5,6] Permanent neurological deficits result from thrombosis in 10% of patients at 12 months of follow-up. However, the majority of patients may be expected to return to neurologic function at or near baseline. It is, in fact, remarkable that venous hemorrhage is so much better tolerated than arterial parenchymal bleed. It is notable that patients with this condition have an increased risk of further venous thromboembolism, including deep vein thrombosis and pulmonary embolism, which usually occurs within the first year following the initial thrombotic event.[1]

3.4 Patient Presentation and Evaluation

CVT may have various presentations, with related syndromes including intracranial hypertension alone, focal neurologic deficits, seizures, and encephalopathy; whether these syndromes present in isolation or in conjunction is dependent on the extent and location of CVT.[1] The syndrome may present with an indolent course, described as chronic, or may present acutely, with severe or multiple symptThe most common presentation of CVT-caused intracranial hypertension is headache.[1] Indeed, a headache, which can manifest as either localized or generalized and may be aggravated by Valsava maneuvers or position change,[1,7] may be present in up to 90% of CVT patients.[1,3]. Headaches may also bear resemblance to low CSF pressure headaches.[4] Initial diagnosis of headache induced by CVT is often a migraine.[1] Papilledema and visual complaints can also be noted based off of the aforementioned intracranial hypertension.[1]] In addition, CVT has also been highlighted as being associated with nausea and vomiting, and may in fact present with intracerebral hemorrhage.[4] Focal neurological deficits are noted in 44% of patients with the condition, with motor weakness in up to 40%.[3] Focal or generalized seizures are observed in 30 to 40% of patients.[8,9] Finally, encephalopathy can result from thrombosis of the straight sinus and its branches or from severe cases that can lead to parenchymal hemorrhages, causing herniation, coma, and death.[1,2]

With respect to the evaluation of patients, there are some fundamental tests or warning flags that should be considered when examining a patient with symptoms that point toward CVT. The AHA/ASA 2011 Scientific Statement on diagnosis and management of CVT recommends imaging of the cerebral venous system in patients with suspected CVT.[10] For suspected CVT patients, head CT is the most frequently performed imaging study. Signs of the condition on CT include hyperdensity in the area of a sinus or cortical vein, and/or filling defects especially in the superior sagittal sinus.[10] Although minor radiation exposure and contrast nephropathy are concerns, computed tomographic venography can provide another reliable method for examining patients with suspected CVT. A major benefit of this approach is that thrombi of heterogeneous densities can be detected, meaning it allows for the diagnosis of subacute or chronic CVT.[1,11] The atypical nonarterial distribution of bleeds and the fact that the edema associated with the bleed is disproportionate to the size of the bleed should lead one to consider CVT. MRI of the head combined with MR venography is the most sensitive study for the detection of CVT.[1,12] ▶ Table 3.1 shows the general signs of acute, subacute, and chronic CVT. MR with T2-weighted imaging and MR venography is recommended by the AHA//ASA 2011 Scientific Statement as the imaging test of choice for the assessment of individuals with suspected CVT.[10] In uncommon cases when there is a high clinical suspicion of the condition, but previous evidence through either MR or CT venography is inconclusive, invasive diagnostic techniques (e.g., cerebral intra-arterial angiography with venous phase imaging and direct cerebral venography) can be used.[10]

A complete blood count is recommended to look for polycythemia as an etiologic factor.[4] A decreased platelet count would support thrombotic thrombocytopenic purpura, which is a major risk factor for CVT. Screening for a patient with a prothrombotic state is also highly recommended because of the high frequency of thrombophilias among patients who develop CVT. This screening includes evaluation for the factor V Leiden mutation, prothrombin gene mutation 20210, lupus anticoagulant, anticardiolipin antibodies, hyperhomocysteinemia, and deficiencies of protein C, S, and antithrombin.[1]

An elevated D-dimer level supports the diagnosis of the disorder. However, the diagnosis of CVT should not be excluded based on a normal D-dimer level if the patient has a clinical presentation that is otherwise indicative of CVT.[13,14] In a study of 239 patients with suspected CVT, D-dimer testing was performed in 98 patients; 9% of the time, a false-positive was noted, while 24% of the time a false-negative was noted.[1,8]

3.5 Management and Treatment Options

Anticoagulation is the principal treatment provided to patients with CVT. Its purpose is to prevent the propagation of the thrombus, as well as to help recanalize occluded sinuses.[10] Two randomized controlled trials comparing immediate anticoagulation with placebo treatment were carried out to analyze the administration of anticoagulant therapy for treatment of CVT. In one trial of anticoagulation versus placebo, patients were randomized 50:50. In the placebo group, one patient completely recovered, while six suffered neurological deficits and three died by 3 months. Of the 10 patients treated with anticoagulation, 8 recovered completely, and 2 had slight residual neurological deficits in the span of 3 months. Furthermore, 2 patients in the placebo group suffered intracranial hemorrhage, compared to none in the treatment group. In fact, the study was terminated after 20 patients, despite a planned 60 patients, due to an early treatment benefit.[1,15] In the second randomized trial of 59 patients, the low-molecular-weight heparin nadroparin was compared with placebo for 3 weeks, followed by 3 months of oral anticoagulation in those in the treatment arm of the study.[1,16] The results of this study showed 13% of patients in the nadroparin group having poor outcomes, versus 21% in the placebo group. Despite concern relating to use of anticoagulation in CVT patients presenting with hemorrhagic infarction, it should be noted that both of these randomized trials documented no extension of existing cerebral hemorrhages prior to therapy, nor the development of novel cerebral hemorrhages. [1,15,16] Based on available literature, regardless of concomitant intracranial hemorrhage related to CVT in patients on presentation, anticoagulation is recommended for CVT patients without contraindications.[1] In particular, either dose-adjusted intravenous unfractionated heparin with an at least doubled activated partial thromboplastin time, or subcutaneously administered low-molecular-weight heparin as a bridge to oral anticoagulation with a vitamin K antagonist may be used for immediate anticoagulation. [1] Furthermore, low-molecular-weight heparin should be preferred in cases of CVT that are uncomplicated. [4]

For patients with large and extensive CVT, patients for whom other management approaches have not stopped the evolution of intracranial pressure, or for the relatively small number of patients who decline despite anticoagulation therapy, catheter-directed fibrinolytic therapy (with or without mechanical thrombus disruption) may be considered at centers with appropriate experience. It should be highlighted, though, that the relevant accessible data is slim.[1,10] A possible clinical benefit of fibrinolysis was shown in a systematic review of 169 patients with severe presentation of CVT. However, following fibrinolysis, intracranial hemorrhages occured in 17% of cases; in 5% of cases, they were associated with clinical deterioration.[1,17] A different systematic review documented 12 deaths subsequent to fibrinolysis, as well as 15 major bleeding complications, 12 of which were intracranial hemorrhages, in 156 CVT patients.[1] Endovascular thrombolysis can also be used for patients with a poor prognosis after anticoagulant treatment. In a study of 20 patients with sinus thrombosis treated with urokinase, which was infused into the sinuses via a transjugular catheter, 12 patients completely recovered, while 6 died and 2 survived with deficits.[18]

One case report documented the use of suction thrombectomy with the 5 max Penumbra catheter (Penumbra, Inc., Alameda, CA) in combination with the Solitaire FR clot retrieval device (Medtronic, Mineeapolis, MN) to attain complete revascularization of an occluded sinus. This approach led to the stopping of cerebral edema progression and the patient ultimately recovered well following prolonged intensive medical therapy. The authors of the case report noted that the clot retrieval properties of the Solitaire device working in conjunction with the newest generation Penumbra catheters may enable swifter, safer, and more efficient revascularization relative to existing endovascular treatments for the treated condition.

Finally, catheter-based rhyolitic thrombectomy is another option for treating CVT. In one study, four procedures were performed in two patients, and this technique was used successfully in all four procedures.[19] The device is stiff, however, and needs a retrograde jugular approach to overcome its short working length and navigate it through the tortuous sigmoid jugular region.

In terms of surgical intervention, surgical thrombectomy is reserved for a very rare circumstance in which all other options have been exhausted and clinical deterioration continues to occur.[10] Decompressive surgery (e.g., craniotomy or hematoma evacuation) has been associated with improved clinical outcomes.[20]

3.6 Preparation for Procedure

Careful evaluation of preprocedural imaging is critical to success. The patient's individual venous anatomy should be studied for accurate navigation of the sinuses, and the dominant venous drainage pathway should be identified and targeted for access.

Ensuring that comprehensive conversations happen prior to the procedure, involving the entire care team and the patient/family, is critical due to the high risk of these procedures. Expectations should be clearly established with all parties. These patients have high morbidity and mortality and require aggressive high-risk care. As such, the key to performing safe and effective intervention in these patients is to have complete institutional medical alignment.

3.7 Technical Tips and Tricks and Details of the Procedure

Transvenous navigation is more relaxing than transarterial navigation because of the resilience of the vein wall. However, there is still a limit to the force that can be applied to a dural sinus wall.

3.8 Postprocedural Management and Follow-up

It is key to ensure that the patient is adequately anticoagulated postprocedure to avoid rethrombosis. Anticoagulation therapy with an oral vitamin K antagonist for 3 to 6 months in patients with provoked CVT and 6 to 12 months in those with unprovoked CVT is recommended.[10] Patients with recurrent CVT or initial CVT in the setting of severe thrombophilia should be considered for indefinite duration of anticoagulation.[10] Women who were being administered hormonal contraceptive therapy, and have experienced CVT in that context, should be encouraged to consider other methods for contraception that are nonestrogen based.[4] AHA/ASA 2011 Scientific Statement recommends regular clinical follow-up coupled with follow-up imaging to assess for durability of recanalization 3 to 6 months after diagnosis.[10]

References

[1] Piazza G. Cerebral venous thrombosis. Circulation. 2012; 125(13):1704–1709

[2] Stam J. Thrombosis of the cerebral veins and sinuses. N Engl J Med. 2005; 352 (17):1791–1798

[3] Ferro JM, Canhão P, Stam J, Bousser MG, Barinagarrementeria F, ISCVT Investigators. Prognosis of cerebral vein and dural sinus thrombosis: results of the International Study on Cerebral Vein and Dural Sinus Thrombosis (ISCVT). Stroke. 2004; 35(3):664–670

[4] McElveen WA. Cerebral venous thrombosis. In: Alway D, Cole JW, eds. Stroke Essentials for Primary Care: A Practical Guide. New York, NY: Humana Press; 2008:183–192

[5] Dentali F, Gianni M, Crowther MA, Ageno W. Natural history of cerebral vein thrombosis: a systematic review. Blood. 2006; 108(4):1129–1134

[6] Canhão P, Ferro JM, Lindgren AG, Bousser MG, Stam J, Barinagarrementeria F, ISCVT Investigators. Causes and predictors of death in cerebral venous thrombosis. Stroke. 2005; 36(8):1720–1725

[7] Agostoni E. Headache in cerebral venous thrombosis. Neurol Sci. 2004; 25 Suppl 3:S206–S210

[8] Tanislav C, Siekmann R, Sieweke N, et al. Cerebral vein thrombosis: clinical manifestation and diagnosis. BMC Neurol. 2011; 11(1):69

[9] Ferro JM, Canhão P, Bousser MG, Stam J, Barinagarrementeria F, ISCVT Investigators. Early seizures in cerebral vein and dural sinus thrombosis: risk factors and role of antiepileptics. Stroke. 2008; 39(4):1152–1158

[10] Saposnik G, Barinagarrementeria F, Brown RD, Jr, et al. American Heart Association Stroke Council and the Council on Epidemiology and Prevention. Diagnosis and management of cerebral venous thrombosis: a statement for healthcare professionals from the American Heart Association/American Stroke Association. Stroke. 2011; 42(4):1158–1192

[11] Khandelwal N, Agarwal A, Kochhar R, et al. Comparison of CT venography with MR venography in cerebral sinovenous thrombosis. AJR Am J Roentgenol. 2006; 187(6):1637–1643

[12] Bousser MG, Ferro JM. Cerebral venous thrombosis: an update. Lancet Neurol. 2007; 6(2):162–170

[13] Crassard I, Soria C, Tzourio C, et al. A negative D-dimer assay does not rule out cerebral venous thrombosis: a series of seventy-three patients. Stroke. 2005; 36(8):1716–1719

[14] Kosinski CM, Mull M, Schwarz M, et al. Do normal D-dimer levels reliably exclude cerebral sinus thrombosis? Stroke. 2004; 35(12):2820–2825

[15] Einhäupl KM, Villringer A, Meister W, et al. Heparin treatment in sinus venous thrombosis. Lancet. 1991; 338(8767):597–600

[16] de Bruijn SF, Stam J. Randomized, placebo-controlled trial of anticoagulant treatment with low-molecular-weight heparin for cerebral sinus thrombosis. Stroke. 1999; 30(3):484–488

[17] Canhão P, Falcão F, Ferro JM. Thrombolytics for cerebral sinus thrombosis: a systematic review. Cerebrovasc Dis. 2003; 15(3):159–166

[18] Stam J, Majoie CB, van Delden OM, van Lienden KP, Reekers JA. Endovascular thrombectomy and thrombolysis for severe cerebral sinus thrombosis: a prospective study. Stroke. 2008; 39(5):1487–1490

[19] Chow K, Gobin YP, Saver J, Kidwell C, Dong P, Viñuela F. Endovascular treatment of dural sinus thrombosis with rheolytic thrombectomy and intra-arterial thrombolysis. Stroke. 2000; 31(6):1420–1425

[20] Ferro JM, Crassard I, Coutinho JM, et al. Second International Study on Cerebral Vein and Dural Sinus Thrombosis (ISCVT 2) Investigators. Decompressive surgery in cerebrovenous thrombosis: a multicenter registry and a systematic review of individual patient data. Stroke. 2011; 42(10):2825–2831

4 Acute Deep Venous Thrombosis: Sporadic and Compressive

Kyle Cooper, Minhaj S. Khaja, and Bill S. Majdalany

Summary

Acute deep venous thrombosis (DVT) may be sporadic, or can result from compressive phenomena, which are recognized as distinct anatomic syndromes. The management of DVT in the acute stage is increasingly of interest to interventional radiologists, as improvement in customized devices has allowed for better outcomes of intervention. This chapter reviews the evaluation of patients with acute DVT, and discusses the management of patients appropriate for pharmacomechanical catheter-directed therapy, with a discussion of management of underlying compressive syndromes. The reader can be expected to become familiar with relevant anatomic variants and their management, as well as developing an understanding of the pharmacologic and device-based interventions available for this patient population. A discussion of the details of procedural management, as well as postprocedural follow-up, is included in the chapter.

Keywords: deep venous thrombosis, venous thoracic outlet syndrome, thrombolysis, thrombectomy, Paget–Schroetter syndrome, May–Thurner syndrome, iliac vein compression

4.1 Introduction

Deep venous thrombosis (DVT) is a common medical problem with varying underlying etiologies and multiple immediate and long-term sequelae. Nearly 600,000 hospitalizations in the United States are attributable to DVT annually. Advances in the detection and treatment of DVT hold the potential to significantly impact a patient's quality of life both in the acute setting and over time. Herein, the evaluation and treatment of DVT is reviewed, including a review of two common syndromes that predispose to DVT: iliac vein compression syndrome (commonly known as May–Thurner syndrome [MTS]) and Paget-Schroetter syndrome (PSS), also known as axillosubclavian venous effort thrombosis.

4.2 Sporadic Deep Venous Thrombosis

DVT most commonly affects veins of the lower extremities; however, the veins of the upper extremities, neck, central thorax, pelvis, and inferior vena cava (IVC) may also be involved. While the visceral and portal venous systems are located deep within the body, the term DVT is generally not used to describe thrombosis in these vessels. In the upper and lower extremities, the deep veins accompany their similarly named arterial counterparts. Symptoms manifest as a direct result of venous obstruction, or due to venous insufficiency as a result of valvular incompetence and decreased venous compliance, both of which are common in recanalized veins previously affected by DVT.

4.2.1 Case Vignette

Patient Presentation

A 46-year-old man presents with new right lower extremity swelling, chest pain, and shortness of breath.

Physical Exam

The patient presented with 2–3 right lower extremity edema, cyanosis, and warmth to the knee. Prominent bulging superficial veins were present in the upper thigh. He exhibited normal lower extremity motor and sensory exams, but displayed pain with deep palpation and during forced dorsiflexion of the right ankle (positive Homan's sign). He was hemodynamically stable. Chest pain was noted on deep inspiration.

Imaging

CT of the chest and abdomen with contrast revealed acute right lower lobe pulmonary emboli and right lower extremity DVT extending to the right common iliac vein (▶ Fig. 4.1a). Lower extremity duplex ultrasound revealed hypoechoic occlusive material within noncompressible lower extremity veins extending from the external iliac to the central aspect of the femoral vein consistent with acute DVT (▶ Fig. 4.1b; ▶ Fig. 4.1c; ▶ Fig. 4.1d). The right popliteal vein and the left lower extremity veins were patent.

Specifics of Consent

Given his symptoms, the patient requested aggressive treatment for his DVT. The risks of venous injury, bleeding, infection, pulmonary embolism (PE), and recurrent thrombosis were all discussed and the patient agreed to proceed.

Details of Procedure

At the time of initial evaluation, anticoagulation was initiated with intravenous heparin. Placement of an IVC filter was discussed for further pulmonary embolus prophylaxis. Right internal jugular vein was accessed under ultrasound guidance and IVC venography was performed prior to deployment of an infrarenal IVC filter. The filter sheath was exchanged for a 9-French sheath, which was positioned below the filter in the IVC. A hydrophilic wire was navigated peripheral to the common femoral vein and right lower extremity, and pelvic venography was performed. Occlusive thrombus was noted extending from the right common femoral to the common iliac vein (▶ Fig. 4.2a). A multiside hole thrombolysis catheter was laid along the extent of thrombus (▶ Fig. 4.2b). Overnight catheter-directed thrombolysis (CDT) was initiated with alteplase at 1 mg/h. By the next day, the thrombus load had reduced significantly. Venoplasty was undertaken with a 10-mm balloon across the length of the vein (▶ Fig. 4.2c; ▶ Fig. 4.2d). The thrombus completely resolved the following day.

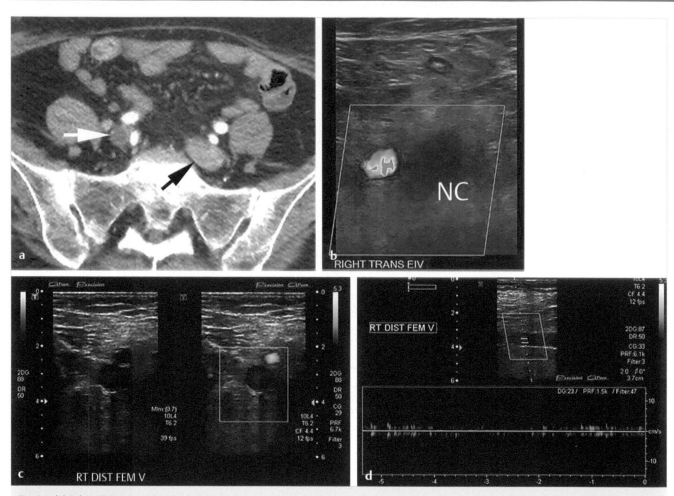

Fig. 4.1 **(a)** Pelvic CT image with venous phase intravenous contrast reveals a globular nonenhancing area in the right common iliac vein (*white arrow*), which is acute thrombus. In contrast, the left common iliac vein is symmetrically filling with contrast and is higher attenuation (*black arrow*). **(b)** Transverse color Doppler ultrasound image of the right external iliac vein demonstrating hypoechoic material within the vein and noncompressibility consistent with acute DVT. **(c)** Transverse grayscale and color ultrasound image of the right femoral vein, demonstrating hypoechoic material within the vein and absence of flow consistent with acute DVT. **(d)** Longitudinal grayscale Doppler ultrasound image of the right femoral vein, demonstrating absent flow consistent with acute DVT.

Final venography demonstrated brisk anterograde venous flow without residual thrombus (▶ Fig. 4.2e; ▶ Fig. 4.2f).

Follow-up

At the conclusion of the procedure, compression stockings were applied and the patient was continued on therapeutic anticoagulation. At discharge 2 days later, his lower extremity swelling had considerably improved. At a follow-up clinic visit 4 weeks after discharge, the patient had returned to baseline. A same-day duplex ultrasound revealed no evidence of recurrent DVT.

4.3 Epidemiology and Scope of the Problem

As many cases of DVT are likely subclinical, precise epidemiologic data are difficult to obtain. The incidence is estimated at 45 to 117 cases per 100,000 person-years for isolated DVT without PE. DVT is often combined with PE into a larger category known as "venous thromboembolism" (VTE) for statistical

tracking; the estimated incidence of VTE is 104 to 183 cases per 100,000 person-years. In the United States, VTE affects approximately 0.96 to 3.0 per 1,000 individuals per year, which equates to over 1 million patients in this country annually.[1] The vast majority of cases are diagnosed in older patients, with the incidence rising dramatically over the age of 60. The overall incidence of VTE ranges from 1 per 10,000 at age 20 up to 10 per 1,000 by age 80. DVT is diagnosed in men slightly more often than in women (1.2:1 ratio), although under the age of 45, women are more commonly affected. Isolated DVT without PE is more common in younger patients, with concomitant PE seen more frequently beginning in the seventh decade.[2]

The high incidence and frequent morbidity associated with DVT burdens the health care system significantly. DVT is a frequent complication of patient hospitalization; it is the second most common reason for prolonged hospital stays, and is the third most common cause of excess hospital-related mortality. More than half of all cases of DVT are encountered in the hospital setting, with 25% occurring in the perioperative setting. The average length of stay for patients with isolated DVT ranges from 4.9 to 7 days, increasing to 7.4 to 9 days in patients with

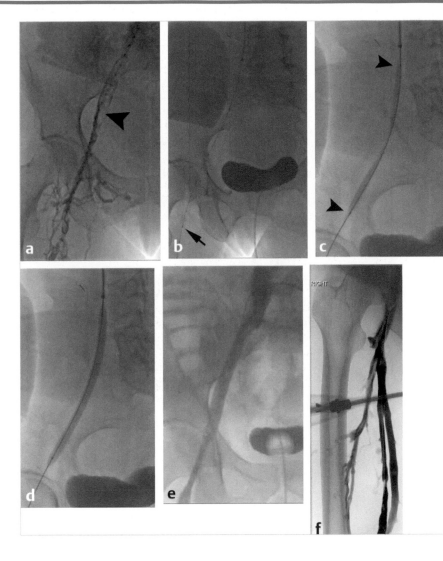

Fig. 4.2 **(a)** Right lower extremity venogram, demonstrating a lobular, occlusive thrombus (*arrowhead*) extends from the right common femoral vein to the right common iliac vein. Collateral veins are present in the vicinity of the common femoral vein. **(b)** Spot-image radiograph with a multiside hole thrombolysis catheter (*arrow*) extending along the length of the thrombus. **(c)** Spot-image radiograph of right iliac venoplasty to help clear any residual thrombus (*arrowheads* demarcate full length of balloon). **(d)** Spot-image radiograph of the right iliac venoplasty, demonstrating complete resolution of the waist with the balloon at full profile. **(e)** Completion right lower extremity venogram, demonstrating resolution of right iliofemoral DVT with brisk antegrade flow. **(f)** Completion right lower extremity venogram, revealing brisk antegrade flow through the duplicated femoral vein moieties, with no significant residual thrombus within either lumen and free flow into the common femoral vein.

concomitant PE. Readmissions are common in this population and subsequent stays are often longer than the initial admission. Current cost estimates for a primary admission for DVT range from $3,000 to $6,000 and are significantly higher for readmissions for the same problem.[1] However, the economic burden does not end at the time of discharge. Recurrent thromboembolic disease is common, and therefore frequent follow-up and long-term anticoagulation are needed to prevent a repeat event. Data from 2004 suggest the total cost of care for a first-event DVT without PE exceeds $33,000, taking all factors into account; this cost has undoubtedly increased.[3]

Unfortunately, even with successful management of an initial DVT, long-term sequelae are common. Aside from recurrent DVT, patients may develop lower extremity venous insufficiency, with an estimated 25 to 50% leading to formation of varicose veins, skin changes and ulcerations, and chronic debilitating symptoms associated with postthrombotic syndrome (PTS). The societal cost, including lost productivity, personal disability, and long-term health care, can be staggering.

4.3.1 Patient Presentation and Evaluation

A detailed history and physical examination are critical during the initial evaluation of a patient with suspected DVT. The most common presenting symptoms, regardless of location, are edema and pain. The modified Wells' criteria for DVT serve as a tool to guide clinicians as to the likelihood of DVT in a patient presenting with symptoms suggestive of the diagnosis.[4] At least one component of the classic "Virchow's triad"—venous stasis, vessel wall injury, and hypercoagulability—is typically identified through a thorough history and laboratory evaluation. A discussion of these three variables follows.

Venous stasis refers to decreased flow through the deep veins, which occurs with decreased extremity movement. DVT can be caused by a prolonged bedbound state, immobilization, limb paresis, or long-distance travel. Trauma patients are particularly susceptible to several of these factors and are at high risk for DVT. Pregnant patients experience compression on their pelvic veins, preventing venous return. Morbidly obese patients are also at an increased risk, likely due to a combination of factors.

Vessel wall or endothelial injury can refer to a number of perturbations to the normal antithrombotic nature of venous endothelium. When the vein wall is damaged, prostaglandin and nitric oxide levels are decreased, thromboplastin is released, and subendothelial collagen and von Willebrand factor are exposed—each encouraging platelet adhesion to the site of injury. Inflammatory cytokines, including interleukin-1 and tumor necrosis factor alpha, are released at the site of vessel wall damage, causing the synthesis and release of tissue factor.[5] Platelet adherence stimulates the release of thromboxane A2 and ADP, which cause further recruitment and aggregation of circulating platelets, bound to one another by fibrinogen. Aggregated platelets and polymerized fibrin combine to form thrombus. Factors that can cause endothelial dysfunction or damage to the vessel wall and lead to this cascade include direct venous trauma (including venipuncture and central venous access placement), hypertension, turbulent flow (particularly across valves, which is more pronounced in valves damaged by prior DVT or phlebitis), circulating toxins from cigarette smoke, radiation injury, bacterial endotoxins, hypercholesterolemia, and hyperhomocysteinemia.

Hypercoagulability can occur in a variety of inherited and acquired conditions, each carrying varying degrees of increased risk for the development of DVT. Deficiencies in protein C, protein S, and antithrombin, activated protein C resistance, prothrombin G20210A, and factor V Leiden mutations, antiphospholipid antibody syndrome, elevated plasma levels of factor VIII or fibrinogen, use of oral contraceptives, pregnancy, and other hormonal factors are all causes of increased thrombus generation. Hypofibrinolysis is seen in patients with elevated levels of the primary inhibitor of tissue plasminogen activator (PAI-1), as well as in patients with elevated levels of thrombin-activatable fibrinolysis inhibitor (TAFI); the end result is an inability to break down early foci of thrombus, leading to DVT. Several other conditions including cancer (particularly myeloproliferative neoplasms), paroxysmal nocturnal hemoglobinuria, Behçet's disease, and multiple autoimmune disorders have all been found to have an association with increased DVT.[6] Evaluation for thrombophilia may be warranted, particularly in unprovoked DVT in younger patients. Extensive panels of tests to determine hypercoagulable states exist to help identify the most common conditions. This topic is discussed in detail in Chapter 2 of this book.

On physical examination, focal or diffuse edema and pain with deep palpation are often present. When present, the classic physical exam finding of pain upon dorsiflexion of the calf (Homan's sign) is helpful in the diagnosis of lower extremity DVT, but is only noted in 50% of cases. Upper or lower extremity DVT may cause erythema or bluish discoloration of the skin at and upstream from the level of the thrombus. The affected limb is typically warm, and prominent superficial veins are common. The presence of a central line on the same side as the patient's symptoms should raise suspicion for DVT, whether in the upper or lower extremity.

Initial noninvasive testing consists primarily of a duplex ultrasound evaluation. Sonographic findings of acute thrombosis include noncompressibility of the vein, venous expansion, absence of flow on spectral waveform analysis and color Doppler imaging, increased flow through collateral veins, and hypoechoic intraluminal filling defects; in hyperacute thrombosis, the thrombus may even be sonolucent. Diminished augmentation of flow with distal tissue compression is often noted when evaluating segments central to the level of the DVT. Venous Doppler waveforms normally exhibit phasicity, which is a result of both cardiac and respiratory variation; examination of a venous segment peripheral to an area of occlusive thrombus will reveal partial or complete loss of phasicity.[7] In the upper extremities, venous waveforms also characteristically demonstrate significant transmitted cardiac pulsatility, which is lost in the setting of central occlusion.

Computed tomography venography (CTV) and magnetic resonance venography (MRV) both provide excellent evaluation of the venous system when imaging is acquired following a sufficient postinjection delay (~120 seconds).[8] These modalities are generally reserved for thoracic and abdominopelvic evaluations in suspected central DVT, or to identify/exclude central venous compression syndromes. Findings of DVT on both CTV and MRV include vein expansion, nonopacification of involved vessels, luminal filling defects, vessel wall enhancement, perivascular edema, and increased flow through collateral veins. On noncontrast CT, increased attenuation can often be seen within the lumen of thrombosed veins. On MRI, signal characteristics within the lumen of thrombosed vessels vary significantly depending on the acuity of the DVT, with T1 and T2 signal in general increasing over time after the first 1 to 2 days. Noncontrast time-of-flight MRV sequences are also available for patients who cannot receive contrast, with thrombosed vessels showing decreased or absent flow-related signal.

Since the introduction of heparin in the 1930s, systemic anticoagulation has been the primary method of treatment for DVT.[9] Anticoagulants prevent propagation of thrombus and decrease the risk of central embolization; however, in general, these medications lack sufficient thrombolytic effect for active thrombus dissolution.[10] Over the past two decades, minimally invasive techniques including CDT, mechanical thrombectomy, and pharmacomechanical thrombectomy have emerged, allowing more rapid clearing of thrombus. Multiple factors are used to determine which therapeutic strategy may best be indicated for a particular patient; however, a lack of sufficient long-term evidence necessitates a highly individualized algorithm. Factors to consider when deciding which patients will benefit from more aggressive therapy for DVT include potential for development of PTS, the risks of hemorrhagic complications, and the presence of (or risk for) PE. While PTS and PE may lead to decreased quality of life, cardiopulmonary compromise, or even death, the risks of interventional DVT therapy are not insignificant, and therefore an intervention is currently considered to be unwarranted in a patient with an incidentally discovered thrombosis and/or minimal or absent symptoms.[11] Conversely, patients with severe acute symptoms should be strongly considered for aggressive therapy (especially those with phlegmasia cerulea dolens, representing peripheral ischemia due to venous thrombosis, compartment swelling, and arterial compression). The patient's age should also be taken into account, given the risk of long-term complications of DVT (particularly iliofemoral DVT) increases over time. A short life expectancy is a relative contraindication to catheter-directed therapy; however, this assessment should take into account the patient's activity level and quality of life prior to the diagnosis of DVT.

The location of thrombosis is also an important data point when weighing the risk–benefit ratio of aggressive versus conservative therapy for DVT management. Approximately 4% of all documented DVTs involve the upper extremities, of which more than 75% are considered "secondary" or "provoked" (e.g., catheter-related).[12] The incidence of PE in these patients is small; however, upper extremity PTS is approximately 15%.[13] Patients with brachiocephalic and subclavian vein involvement tend to be the most symptomatic and have the highest risk for upper extremity PTS.

In cases of lower extremity DVT, it is relatively uncommon to develop only a single level of thrombus; when present, these clots tend to produce mild symptoms or are completely asymptomatic. Isolated caval thromboses are the least likely to produce symptoms in isolation, but are the most likely to produce PE. The risk of both PE and PTS decreases in more distal segments, such that it is relatively rare to develop either from calf thrombosis alone, particularly when involving only a single calf vein. The iliac and popliteal veins appear to comprise the most critical levels, with occlusions involving these segments producing the most symptoms in isolation and contributing the greatest risk of subsequent PTS; when either is combined with multilevel thrombosis involving additional segments, symptoms and risk of developing PTS increase significantly.[14,15]

Contraindications to long-term anticoagulation in symptomatic patients may not only represent an indication for IVC filter placement to prevent pulmonary embolization in some circumstances, but also include the need for DVT thrombectomy and possibly thrombolysis. A history of frequent falls is a common exclusion therapy for long-term anticoagulation, but does not necessarily preclude thrombolytic therapy during which patients are generally confined to bed and housed in hospital units with higher levels of observation and care. Standardly accepted contraindications to systemic thrombolysis include recent surgery, trauma or childbirth, intracranial lesions, history of hemorrhagic stroke (ever) or ischemic stroke (within the past year), active bleeding, or uncorrectable coagulopathy. In these patients, mechanical thrombus removal may be considered, with pharmacomechanical adjunctive measures employed on a case-by-case basis.

4.3.2 Preparation for Procedure

The initial decision when treating a patient with DVT is whether treatment can be completed in a single session or if overnight CDT will be required. In general, longer segment DVT, with a greater propensity for creating clinically relevant PE, is more commonly treated with CDT, while shorter segment or isolated segment thrombosis may be treated with either CDT or pharmacomechanical thrombectomy. CDT carries with it multiple requirements that may be unexpected to the patient: dietary, activity, and limb restrictions during the infusion, ICU admission, the insertion of a urinary catheter, and procedures on multiple days. These should be discussed in detail during the consent process in order to appropriately set expectations. If thrombolysis is expected, placement of multiple secure peripheral intravenous accesses and insertion of a urinary catheter is recommended prior to initiation of thrombolysis. Preprocedural assessment evaluating the safety of moderate sedation should be performed; involvement of anesthesiology support should be considered in all patients with American Society of Anesthesiology Physical Status (ASA-PS) scores ≥ 4 or Mallampati scores of ≥ 3.[16]

Baseline laboratory studies are required prior to initiating DVT intervention. A complete blood count (CBC) should be obtained; a baseline hemoglobin ≥ 8 g/dL is advised, and can be compared to future values for evidence of bleeding. For most operators, a platelet count ≥ 50 K/μL is considered a safe

threshold for venous puncture and lysis initiation. Determination of coagulation status, specifically partial thromboplastin time (PTT) and prothrombin time (PT)/international normalized ratio (INR), is also necessary prior to intervention, particularly if pharmacologic thrombolysis is anticipated. PTT ≤ 30 seconds and INR ≤ 1.5 are typical thresholds prior to initiating thrombolysis, as significantly elevated values of either are predictive of increased bleeding risk during thrombolysis[17] Type and crossmatch may be considered in patients who are vulnerable to complications of bleeding. A creatinine value or estimated glomerular filtration rate should be obtained prior to angiography; the normal range varies according to patient size, lean body weight, and local reference values. An abnormal value does not necessarily preclude intervention, but renal protective measures such as pre- and postprocedural hydration, minimization of contrast load, the use of alternative contrast agents such as CO_2, and adjunctive use of intravascular ultrasound (IVUS) should be entertained in patients with renal compromise who are not already on dialysis.

The selection of an appropriate access site is an important factor in procedural success as well as both patient and operator comfort, and should be determined beforehand to guide room setup and patient positioning. Ideally, the access into the venous system should allow treatment of the entire thrombus burden. This is often possible by using a combination of both anterograde and retrograde approaches, dependent on DVT location and extension. Peripheral access (using the veins of the calf or forearm) is desirable. It is relatively easy to perform with ultrasound, due to the superficial location of the structures, and safe, since the veins can be easily compressed upon procedure completion. Unfortunately, peripheral veins are relatively small, which can make cannulation difficult and limit the size of devices that can be safely delivered. Superficial veins are prone to spasm, complicating access and occasionally preventing advancement of devices through these vessels, even over a wire. The popliteal and brachial veins are larger and can accommodate the majority of devices and sheaths required for most procedures. Accessing these vessels may require puncture of a thrombosed segment, as the DVT may extend across these segments. This approach via a thrombosed vein may leave portions of the DVT untreated; however, by establishing flow central to the thrombosis, symptomatic improvement is often accomplished. For popliteal vein access, prone or "frog-leg" positioning is required. The advantage of the latter is that this allows access to the jugular veins without repositioning, if necessary, and is generally better tolerated by the patient for longer procedures. Common femoral vein access can be used in the treatment of iliofemoral, iliocaval, central thoracic, jugular, or upper extremity DVT; rarely, it can also be applied for both contralateral ("up-and-over") or ipsilateral (anterograde) lower extremity treatment. These veins are large and generally quite forgiving, and this approach is familiar to interventional staff and relatively conducive to most room setups. Central greater saphenous vein access is an option in most cases where common femoral access is applicable, and has several advantages: if damaged or thrombosed, the consequences to the patient are often less severe, there is less chance of missing a segment of disease within the common femoral vein that could compromise inflow when treating iliofemoral disease, and the superficial venous system is generally exposed to less pressure and therefore it is easier to obtain hemostasis at the termination of the procedure. Internal or even external jugular venous access can be utilized for therapies involving all four extremities as well as for caval thrombosis, and is frequently combined with more peripheral accesses for more complex procedures, particularly when some degree of chronic occlusion is also present. With all access points, it is important to note that approaching a limb vein from a central location may require navigation of valves in order to pass a wire, whereas a peripheral approach mitigates this issue.

The most common thrombolytic agent currently used in the United States is alteplase, which is a recombinant form of human tissue plasminogen activator (tPA). Other modified recombinant agents used throughout the world include reteplase and tenecteplase. Historically, streptokinase and urokinase were also used for thrombolysis; however, these agents are now used infrequently. The concentration of tPA used depends on the context of the intervention, ranging from high concentrations for pulse-spray thrombectomy to more dilute preparations used for overnight pharmacologic thrombolysis.

Equipment that may be helpful throughout the procedure should ideally be gathered prior to beginning the intervention. Devices that may be utilized include a variety of sheaths, directional and balloon catheters, wires (both hydrophilic and standard, including exchange lengths), infusion pumps, an ultrasound-enhanced thrombolysis unit, thrombolysis infusion catheters, rheolytic thrombectomy, IVUS catheters and the IVUS display unit, and any of a number of mechanical or pharmacomechanical devices and their associated catheters.

4.3.3 Technical Tips and Tricks and Procedural Details

Once an access site has been selected, ultrasound-guided access is favored to decrease the risk of bleeding, particularly if thrombolysis is planned. Micropuncture access using a 21-gauge needle is favored over 18-gauge needle access, with single-wall technique preferred by the authors. If a peripheral access vessel was selected, initial venography can be performed through the micropuncture dilator for an initial assessment of thrombus burden, flow characteristics, and variant anatomy. As with any interventional procedure, initial sheath size is selected based on the required diameter for insertion of the instruments planned for intervention; sheath length is chosen according to the depth of the access vessel and the distance to the area of intervention from the venotomy site. Ideally, the sheath tip should terminate relatively close to the area of intervention to facilitate intermittent venography via the sheath after interventions. Anticoagulation should be continued throughout and following the procedure.

Often, a Bentson wire or J-tipped wire will easily traverse acute and subacute thrombus (the "wire test"). A standard angled-tip hydrophilic wire can be used to navigate through firm organized thrombus, chronic occlusions, and venous stenoses when standard wires fail to pass. A 4- or 5-French end-hole catheter with an angled tip can help support the wire for increased pushability. After removing the wire, an injection of contrast can be performed through the catheter as it is pulled back to define the full extent of DVT once it has been traversed.

The procedure then varies depending on the chosen method of thrombus removal.

For pharmacologic thrombolysis, the length of the thrombus must be measured to select an infusion catheter with an appropriate treatment length. A standard or ultrasound-enhanced infusion catheter approximating the length of the DVT is placed across the thrombosed segment, attempting to place as many side holes as possible within the thrombus so thrombolytic is not injected directly into the systemic circulation. It is important to have the most proximal and distal side holes within a patent vessel, if possible, to treat the ends of the thrombus. CDT is then initiated; progress must be monitored no less frequently than every 24 hours by performing a "lysis check" venogram. Typical tPA infusion rates range from 0.5 to 1.0 mg/h, and usually a fixed rate of heparinized saline (~300–500 units/h) is administered through the side-port of the access site sheath to prevent sheath thrombosis. Many operators elect to maintain low-dose, subtherapeutic heparin infusion without adjusting according to PTT nomograms, due to concerns for increased risk of bleeding with therapeutic heparinization. However, there is a trend toward utilizing therapeutic heparinization during thrombolysis, and there is no definitive consensus in this regard. Close clinical follow-up during the infusion is imperative. At most institutions, patients undergoing thrombolytic therapy require admission to an intensive care or step-down unit familiar with management of patients undergoing thrombolysis. This is necessary predominately to monitor for signs of access site or remote bleeding, as well as to closely monitor progress in the affected limb. Many institutions vary in their practice of following serum fibrinogen values and blood counts during lysis, and this is discussed in detail below.

Mechanical thrombectomy comprises a broad range of techniques utilized to disrupt, dislodge, and remove thrombus from the vein. Inflation of a noncompliant balloon within a segment of thrombus can help macerate the thrombus, which is occasionally performed prior to thrombolysis to help expose an increased amount of thrombus surface area to the thrombolytic agent. High-pressure angioplasty is generally not necessary for this purpose, although not uncommonly one or more venous stenoses are encountered. If visualized, this stenosis can be angioplastied early in the procedure to encourage outflow following debulking of the clot. Passage of a nominally inflated balloon sized 1:1 to the vessel in question in a peripheral-to-central direction can also be used to displace thrombus into the central veins, as with arteriovenous fistula thrombectomy. However, caution should be taken when treating a large thrombus burden as this clot embolizes to the lungs.

A multitude of mechanical thrombectomy devices currently exist on the market (over 30 as of 2016), a full discussion of which is beyond the scope of this chapter. The prototypical device in this class is the Arrow-Trerotola Percutaneous Thrombolytic Device (Teleflex, Wayne PA), which is commercially available in both over-the-wire (OTW) and non-OTW varieties. Both device types are available in 65 and 120 cm lengths. The device is unsheathed within the thrombus and activated, causing rapid rotation of the fragmentation basket and maceration of the thrombus. Many other currently available devices are a variation on this theme. The major limitation in these devices is the lack of thrombus removal and the potential for clinically significant distal embolization. In general, the authors reserve the use of these devices for tough, refractory thrombus, particularly material adherent to the vessel wall that is unsuccessfully treated using other methods.

The AngioJet peripheral thrombectomy system (Boston Scientific, Marlborough, MA) is a mechanical rheolytic thrombectomy device that can be utilized to both disrupt and remove acute and subacute thrombus from the vessel. The device is advanced over a guidewire through the thrombus and can be used in two modes: pulse-spray mode, which administers rapid bursts of a user-defined solution into the vein without aspirating, and thrombectomy mode, which simultaneously infuses and aspirates. In pulse-spray mode, typically a 50- to 100-mL solution of 25 to 50% tPA is administered into the thrombus by slowly advancing it over the wire while the device is activated to lace the thrombus with tPA. The medication is typically allowed to dwell for 10 to 30 minutes. This administration facilitates softening and partial dissolution of the thrombus, which can then be removed by using the thrombectomy mode. If the patient is at a high risk of bleeding, pulse-spray can also be performed with saline. A variety of catheter diameters and lengths are available, ranging from 3 to 8 French and from 50 to 150 cm. Each catheter is connected to the same base unit that drives infusion and aspiration. Contrast can be injected through a side-port intermittently to monitor treatment progress. In using the Angiojet, systemic heparinization is recommended after gaining venous access in order to prevent acute rethrombosis. Up to 60 mL/min can be aspirated using this device, and therefore it should be used sparingly in flowing blood. Transient hemolysis can occur during treatment, and therefore the device should not be used for more than 480 seconds of total treatment time (or 240 seconds in flowing blood) due to risk of renal injury. Patients and caregivers should be warned that most patients will experience some degree of hemoglobinuria following the use of this device, and hydration afterward is recommended. This system is far more effective when treating acute thrombus and is relatively limited for the treatment of organized, chronic DVT.

Peripheral suction thrombectomy using the Indigo device (Penumbra, Alameda, CA) is a relatively recent addition to the thrombectomy armamentarium. The system consists of 4.1- to 8-French suction catheters (ranging in length from 85 to 115 cm), a catheter-specific wire-mounted separator device, a collection canister, and the MAX pump unit. The catheters are made of a reinforced material that prevents collapse during suction, and the catheter tips are available in straight and angled varieties. The catheter is advanced over a wire through the hemostatic valve of the sheath and positioned in the area of the thrombus. The wire is removed and the separator wire is advanced through a rotating hemostatic valve attached to the back end of the catheter. The suction tubing is connected to the side-port of the rotating hemostatic valve. The catheter is manipulated through the thrombus while suction is applied. The operator intermittently pulls the separator device back into the catheter to clear thrombus adhered to the catheter tip. Close attention must be paid to the rate of aspirate obtained in the collection canister, as a large amount of blood can be removed when the thrombus has cleared and blood flow is restored. For this reason, the authors recommend a type and screen prior to use of this device, as well as a hemoglobin and hematocrit level before and after the procedure. Similar to the

AngioJet, this device is much more useful for acute and subacute thrombus, and its usefulness for chronic DVT is relatively limited.

In some settings, a large volume of thrombus may be present in a larger vessel that does not cause complete occlusion (e.g., free-floating thrombus extending above an IVC filter). In these settings, thrombectomy can be risky because of the potential for a relatively large amount of blood loss, and the risk of embolizing substantial thrombus to the lungs. The AngioVac venous drainage system (AngioDynamics, Latham, NY) is an excellent option in these situations, as the material removed is passed through a filter to trap solid material such as thrombus, with the remaining blood products returned to the patient through an extracorporeal bypass circuit. The AngioVac circuit can be connected to any centrifugal bypass pump console, but requires a perfusionist to monitor the extracorporeal bypass process. The 22-French, coil-reinforced cannula has a tip that assumes a funnel-shaped configuration once the balloon is inflated, allowing it to fill the cross-sectional area of the vessel and decrease the likelihood of embolization past the catheter tip. The device is highly efficient and can remove large amounts of thrombus en bloc, without the fear of massive blood loss. Catheter clogging is rare. Potential limitations include the need for an available perfusionist, the large access sheath required for catheter delivery, and the need for an additional venous access site for the return of blood products to the patient.

Regardless of the device used, once the thrombus has been treated, venography should be performed in order to monitor treatment progress and evaluate for underlying venous stenosis, which may have predisposed the patient to the thrombosis. Adjunctive treatments may include balloon angioplasty and/or stenting. Following treatment, therapeutic anticoagulation should be initiated for all patients in whom it is safe.

The use of caval filtration during DVT treatment is controversial. Clinically significant PE has been reported as high as 5% during catheter-directed DVT therapy, with up to 10% of in-hospital deaths following treatment attributed to PE.[18] In one recent study, more than 40% of patients that underwent prophylactic IVC filter placement prior to aspiration thrombectomy demonstrated thrombotic material within the filter during the caval venogram prior to filter retrieval.[19] Until further evidence is compiled, the placement of a caval filter is at the discretion of the operator. The decision should take into account the respiratory status of the patient, preexisting PE, the location and volume of thrombus being treated, and the specific method of therapy. At the authors' institution, IVC filters are used sparingly during DVT interventions, primarily in the setting of large-volume iliocaval thrombus. Superior vena cava (SVC) filter placement is far less common than IVC filters; the authors feel that filters are generally unnecessary during DVT interventions above the heart.[20]

4.3.4 Potential Complications or Pitfalls

Significant complications of DVT intervention are rare. During thrombolysis, the most common and potentially most severe complications are related to bleeding. Minor bleeding complications, such as oozing at the puncture site or local hematoma formation, are around twice as common in patients undergoing thrombolysis than in those receiving systemic anticoagulation alone, with a relative risk of 2.2.[21] Access site bleeding should initially be managed using conservative measures: application of pressure to the site of bleeding and/or the use of hemostatic adjuncts such as hemostatic pads or powder.

Close hemodynamic monitoring and frequent measurement of blood counts is suggested during thrombolytic therapy, to aid in early identification of bleeding in nonvisible locations, such as the retroperitoneum. Early identification of bleeding also guides the need to cease therapy or search for an obscure site of bleeding with additional imaging. Routine serum fibrinogen value monitoring is controversial; however, most investigators still report its use as a tool to alert clinicians of a potential increase in the risk of bleeding complications. There are conflicting data regarding the specific level of serum fibrinogen below which bleeding risk becomes prohibitive.[22,23] Rapid decreases in fibrinogen level (e.g., > 50% decrease from baseline) may prompt a decrease in the dose of tPA administration, more frequent fibrinogen monitoring, and the consideration of a venographic assessment earlier than originally planned. Fibrinogen levels below 100 mg/dL should prompt the consideration of temporary or complete cessation of therapy, and potentially the administration of cryoprecipitate. Aggressive resuscitative measures should be initiated in patients with signs of significant remote bleeding, including the administration of packed red blood cells, platelets, and plasma, as appropriate.

Intracranial bleeding has been reported in up to 2.5% of patients undergoing thrombolysis, and can be potentially devastating. Any new focal neurologic signs should be considered an intracranial bleed until proven otherwise; immediate interruption in thrombolysis and a noncontrast CT of the head are prudent. PE is another concern for patients undergoing treatment of DVT, particularly those with iliocaval thrombus. No statistically significant increase in PE has been reported for patients undergoing thrombolysis alone, but up to 2.5% of patients undergoing pharmacomechanical thrombectomy may develop clinically significant PE.

4.3.5 Postprocedural Management and Follow-up

Upon treatment completion, eligible patients should be started on therapeutic anticoagulation to avoid rethrombosis. Bed rest should be maintained for at least 2 hours to mitigate the risk of hematoma formation. A repeat CBC and coagulation panel should be obtained to exclude significant blood loss and to document appropriate anticoagulation levels. A creatinine level 24 to 48 hours after therapy should be obtained in order to monitor for acute kidney injury related to contrast load or as a complication of rheolytic thrombectomy. Venous duplex ultrasound should be obtained the following day to document a new baseline and to exclude acute rethrombosis. Lower extremity compression stocking therapy is recommended, using a 30 to 40 mm Hg compression if tolerated (preferably thigh-high or chaps style) for 3 to 6 months following treatment. Patients should be transitioned to oral anticoagulation according to patient preference. For patients requiring stenting, antiplatelet therapy using aspirin and clopidogrel may be indicated. In the

authors practice, clopidogrel is generally discontinued after 2 to 3 months, but aspirin is continued for life. Outpatient follow-up is variable, but the authors' preference is for follow-up at 1, 3, and 6 months at a minimum, with outpatient duplex generally reserved for new or recurrent symptoms only.

4.3.6 Outcomes

Thrombolytic therapy has been consistently shown to accelerate the resolution of DVT and decrease the risk of PTS. A recent Cochrane review of 17 studies including 1,103 patients demonstrated a significantly higher rate of complete thrombus resolution in patients undergoing thrombolysis at early (risk ratio [RR]: 4.91) and intermediate (RR: 2.37) follow-up intervals. Rates of PTS were substantially lower in these patients (RR: 0.64), and leg ulcerations were also less common (RR: 0.48).[24] Immediate treatment failure (defined as less than 50% thrombus resolution) is rare and is most commonly associated with recent surgery (odds ratio [OR]: 19.6) and phlegmasia cerulea dolens (OR: 3.12). Although not statistically significant, there was a trend toward lower treatment success rates in men and in elderly patients.[25] Bleeding complications were uncommon, with higher bleeding risk associated with higher cumulative thrombolytic dose and longer durations of therapy.

The multicenter PEARL registry, documenting outcomes in patients undergoing treatment using the AngioJet, revealed 3-, 6-, and 12-month rates of freedom from rethrombosis of 94, 87, and 83%, respectively. One limitation of this registry is that the specific protocols of use varied significantly.[25] Given the relative novelty of the Penumbra Indigo device for use in the periphery, long-term efficacy and safety data are also notably absent. Anecdotally, patency and safety of these technologies approaches that of pharmacologic thrombolysis, with shorter procedure times and fewer bleeding complications, as well as considerably higher rates of patient tolerance and immediate treatment satisfaction.

In an effort to improve the quality of evidence and more precisely determine if pharmacomechanical CDT (PCDT) will reduce the frequency of PTS, the National Institutes of Health sponsored a phase III, multicenter, randomized, open-label, controlled clinical trial titled: Acute Venous Thrombosis: Thrombus Removal with Adjunctive Catheter-Directed Thrombolysis Trial, ATTRACT. Researchers randomized 692 patients with acute suprapopliteal DVT (femoral, common femoral, and/ or iliac veins) to anticoagulation and compression stockings or PCDT in addition to anticoagulation and compression stockings. Enrollment was completed by January 2015 and patients were followed for 2 years. While the full results of the study have not been released, partial results were announced at the 2017 Society of Interventional Radiology (SIR) Annual meeting by Dr. Suresh Vedantham, the principal investigator. PTS occurrence was approximately the same in both treatment groups, without difference in primary outcome. However, patients who underwent PCDT were 25% less likely to develop moderate-to-severe PTS. Initial impressions of the data suggest that patients with iliofemoral DVT will likely benefit from PCDT, more so than patients with femoral-popliteal DVT. As more data are released, this study will serve as a basis for future evidence-based guidelines.

4.4 Pearls of Wisdom

- CDT and pharmacomechanical thrombectomy should be considered in all patients with DVT, particularly if the patient has severe symptoms, is young, and/or has proximal occlusions (iliofemoral or brachiocephalic/subclavian segments).
- Rethrombosis can occur in the immediate posttreatment period. Ideally, patients should be anticoagulated for at least a few weeks to months. Compression stocking therapy following thrombolysis for lower extremity DVT may decrease the risk of PTS.
- IVC filter use is controversial during CDT and PMT, and is at the discretion of the operator, taking into account the presence of coexisting PE, respiratory status, thrombus volume, and location and the likelihood of large volume embolization.

4.5 Unanswered Questions

Anticoagulation therapy is not the only tool used in the treatment of DVT. Thrombolysis and thrombectomy are superior to anticoagulation in regard to the speed of thrombus resolution, but which therapy to use remains obscure. The questions of optimal thrombolytic dose, the length of therapy prior to angiographic recheck, the use of concomitant, and type and duration of follow-up anticoagulation all have yet to be answered. Preliminary results from the ATTRACT trial suggest that PTS occurs in patients with lower extremity DVT, regardless of treatment paradigm (standard therapy or PCDT). The severity of symptoms appears to be decreased in patients who undergo thrombolysis for iliofemoral DVT, but does not appear to be diminished in patients undergoing thrombolysis for femoropopliteal DVT. Additionally, more targeted investigations of these therapies would add significantly to the literature.

4.6 May–Thurner Syndrome

MTS is the most commonly used eponym for compression of the left common iliac vein by the right common iliac artery, anteriorly, and the vertebral column, posteriorly. Pulsations from the overlying artery and chronic compression of the left common iliac vein predispose to vascular thickening, intimal proliferation, and adhesions that can result in venous obstruction. Historically, Virchow noted that iliofemoral DVT was five times more likely in the left leg as compared to the right as early as 1851.[26] McMurrich in 1908, Ehrich and Krumbharr in 1943, and May and Thurner in 1956 noted that 22 to 30% of studied cadavers had venous obstructions, termed "spurs," in the left common iliac vein, attributable to the overlying right common iliac artery—the anatomic variant responsible for Virchow's observation.[27,28,29] Cockett and Thomas further defined the anatomical relationship and noted that patients with left common iliac vein "spurs" could be asymptomatic due to venous collateral formation, though the "spurs" were irreversible and predisposed to venous thrombosis and lower extremity venous disease.[30] MTS patients may present with or without DVT, stigmata of PTS, left leg edema, or left leg pain. A thorough workup with history, physical examination, and imaging studies can lead to early diagnosis and prompt treatment to help avoid venous complications in these patients.

4.6.1 Case Vignette

Patient Presentation

A 26-year-old woman presented with a 1-week history of progressive left lower extremity swelling and pain. She has no prior medical history, family history of DVT, or hypercoagulable risk factors, does not smoke, and does not take oral contraceptives.

Physical Exam

Isolated left lower extremity swelling was noted, extending from the foot to the thigh, with cyanotic discoloration and diffuse tenderness throughout. The right lower extremity was unremarkable.

Imaging

Lower extremity duplex ultrasound imaging demonstrated expanded, noncompressible left lower extremity veins with intraluminal hypoechoic material consistent with acute lower extremity DVT (▶ Fig. 4.3a, ▶ Fig. 4.4b). The thrombus extended from the left external iliac vein to the infrapopliteal veins. The

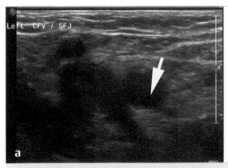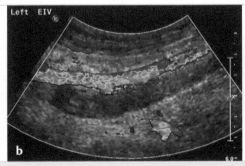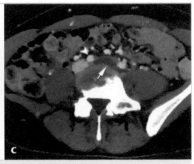

Fig. 4.3 (a) Transverse grayscale ultrasound image of left common femoral vein, revealing occlusive hypoechoic material within the vein (*arrow*) consistent with acute DVT. **(b)** Longitudinal color Doppler ultrasound image of left external iliac vein, demonstrating occlusive hypoechoic material within the vein and absence of flow consistent with acute DVT. **(c)** Axial computed tomography venogram (CTV) image demonstrating an occlusive filling defect within the left common iliac vein (*arrow*) consistent with DVT. Note the compression of the vein by the overlying right common iliac artery (*arrowhead*).

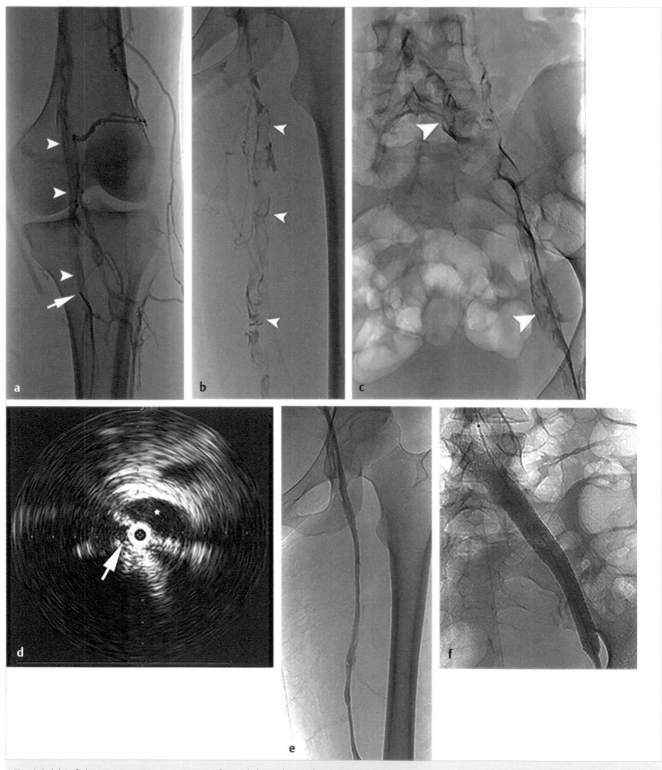

Fig. 4.4 (a) Left lower extremity venogram performed through a catheter (*arrow*) inserted through a posterior tibial vein sheath, revealing partially occlusive filling defects (*arrowheads*) throughout the popliteal vein, consistent with DVT. **(b)** Left lower extremity venogram demonstrates occlusive filling defects throughout the femoral and common femoral veins (*arrowheads*), consistent with DVT. **(c)** Left lower extremity venogram demonstrates occlusive within the left common and external iliac veins (*arrowheads*), consistent with DVT. **(d)** Intravascular ultrasound (IVUS) image obtained within the left common iliac vein demonstrating severe compression of the vein (*arrow*) by the overlying artery (*star*). **(e)** Left lower extremity venogram postlysis reveals complete resolution of thrombus within the left popliteal, femoral, and common femoral veins. **(f)** Left iliac venogram following successful lysis and stenting reveals widely patent left common iliac vein in the area of previously demonstrated compression.

right lower extremity evaluation was normal. Given the unilateral left DVT, MTS was suspected. A CT venogram was performed, which revealed expanded, nonenhancing left-sided veins extending from the left popliteal vein to the IVC, with compression of the left common iliac vein by the overlying right common iliac artery (► Fig. 4.3c).

Specifics of Consent

Given the iliofemoral venous involvement, the relatively high risk of PTS even with anticoagulation and eventual clot resolution was discussed with the patient. She was screened for thrombolytic contraindications. The potential risk of severe bleeding during thrombolysis, including intracranial bleeding, PE, and death, was discussed. As the DVT was presumed to have been caused by the left common iliac vein compression, the anticipated need for iliac stenting and future implications were discussed.

Details of Procedure

Initial access was performed through the posterior tibial vein at the level of the ankle under ultrasound guidance. Left lower extremity venography was performed, demonstrating diffuse thrombus from the posterior tibial vein through the IVC (► Fig. 4.4a; ► Fig. 4.4b; ► Fig. 4.4c). As a catheter would not pass cranially, a wire was passed from below into the IVC and snared from a right internal jugular access. This through-and-through access was used to deliver a multiside hole infusion catheter across the thrombosed iliofemoral segment to the popliteal vein. Overnight thrombolysis was performed using tPA at a rate of 1.0 mg/h. The thrombus was completely resolved by the following day. IVUS was used to both confirm and delineate the compression of the left common iliac vein by the overlying right common iliac artery (► Fig. 4.4d). A 16 mm × 8 cm self-expanding stent was placed across the area of narrowing, extending from the IVC to below the internal iliac vein. Completion venogram showed brisk anterograde venous flow from the popliteal vein to the IVC (► Fig. 4.4e; ► Fig. 4.4f).

Follow-up

Following the procedure, the patient was discharged on enoxaparin and clopidogrel. One-week follow-up in the clinic revealed complete resolution of her left leg swelling and pain. She was transitioned to warfarin for 6 months and maintained on clopidogrel for a total of 2 months. She had no recurrence of symptoms through 2-year follow-up.

4.7 Epidemiology and Scope of the Problem

MTS is most commonly described in younger and middle-aged women, particularly during pregnancy or after immobilization. Cadaveric studies revealed 50% compression of the left common iliac vein by the right common iliac artery in 22 to 32% of all subjects. More recently, Kibbe et al reviewed CT imaging of emergency department patients for all indications and found 24% of patients exhibited at least 50% compression of the left common iliac vein.[31] In symptomatic individuals, compression is present in greater than 90%.[32] While the true incidence is not known, 50 to 60% of left-sided iliofemoral DVT have the venous spurs typical of extrinsic compression.[32,33]

4.7.1 Patient Presentation and Evaluation

There are three stages of MTS. Stage I represents asymptomatic left common iliac vein compression; stage II is defined by the formation of an intraluminal spur; and stage III demonstrates left iliac vein DVT, distal to the compression. Patients may present acutely with sudden onset of left leg swelling with DVT. Less dramatic presentations of chronic symptoms may include DVT, edema, pain, varicose veins, pigment changes, or other stigmata of PTS.[34] Patient history should include screening for risk factors for DVT and inquiring about prior potential DVT events. Clinical assessment tools such as CEAP (a comprehensive classification system for chronic venous disorders) or others are utilized for standardization. Laboratory evaluations include a CBC, basic metabolic panel, coagulation profile, and a hypercoagulability workup, as necessary. Imaging evaluation begins with lower extremity ultrasonography to evaluate for DVT and venous reflux, and venous-phase cross-sectional imaging of the pelvis is also commonly performed. Either CT or MRI is able to demonstrate the relationship of the common iliac veins and arteries relative to the spine. Moreover, DVT in the pelvic veins and collateral venous outflow may be visualized with either modality.

4.7.2 Preparation for Procedure

Preprocedural medications may include a single dose of an antibiotic to cover skin flora, but no other medications are necessary. The procedure can be performed with intravenous sedation, unless comorbid conditions warrant general anesthesia. If thrombolysis is expected, placement of multiple secure peripheral intravenous accesses and insertion of a urinary catheter is suggested prior to initiation of thrombolysis. Patient positioning can be either supine or prone, based on level of thrombus extension; however, supine positioning may be more desirable for purposes of patient comfort and for access to the internal jugular vein, if needed.

After the patient is positioned on the angiography table, sterile preparation and draping is performed for each potential access site (most commonly the left groin and either the right groin or right neck). IVUS is quite helpful in venous interventions and the authors recommend having IVUS capability for use in all suspected MTS patients. Otherwise, no special equipment is needed beyond the standard repertoire found in interventional suites. As with any endovascular procedure, the operator should be mindful of contrast usage and radiation dose.

4.7.3 Technical Tips and Tricks and Procedural Details

The left greater saphenous vein is useful for access, as it is superficial and easily compressed for hemostasis, decreases instrumentation of the deep venous system, and frequently remains patent despite thrombus load in the deep venous system. After placement of a sheath, venography is performed, which may reveal a flattened left common iliac vein, cross pelvic or lumbar collaterals, or filling defects consistent with DVT. A hydrophilic guidewire and directional catheter are navigated to the area of suspected compression and are used to traverse the stenosis into the IVC. In the setting of a chronic occlusion or a long segment lesion, intermittent contrast injection and oblique images may be necessary to confirm an intravascular anatomic course of the catheter.

After the catheter has crossed into the IVC, the wire is exchanged for a stiff, nonhydrophilic working wire and IVUS is performed; IVUS accurately delineates the degree of left common iliac vein compression, the length of the stenosis, and the presence of an intraluminal spur or thrombus. Additionally, IVUS allows for precise measurement of the luminal area of the normal venous segments, allowing selection of appropriately sized balloons and stents. Fluoroscopic correlation of the length of the stenosis is performed, and compared with venography, in preparation for stenting. The stent should extend into the IVC to adequately treat the compression and prevent early restenosis. To help with accurate stent placement, frequently a second venous access, either the right internal jugular or right greater saphenous vein, is established. A wire is passed into the IVC, and a catheter is placed adjacent to the point in the IVC where the stent is expected to land. For common iliac veins, the most frequently used sizes are 14- to 18-mm diameter self-expanding stents. Predilation of the stenotic segment, up to the nominal size of the stent, is helpful and suggested to facilitate stent placement and to establish flow prior to deployment. After deploying the stent, venoplasty is repeated to ensure immediate maximum expansion of the stent.

Completion venography and IVUS is performed in order to evaluate if additional stenting is warranted. Specific attention is paid to the degree of stent apposition to the wall within the nonadjacent nonstenotic venous segments in order to be certain that the stent is appropriately sized. Attention is also paid to the flow dynamics by assessing for brisk anterograde flow and collapse of collaterals. It is important that the proximal and distal ends of the stent lie in normal venous segments and that there is brisk inflow to maintain stent patency. After concluding the procedure and achieving hemostasis, therapeutic anticoagulation is immediately initiated. The authors prefer initiation with enoxaparin with transition to an oral agent at the first follow-up clinic visit.

4.7.4 Potential Complications or Pitfalls

Major complications after MTS treatment are uncommon but generally include those typical to venous angioplasty and stenting. These specifically include bleeding from the access site, venous rupture with bleeding in the retroperitoneum, stent migration, stent fracture, or early in-stent thrombosis. Stent thrombosis is more common in patients who have presented with left common iliac vein thrombosis as opposed to nonthrombotic MTS. Reviewing retrospective case series comprising 130 patients who underwent CDT and stenting for MTS revealed transfusion rates from 4 to 14%, PE risk of 1%, and intracranial hemorrhage < 1%.[35] Some patients also report

transient left flank pain that usually resolves within 1 to 2 weeks and only requires treatment with over-the-counter analgesics.

4.7.5 Postprocedural Management and Follow-up

If admitted overnight, the vast majority of patients are discharged the following day. Therapeutic anticoagulation and dual antiplatelet therapy (aspirin 81 mg and clopidogrel 75 mg) is initiated. Clopidogrel is continued for 2 months and aspirin therapy indefinitely. The duration of therapeutic anticoagulation is made on a case-by-case basis, but is no less than 6 months. The first follow-up visit is 2 weeks after treatment, where CEAP scoring and lower extremity ultrasonography are repeated. Subsequent visits are planned at 6, 12, and 24 months. If symptoms return, the authors proceed to venography. Compression stockings are encouraged for all patients, particularly if there is a history of DVT, edema, or venous reflux.

4.7.6 Outcomes

Historically, treatment for patients involved surgical thrombectomy; however, nearly 70% of patients developed reocclusion. Endovascular treatment with placement of a venous stent was initially described in 1995.[36] The combination of thrombolysis/thrombectomy with angioplasty and stent placement was also described in the late 1990s, and has become a standard approach.[37,38,39,40,41] Several papers have been published describing outcomes for endovascular treatment of MTS with left iliac venous thrombosis and/or symptoms of chronic venous disease. The technical success rate of venous stenting for chronic postthrombotic iliac vein obstruction approaches 90%, with nearly 100% success in the setting of acute thrombosis. In patients presenting with thrombosis, primary, primary assisted, and secondary stent patency rates at 6 to 10 years range from 57 to 83%, 80 to 89%, and 86 to 93%, respectively. In the setting of patients presenting with nonthrombotic MTS, primary, primary assisted, and secondary patency rates at 6 years are 79, 100, and 100%, respectively.[42,43,44] Clinical improvement with partial or complete relief of symptoms is expected in > 80% of patients, and in some reports, exceeds 90%.[45]

4.8 Pearls of Wisdom

- Cross-sectional imaging is helpful in the evaluation of patients to visualize the severity and extent of compression, and can exclude alternative diagnoses. Cross-sectional imaging is also helpful for preprocedure planning.
- Large, self-expanding stents should be used with predilation of the stenotic segment. Venography and IVUS measurements of the adjacent normal venous segments can aid with the selection of the stent diameter.
- Stenting across to the confluence of the common iliac veins can be challenging, but is necessary in most patients with MTS. Precise delineation of the stenosis should be confirmed with IVUS. Extending the stent into the IVC helps avoid early restenosis and usually will not adversely affect venous drainage from the other leg. If there is concern for

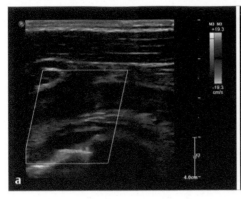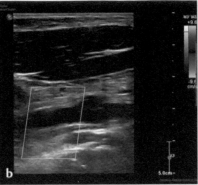

Fig. 4.5 (a) Longitudinal color Doppler ultrasound image of left subclavian vein, demonstrating absent flow and occlusive hypoechoic material within the vein consistent with acute DVT. (b) Longitudinal color Doppler ultrasound image of left axillary vein, demonstrating absent flow and occlusive hypoechoic material within the vein consistent with acute DVT.

compromise of flow in the right iliac system, predeployment venography from the right common iliac vein can be performed to confirm landmarks, and should kissing stents be necessary a wire can be left in the right-sided common iliac vein to aid appropriate placement of the left-sided stent.

4.9 Unanswered Questions

Compression of the left common iliac vein by the right common iliac artery is a common occurrence, though it is difficult to predict which patients will progress to MTS. Establishment of standardized diagnostic criteria is needed as timely diagnosis and prompt endovascular treatment can effectively mitigate the long-term consequences of this entity. Endovascular treatment results in high technical and clinical success rates in patients who present with acute or chronic symptoms. Postprocedure management with either anticoagulation, antiplatelet agents, or both and the duration for such treatment remains an area of controversy and has not been rigorously evaluated.

4.10 Paget–Schroetter Syndrome

PSS, also known as axillosubclavian vein effort thrombosis or venous thoracic outlet syndrome, most commonly occurs with strenuous and repetitive activity of the upper extremities. Cruveilhier described spontaneous axillosubclavian vein thrombosis in 1816, Paget expanded on this description in 1875, and Schroetter linked muscular effort to venous injury in 1884.[46,47,48] The first review of PSS was ultimately published in 1949.[49,50] Presently, it is estimated that PSS is the etiology in 30 to 40% of spontaneous axillosubclavian venous thrombosis and in up to 10 to 20% of all upper extremity deep venous thromboses.

4.10.1 Case Vignette
Patient Presentation

A 25-year-old woman presented with acute-onset left upper extremity swelling and pain. She has been healthy all her life, has no personal or family history of DVT, has no known hypercoagulable risk factors, does not smoke, and does not take oral contraceptives. The patient reported that she is physically active most days of the week, but does not participate in any upper extremity exercise regularly. The patient recalled that she recently completed painting the walls of her house.

Physical Exam

Isolated left upper extremity swelling was noted, extending from the wrist to the shoulder, with mild cyanotic discoloration, decreased range of motion at the elbow secondary to pain, and diffuse tenderness to palpation. Her pulse exam was normal, both with the arm adducted and abducted at the shoulder. The right upper extremity was unremarkable.

Imaging

Upper extremity duplex ultrasound was performed, which demonstrated expanded, noncompressible left upper extremity axillary and subclavian veins with intraluminal hypoechoic material, consistent with acute DVT (► Fig. 4.5a; ► Fig. 4.5b). The radial, ulnar, cephalic, brachial, and basilic veins were patent. The right upper extremity veins were normal.

Specifics of Consent

The patient had a history of heavy menses and also a history of a Chiari 1 malformation and was unwilling to accept the potential risk of severe bleeding associated with thrombolytic therapy; the authors elected not to perform thrombolysis in this patient. The risks of pharmacomechanical thrombectomy and venoplasty, including the inability to maintain venous patency, venous rupture, recurrent thrombosis, PE, and death, were all discussed. The patient was fully aware that she would require surgical intervention following thrombolysis and venoplasty should the diagnosis of PSS be confirmed angiographically. Alternative therapies such as anticoagulation, primary surgical decompression, or conservative therapy alone were also offered.

Details of Procedure

The patient was placed on the angiographic table in the supine position. The left upper extremity, left neck, and right groin were prepared in a sterile fashion. Ultrasound-guided access was performed in the left basilic vein, and a 6-French sheath was placed. A 5-French direction catheter and hydrophilic guidewire were navigated to the left shoulder region. Left upper extremity and central venography was performed, demonstrating occlusion of the subclavian and central axillary veins with rounded filling defects consistent with acute thrombosis, as well as extensive collateral vein formation bypassing the

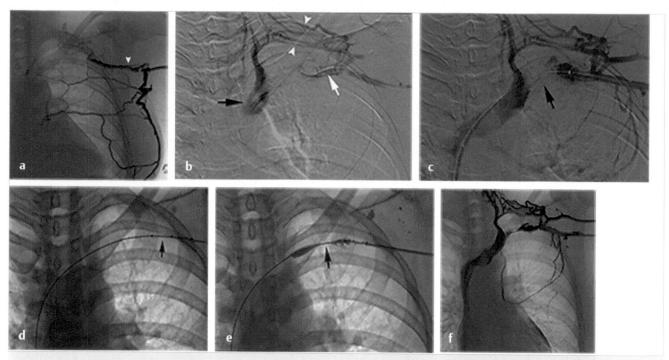

Fig. 4.6 (a) Left axillary venogram (*arrowhead*: catheter tip) revealing complete occlusion of the left subclavian and distal axillary veins. (b) Left subclavian venogram demonstrating filling defects within the axillary (*white arrow*) and reconstituted brachiocephalic (*black arrow*) veins. Note the collaterals (*arrowheads*). (c) Left subclavian venogram after wire crossing of occluded left subclavian vein (*arrow*). (d) Spot-image radiograph revealing AngioJet rheolytic thrombectomy device (*arrow*). (e) Spot-image radiograph revealing significant waist during balloon venoplasty (*arrow*). (f) Left axillary venogram demonstrating patency of the left subclavian vein, but with persistent stenosis and collaterals.

occluded segment from the axillary vein to the brachiocephalic vein and the SVC (▶ Fig. 4.6a; ▶ Fig. 4.6b). The wire and catheter were used to cross into the SVC and ultimately the IVC (▶ Fig. 4.6c). Pulse-spray thrombolysis with tPA was then performed using the AngioJet device, followed by thrombectomy of the involved segment (▶ Fig. 4.6d). Balloon angioplasty of the treated vein was performed using a 10 mm × 40 mm angioplasty balloon (▶ Fig. 4.6e).

Postvenoplasty angiogram revealed a residual stenosis in a patent left subclavian vein with antegrade flow to the SVC (▶ Fig. 4.6f). This was resistant to further balloon venoplasty. In anticipation of upcoming decompressive surgery, no stent was placed.

Follow-up

Anticoagulation was initiated immediately with enoxaparin. The patient proceeded to thoracic outlet decompression surgery 5 days later, where partial first rib resection and scalenectomy was performed. She was continued on anticoagulation therapy for 3 months, with no recurrence in her symptoms and no residual DVT on subsequent duplex ultrasound. She remained symptom-free at her 6-, 12-, and 24-month appointments.

4.11 Epidemiology and Scope of the Problem

PSS is most common in young adulthood, with a 2:1 predilection for men given the additional muscular bulk and bony mass. The right side is affected more often than the left, likely a function of the increased prevalence of right-hand dominance. More than 85% of patients report a history of recent vigorous exercise involving the upper extremities, or a career or hobby involving a great deal of arm abduction—painters, auto mechanics, baseball pitchers, badminton players, or weight lifters, for example. The approximate incidence of this condition is 1 to 2 per 100,000 person-years, or approximately 3,000 to 6,000 patients in the United States each year.[51]

4.11.1 Patient Presentation and Evaluation

Patients with venous compression alone but not thrombosis may complain of episodic arm discoloration and swelling, usually incited by arm abduction. Over time, repetitive trauma to the vein is suspected to cause inflammation within and around the vein, resulting in fibrosis, adherence to surrounding structures, and intimal hyperplasia. This causes stretching and tearing of the vein as further repetitive motion occurs. Venous stasis during periods of compression and endothelial injury caused by the trauma may result in the initiation of upper extremity DVT, which may propagate peripherally. Acute DVT at this location often produces sudden onset of severe symptoms, as the normal collateral pathways through the cephalic and profunda brachii venous branches are generally insufficient to provide complete drainage of the arm. Pain, swelling, and cyanosis are noted, similar to any other DVT. Dilated superficial veins on the arm, ipsilateral chest, and neck are often identified on physical examination.

PSS should be suspected in all cases of unexplained axillosub-clavian DVT, especially in young, healthy individuals. The thrombus can usually be identified using ultrasound, either through direct visualization or through indirect physiologic evidence such as decreased pulsatility and phasicity on Doppler evaluation of more peripheral veins. Cross-sectional imaging, including CT or MR venography, can be obtained if there is a question of the diagnosis, and may better delineate the site of maximum compression, associated collateral pathways, and any aberrant anatomy that may be responsible for the venous compression.

4.11.2 Preparation for Procedure

Preprocedural medications may include a single dose of an anti-biotic to cover skin flora, but generally no other medications are necessary. The procedure can be performed with intravenous moderate sedation, unless comorbid conditions warrant general anesthesia. If thrombolysis is expected, placement of multiple secure peripheral intravenous accesses and placement of a urinary catheter is suggested prior to initiation of thrombolysis. Patients are positioned supine with sterile preparation and draping of the access sites, which include the arm of the affected upper extremity, the ipsilateral neck, and, if needed, the ipsilateral groin. IVUS is quite helpful in venous interventions and the authors recommend its use routinely. Otherwise, no special equipment is needed beyond the standard devices found in interventional suites. As with any endovascular procedure, the operator should be mindful of contrast usage and radiation dose.

4.11.3 Technical Tips and Tricks and Procedural Details

Generally, access is acquired in the affected extremity peripheral to the thrombus in either the basilic or brachial veins. After placement of a sheath, venography is performed, which may reveal focal or diffuse thrombus, a flattened subclavian vein, or numerous collateral veins bypassing the segment crossing the first rib. A hydrophilic guidewire and directional catheter are navigated to the area of suspected compression and used to cross into the SVC and ultimately into the IVC. If there is a chronic occlusion or a long segment lesion, intermittent contrast injection and oblique images may be necessary to confirm an intravascular anatomic course. After the catheter has crossed into the IVC, hydrophilic wires are exchanged for a stiff nonhydrophilic working wire; pharmacologic thrombolysis or mechanical thrombectomy is performed in standard fashion if acute thrombus is present. IVUS accurately delineates the degree of axillosubclavian compression, the length of stenosis, and the presence of intraluminal webs. Additionally, IVUS allows for accurate measurement of the luminal area of the adjacent normal venous segments. Overdilation of the vein is avoided in order to decrease the degree of posttreatment inflammatory response; generally, a 10-mm balloon will suffice.

After venoplasty, completion venography and IVUS is performed to document flow dynamics, with brisk anterograde flow and decompression of collaterals expected following a successful treatment. Venography can be repeated in abduction to confirm thoracic outlet compression. As the cause of stenosis is related to mechanical extrinsic compressive forces that may cause compression of stents, stenting is not recommended except in extreme cases of refractory, symptomatic stenosis after thoracic decompressive surgery. After concluding the procedure and achieving hemostasis, therapeutic anticoagulation is immediately initiated. The authors prefer initiation of enoxaparin with transition to an oral agent at the first follow-up clinic visit.

4.11.4 Potential Complications or Pitfalls

Major complications after PSS treatment are uncommon but include those typical to thrombolysis and venous angioplasty. Access site bleeding, venous rupture, and early rethrombosis have all been reported. Overall, complication rates are similar to other CDT and venoplasty procedures.

4.11.5 Postprocedural Management and Follow-up

If admitted to the hospital, after overnight observation the vast majority of patients are discharged and instructed to maintain good hydration status, as well as to avoid strenuous activity in the affected extremity. Therapeutic anticoagulation is initiated and maintained until patients undergo decompressive surgery. The duration of therapeutic anticoagulation postsurgery is made on a case-by-case basis, and typically is between 3 and 6 months. If symptoms recur, the authors proceed to venography with possible repeat venoplasty.

4.11.6 Outcomes

Outcomes data for the treatment of PSS are limited to small, retrospective series. Different centers follow different treatment regimens, which have also changed over time making direct comparison between the treatments difficult. A review of 159 patients who underwent first rib resection with limited venoplasty and anticoagulation reported patency rates at 3 years ranging between 92 and 100%.[52] Another published series of 117 patients found that CDT with early decompressive surgery had a superior outcome to later decompressive surgery or in patients who were treated conservatively.[53] Several single-center series with smaller patient populations have been described with conflicting results, making it difficult to draw conclusions from the literature.

4.12 Pearls of Wisdom

- Provocative venography, MRI, or CT imaging can reveal dynamic compression of the axillosubclavian vessels and support the diagnosis of PSS.
- IVUS is helpful to evaluate the venous lumen as well as the severity and extent of compression.
- Overdilation of the vein should be avoided in order to minimize inflammatory changes. Routine stenting is not recommended except in extreme, refractory postsurgical cases as the mechanical compression can result in stent fracture.

- CDT is most successful in the first 2 weeks of thrombosis. A short interval of time, ideally less than 2 weeks, is suggested between thrombolysis and definitive surgical decompression.

4.13 Unanswered Questions

Axillosubclavian vein thrombosis often affects young, fit adults. The potential long-term sequelae can be disabling. While CDT and early surgical decompression is performed at several centers with compelling results, others prefer to reserve surgery for persistent symptoms or perform surgery at a later date. Less aggressive medical centers prefer thrombolysis followed by anticoagulation, which, based on available data, is likely to be inadequate. No large prospective, randomized trials comparing the different treatment strategies are present to provide evidence-based guidelines for management, though increasingly more aggressive approaches are favored.

References

[1] Fernandez MM, Hogue S, Preblick R, Kwong WJ. Review of the cost of venous thromboembolism. Clinicoecon Outcomes Res. 2015; 7:451–462

[2] Heit JA, Spencer FA, White RH. The epidemiology of venous thromboembolism. J Thromb Thrombolysis. 2016; 41(1):3–14

[3] Hawkins D. Economic considerations in the prevention and treatment of venous thromboembolism. Am J Health Syst Pharm. 2004; 61(23) Suppl 7:S18–S21

[4] Wells PS, Owen C, Doucette S, Fergusson D, Tran H. Does this patient have deep vein thrombosis? JAMA. 2006; 295(2):199–207

[5] Jackson SP. The growing complexity of platelet aggregation. Blood. 2007; 109 (12):5087–5095

[6] Smalberg JH, Kruip MJ, Janssen HL, Rijken DC, Leebeek FW, de Maat MP. Hypercoagulability and hypofibrinolysis and risk of deep vein thrombosis and splanchnic vein thrombosis: similarities and differences. Arterioscler Thromb Vasc Biol. 2011; 31(3):485–493

[7] Abu-Yousef MM, Mufid M, Woods KT, Brown BP, Barloon TJ. Normal lower limb venous Doppler flow phasicity: is it cardiac or respiratory? AJR Am J Roentgenol. 1997; 169(6):1721–1725

[8] Cham MD, Yankelevitz DF, Shaham D, et al. The Pulmonary Angiography-Indirect CT Venography Cooperative Group. Deep venous thrombosis: detection by using indirect CT venography. Radiology. 2000; 216(3):744–751

[9] Mannucci PM, Poller L. Venous thrombosis and anticoagulant therapy. Br J Haematol. 2001; 114(2):258–270

[10] Amin VB, Lookstein RA. Catheter-directed interventions for acute iliocaval deep vein thrombosis. Tech Vasc Interv Radiol. 2014; 17(2):96–102

[11] Ginsberg JS, Hirsh J, Julian J, et al. Prevention and treatment of postphlebitic syndrome: results of a 3-part study. Arch Intern Med. 2001; 161(17):2105–2109

[12] Levy MM, Bach C, Fisher-Snowden R, Pfeifer JD. Upper extremity deep venous thrombosis: reassessing the risk for subsequent pulmonary embolism. Ann Vasc Surg. 2011; 25(4):442–447

[13] Elman EE, Kahn SR. The post-thrombotic syndrome after upper extremity deep venous thrombosis in adults: a systematic review. Thromb Res. 2006; 117(6):609–614

[14] Labropoulos N, Waggoner T, Sammis W, Samali S, Pappas PJ. The effect of venous thrombus location and extent on the development of post-thrombotic signs and symptoms. J Vasc Surg. 2008; 48(2):407–412

[15] Monreal M, Martorell A, Callejas JM, et al. Venographic assessment of deep vein thrombosis and risk of developing post-thrombotic syndrome: a prospective study. J Intern Med. 1993; 233(3):233–238

[16] American Society of Anesthesiologists Committee. Practice guidelines for preoperative fasting and the use of pharmacologic agents to reduce the risk of pulmonary aspiration: application to healthy patients undergoing elective procedures: an updated report by the American Society of Anesthesiologists Committee on Standards and Practice Parameters. Anesthesiology. 2011; 114 (3):495–511

[17] Vedantham S, Sista AK, Klein SJ, et al. Society of Interventional Radiology and Cardiovascular and Interventional Radiological Society of Europe Standards

of Practice Committees. Quality improvement guidelines for the treatment of lower-extremity deep vein thrombosis with use of endovascular thrombus removal. J Vasc Interv Radiol. 2014; 25(9):1317–1325

[18] Lee SH, Kim HK, Hwang JK, et al. Efficacy of retrievable inferior vena cava filter placement in the prevention of pulmonary embolism during catheter-directed thrombectomy for proximal lower-extremity deep vein thrombosis. Ann Vasc Surg. 2016; 33:181–186

[19] Kwon SH, Park SH, Oh JH, Song MG, Seo TS. Prophylactic placement of an inferior vena cava filter during aspiration thrombectomy for acute deep venous thrombosis of the lower extremity. Vasc Endovascular Surg. 2016; 50(4):270–276

[20] Mir MA. Superior vena cava filters: hindsight, insight and foresight. J Thromb Thrombolysis. 2008; 26(3):257–261

[21] Watson L, Broderick C, Armon MP. Thrombolysis for acute deep vein thrombosis. Cochrane Database Syst Rev. 2014(1):CD002783

[22] Skeik N, Gits CC, Ehrenwald E, Cragg AH. Fibrinogen level as a surrogate for the outcome of thrombolytic therapy using tissue plasminogen activator for acute lower extremity intravascular thrombosis. Vasc Endovascular Surg. 2013; 47(7):519–523

[23] Lee K, Istl A, Dubois L, et al. Fibrinogen level and bleeding risk during catheter-directed thrombolysis using tissue plasminogen activator. Vasc Endovascular Surg. 2015; 49(7):175–179

[24] Garcia MJ, Lookstein R, Malhotra R, et al. Endovascular management of deep vein thrombosis with rheolytic thrombectomy: final report of the prospective multicenter PEARL (Peripheral Use of AngioJet Rheolytic Thrombectomy with a Variety of Catheter Lengths) registry. J Vasc Interv Radiol. 2015; 26(6):777–785, quiz 786

[25] Avgerinos ED, Hager ES, Naddaf A, Dillavou E, Singh M, Chaer RA. Outcomes and predictors of failure of thrombolysis for iliofemoral deep venous thrombosis. J Vasc Surg Venous Lymphat Disord. 2015; 3(1):35–41

[26] Virchow R. Ueber die Erweiterung Kleinerer Gefäfse—Hierzu Tab. Virchows Arch Pathol Anat Physiol Klin Med. 1851; 3:427–462

[27] McMurrich JP. The occurrence of congenital adhesions in the common iliac veins, and their relation to thrombosis of the femoral and iliac veins. Am J Med Sci. 1908; 135:342–345

[28] Ehrich WE, Krumbhaar EB. A frequent obstructive anomaly of the mouth of the left common iliac vein. Am Heart J. 1943; 26(6):737–750

[29] May R, Thurner J. The cause of the predominantly sinistral occurrence of thrombosis of the pelvic veins. Angiology. 1957; 8(5):419–427

[30] Cockett FB, Thomas ML. The iliac compression syndrome. Br J Surg. 1965; 52 (10):816–821

[31] Kibbe MR, Ujiki M, Goodwin AL, Eskandari M, Yao J, Matsumura J. Iliac vein compression in an asymptomatic patient population. J Vasc Surg. 2004; 39 (5):937–943

[32] Raju S, Neglen P. High prevalence of nonthrombotic iliac vein lesions in chronic venous disease: a permissive role in pathogenicity. J Vasc Surg. 2006; 44(1):136–143, discussion 144

[33] Hurst DR, Forauer AR, Bloom JR, Greenfield LJ, Wakefield TW, Williams DM. Diagnosis and endovascular treatment of iliocaval compression syndrome. J Vasc Surg. 2001; 34(1):106–113

[34] Kim D, Orron DE, Porter DH. Venographic anatomy, technique and interpretation. In: Kim D, Orron DE, eds. Peripheral Vascular Imaging and Intervention. St Louis, MO: Mosby-Year Book; 1992:269–349

[35] Karthikesalingam A, Young EL, Hinchliffe RJ, Loftus IM, Thompson MM, Holt PJ. A systematic review of percutaneous mechanical thrombectomy in the treatment of deep venous thrombosis. Eur J Vasc Endovasc Surg. 2011; 41(4):554–565

[36] Berger A, Jaffe JW, York TN. Iliac compression syndrome treated with stent placement. J Vasc Surg. 1995; 21(3):510–514

[37] Okrent D, Messersmith R, Buckman J. Transcatheter fibrinolytic therapy and angioplasty for left iliofemoral venous thrombosis. J Vasc Interv Radiol. 1991; 2(2):195–197, discussion 198–200

[38] Semba CP, Dake MD. Iliofemoral deep venous thrombosis: aggressive therapy with catheter-directed thrombolysis. Radiology. 1994; 191(2):487–494

[39] Patel NH, Stookey KR, Ketcham DB, Cragg AH. Endovascular management of acute extensive iliofemoral deep venous thrombosis caused by May-Thurner syndrome. J Vasc Interv Radiol. 2000; 11(10):1297–1302

[40] Vedantham S, Vesely TM, Parti N, Darcy M, Hovsepian DM, Picus D. Lower extremity venous thrombolysis with adjunctive mechanical thrombectomy. J Vasc Interv Radiol. 2002; 13(10):1001–1008

[41] O'Sullivan GJ, Semba CP, Bittner CA, et al. Endovascular management of iliac vein compression (May-Thurner) syndrome. J Vasc Interv Radiol. 2000; 11(7):823–836

[42] Neglén P, Hollis KC, Olivier J, Raju S. Stenting of the venous outflow in chronic venous disease: long-term stent-related outcome, clinical, and hemodynamic result. J Vasc Surg. 2007; 46(5):979–990

[43] Hartung O, Loundou AD, Barthelemy P, Arnoux D, Boufi M, Alimi YS. Endovascular management of chronic disabling ilio-caval obstructive lesions: long-term results. Eur J Vasc Endovasc Surg. 2009; 38(1):118–124

[44] Hartung O. Results of stenting for postthrombotic venous obstructive lesions. Perspect Vasc Surg Endovasc Ther. 2011; 23(4):255–260

[45] Hager ES, Yuo T, Tahara R, et al. Outcomes of endovascular intervention for May-Thurner syndrome. J Vasc Surg Venous Lymphat Disord. 2013; 1(3):270–275

[46] Cruveilhier LJB. Essai sur l'anatomie pathologique en général et sur les transformations et productions organiques en particulier [doctoral thesis]. Paris; 1816

[47] Paget J. Clinical Lectures and Essays. London: Longman Green; 1875:292

[48] Von Schrötter L. Nathnagel's Handbuch der speciellen Pathologie und Therapie. Erkrankungen der Gefässe. Vienna, Austria: Holder; 1884

[49] Hughes ESR. Venous obstruction in the upper extremity. Br J Surg. 1948; 36 (142):155–163

[50] Hughes ES. Venous obstruction in the upper extremity; Paget-Schroetter's syndrome; a review of 320 cases. Surg Gynecol Obstet. 1949; 88(2):89–127

[51] Illig KA, Doyle AJ. A comprehensive review of Paget-Schroetter syndrome. J Vasc Surg. 2010; 51(6):1538–1547

[52] Abularrage CJ, Rochlin DH, Selvarajah S, Lum YW, Freischlag JA. Limited venoplasty and anticoagulation affords excellent results after first rib resection and scalenectomy for subacute Paget-Schroetter syndrome. J Vasc Surg Venous Lymphat Disord. 2014; 2(3):297–302

[53] Taylor JM, Telford RJ, Kinsella DC, et al. Long-term clinical and functional outcome following treatment for Paget-Schroetter syndrome. Br J Surg. 2013; 100(11):1459–1464

5 Pulmonary Embolism

Ronald S. Winokur and Akhilesh K. Sista

Summary

Pulmonary embolism (PE) remains a management challenge for the interventional radiologist. There is a spectrum of severity in patient presentation, and the long-term sequelae of PE are poorly understood. Management decisions in patients with submissive PE remain complicated due to incomplete understanding of which patients are most likely to benefit from intervention. This chapter will review the available data regarding evaluation and management of patients with PE, and will discuss the details of catheter-directed therapy in these patients. Outcomes data will also be presented.

Keywords: pulmonary embolism, venous thromboembolism, catheter-directed thrombolysis, chronic thromboembolic pulmonary hypertension, pulmonary embolism response team

5.1 Introduction

Pulmonary embolism (PE) is a major cause of death among hospitalized patients and is considered to be the third most common cause of death in this population. Massive PE carries a mortality rate that can exceed 58% and is typically fatal within 1 hour of presentation.[1] As a result of this major public health concern, the U.S. Surgeon General has issued a call to action to improve outcomes for patients with PE.[2]

Management of PE includes anticoagulation alone, inferior vena cava filtration, adjunctive systemic thrombolysis, catheter-directed thrombolysis (CDT), catheter-directed thrombectomy/thromboaspiration, and/or surgical thrombectomy. The Antithrombotic Therapy for VTE guidelines suggest systemic thrombolytic therapy using a peripheral vein over CDT (Grade 2C level of evidence).[3] The authors comment that patients who have a higher risk of bleeding with systemic thrombolytic therapy, and who have access to the expertise and resources required to do CDT, are likely to choose CDT over systemic thrombolytic therapy. For patients with acute massive PE who have a high bleeding risk, have already failed systemic thrombolysis, or are in shock that is likely to cause death before systemic thrombolysis can take effect (e.g., within hours), catheter-assisted thrombus removal is suggested over no intervention (Grade 2C).[3] In response to the range of therapies, clinical presentations, and comorbidities that face physicians who treat PE, local multidisciplinary pulmonary embolism response teams (PERTs) have been created in order to implement these guideline suggestions and recommendations and to fill in management gaps left by uncertainties in these guidelines. A common PERT mission statement is to manage the intricacies of PE by engaging multiple specialists to deliver coordinated care to PE patients. While the PERT model is gaining a foothold in the medical community, its efficacy has yet to be determined.

5.2 Case Vignette

5.2.1 Patient Presentation

A 23-year-old female with no past medical history is brought in by emergency medical services for possible seizure/syncope. The patient states that she was standing on the escalator and started feeling short of breath, lightheaded, and hot. She syncopized and woke up on the ground. The patient also endorsed dyspnea on exertion for a couple of days during short trips to the bathroom.

She has no prior history of cancer. There is no personal or known family history of clotting disorders. The patient has been taking oral contraceptive pills for 5 years. She has no history of smoking. The patient denies fevers, chills, headache, chest pain, palpitations, abdominal pain, diarrhea, constipation, or dysuria.

5.2.2 Physical Exam

Temperature: 36.7 °C; heart rate: 87 bpm; blood pressure: 111/53 mm Hg; respiratory rate: 20 per minute; pulse oximetry: 99% on RA.

- General: No apparent distress; alert and oriented; well appearing.
- Eyes: External ocular motion intact; pupils equal, round, reactive to light and accommodation.
- CV: Regular rate and rhythm; no murmurs.
- Lungs: Clear to auscultation bilaterally.
- Gastrointestinal: soft; nontender.
- Head/neck: nontender neck; atraumatic.
- Pelvis/back: stable.
- Extremities: no deformity; no calf tenderness.
- Skin: no edema.
- Neuro: alert; cranial nerves II–XII intact; motor WNL; sensation intact.

5.2.3 Noninvasive Testing

- Troponin I: 0.2 ng/mL (normal range 0–0.4 ng/mL).
- B-type natriuretic peptide (BNP): 175 pg/mL (normal range ≤ 100 pg/mL).
- D-dimer: 2.91 µg/mL (normal range 0.27–0.5 µg/mL FEU).

5.2.4 Imaging

CT chest (▶ Fig. 5.1):
- Extensive pulmonary emboli extending from the distal right and left main pulmonary arteries into multiple lobar, segmental and subsegmental branches predominantly in the bilateral lower lobes.
- Findings suggestive of right heart strain with right ventricle: left ventricle (RV:LV) ratio of 1.3.

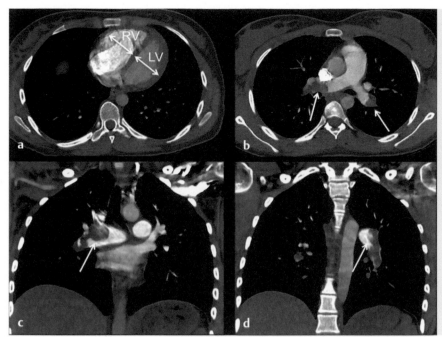

Fig. 5.1 Axial (**a, b**) and coronal (**c, d**) CT images of the chest following contrast injection. (**a**) A dilated right ventricle with an RV:LV ratio of 1.3. (**b–d**) Large filling defects in the main pulmonary arteries (*arrows*).

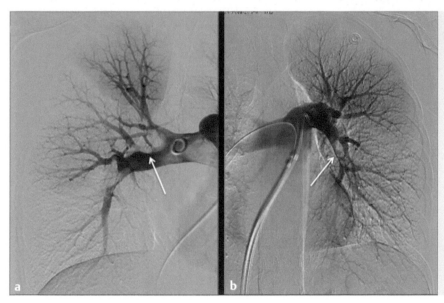

Fig. 5.2 Right (**a**) and left (**b**) digital subtraction pulmonary arteriography showing large bilateral pulmonary emboli (*arrows*).

Transthoracic echocardiogram:
- Dilated RV.
- Reduced RV function.
- Severe tricuspid regurgitation.
- Severe pulmonary hypertension.
- Systemic venous hypertension.
- Normal LV diastolic relaxation.
- Dilated right atrium.
- Flattening of the septum consistent with RV overload.

CT head:
   No CT evidence of acute intracranial abnormality.

5.2.5 Specifics of Consent

Prior to starting the procedure, the nature, purpose, risks, and alternatives of the procedure were explained to the patient, and informed consent was obtained. Procedure-related risks discussed included, but were not limited to, vessel injury during catheterization and major bleeding including life-threatening hemorrhage requiring transfusion and intracranial bleeding.

5.2.6 Details of Procedure

Using ultrasound guidance, the right common femoral vein was accessed at two sites and long vascular sheaths were inserted. A 7-French modified Grollman catheter was advanced into each pulmonary artery. Pressure measurements were 59/19 mm Hg (mean: 33 mm Hg) in the right pulmonary artery and 68/22 mm Hg (mean: 40 mm Hg) in the left pulmonary artery. Digital subtraction pulmonary arteriography was performed (► Fig. 5.2). Based on the findings, UniFuse catheters (Angiodynamics, Latham, NY) were inserted into the largest clot-bearing branches (► Fig. 5.3). Alteplase infusion was initiated without a bolus at 0.5 mg per hour through each catheter and continued for 23 hours at which time the infusion was discontinued and repeat pulmonary arteriography was performed prior to catheter removal (▶ Fig. 5.4). Follow-up pulmonary pressure measurements were 33/13 mm Hg on the right and 29/8 mm Hg on the left.

5.2.7 Follow-up

The patient initially returned for follow-up 1 month following CDT and stated that she no longer had any chest pain or shortness of breath. The chest pain stopped about 3 weeks after her procedure. She was able to attend the gym and run on the treadmill for 1 mile at a slow pace without symptoms. By her 2-month follow-up visit, she was able to run 6 miles without

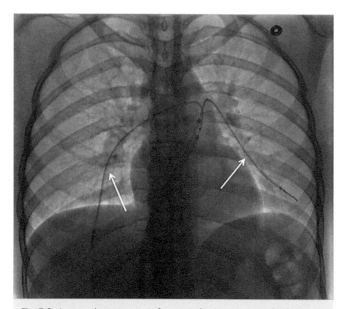

Fig. 5.3 Arrows depicting an infusion catheter traversing both lower lobe pulmonary arteries.

symptoms. She was treated with apixaban for anticoagulation without bleeding complications. An echocardiogram performed at 3 weeks postprocedure showed a dilated RV with normal function. A repeat echocardiogram at 5 months postprocedure showed normal RV size and function.

5.3 Epidemiology and Scope of the Problem

Venous thromboembolism (VTE), encompassing both deep vein thrombosis (DVT) and PE, is a common diagnosis that carries a risk of both short- and long-term morbidity and mortality. The annual event rate of VTE from 1985 to 2009 was shown to be 142 per 100,000 persons, with 30% occurring as a result of PE and 20% with concurrent PE and DVT.[4] In 2008, the U.S. Surgeon General estimated that over 100,000 deaths from PE occur yearly in the United States, and named PE as the most preventable cause of death in hospitalized patients.[2] The reason for this call to action is that in hospital mortality from acute PE still approaches 7% overall and 32% in patients with hemodynamic instability.[4] The long-term consequences of PE manifest as cardiopulmonary dysfunction and/or decreased exercise tolerance, and 1.4 to 4% of survivors develop chronic thromboembolic pulmonary hypertension (CTEPH).[4,5] Late recurrence of VTE has been up to 13% at 1 year, 23% at 5 years, and 30% at 10 years if not treated with extended anticoagulation.[5] Survivors face a higher overall mortality rate up to 30 years later, and PE is a significant cause of death.[6]

5.3.1 Patient Presentation and Evaluation

Patients with PE most often present with dyspnea, chest pain, leg swelling, and/or dizziness.[1,7] The onset of symptoms can be acute or insidious (over a period of days to weeks). Other nonspecific signs/symptoms of PE include tachypnea, tachycardia, palpitations, lightheadedness, fever, cough, wheezing, and rales.

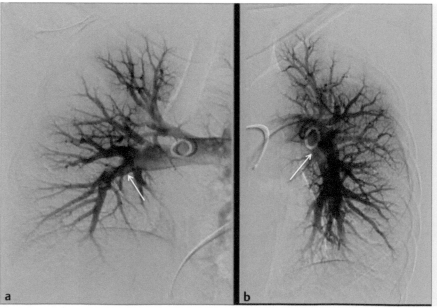

Fig. 5.4 Right (**a**) and left (**b**) digital subtraction pulmonary arteriography showing marked reduction in burden of thrombus (*arrows*).

In the study evaluating the patients treated by the Massachusetts General Hospital (MGH) PERT, 74% of PE patients presented with dyspnea and 33% presented with chest pain. Tachycardia occurred in 57% of PE patients, while tachypnea and hypoxemia occurred in 37 and 55%, respectively. Syncope, a sign suggestive of hemodynamic distress, occurred in 12% of this patient cohort.[7]

The history, imaging, and laboratory biomarker assessment are critical upon arrival to stratify patients by their PE-related mortality. According to the American Heart Association (AHA), the major categories of patients diagnosed with PE are low-risk, submassive, and massive.[8] Patients with a low-risk PE are normotensive, have normal biomarker levels, and have normal RV function. These patients carry a short-term mortality risk of less than 1%.[8] Submassive PE refers to acute PE without systemic hypotension, but with either RV dilation, dysfunction, or myocardial necrosis. RV dilation can be determined by CT or echocardiography and is defined as an RV:LV ratio greater than 0.9.[9] RV dysfunction is defined by RV wall movement on echocardiography, BNP elevation (> 90 pg/mL), N-terminal pro-BNP elevation (> 500 pg/mL), or electrocardiogram (ECG) changes of new complete or incomplete right bundle branch block, anteroseptal ST elevation/depression, or anteroseptal T-wave inversion. Myocardial necrosis is defined by elevation of troponin I (> 0.4 ng/mL) or elevation of troponin T (> 0.1 ng/mL). Approximately one-quarter of hemodynamically stable patients will fall into this group and have a mortality risk of 3 to 15%.[10] Massive PE is the most critical category and carries a mortality rate that ranges from 25 to 65% in recent studies.[8] The criteria for massive PE include acute PE with sustained hypotension (systolic blood pressure < 90 mm Hg for at least 15 minutes or requirement of inotropic blood pressure support), pulselessness, or persistent profound bradycardia (heart rate < 40 bpm with signs and symptoms of shock).

In addition to the AHA guidelines above for classification of PE, clinical scoring systems have been developed to attempt to risk stratify patients, including the Wells score, Geneva score, Pulmonary Embolism Severity Index (PESI) score, and simplified PESI (sPESI) score. The PESI score is validated for the prognostic assessment of patients suffering from PE and identifies patients at low risk for 30-day mortality.[5] The sPESI has also been validated for predicting 30-day mortality and a score of 0 is accurate for identifying low-risk PE patients.[11] The European Society of Cardiology guidelines differentiate PE by mortality risk into high risk, intermediate-high risk, intermediate-low risk, and low risk.[5] Patients with PESI class III–V have a 30-day mortality up to 24.5%[12] and those with a sPESI ≥ 1 have up to 11%.[13] Patients who have a PESI class III–V or sPESI ≥ 1 without both imaging and laboratory signs of RV dysfunction can be classified as intermediate-low risk and will likely not require escalation of therapy.[5] The intermediate-high risk group merits close monitoring for rescue reperfusion therapy if hemodynamic compromise develops.

5.3.2 Preparation for Procedure

Several options exist for catheter-based treatment of PE including CDT with or without ultrasound assistance, catheter-directed mechanical fragmentation, percutaneous thromboaspiration, and percutaneous endovascular thrombectomy (e.g., AngioVac, Angiodynamics, Latham, NY). The choice of procedure and tools will differ based on the severity of the PE; mechanical fragmentation, thromboaspiration, and thrombectomy are usually reserved for patients in extremis or for those who are not candidates for fibrinolytic medications.

CDT involves the insertion of multiside hole infusion catheters into the thrombus within the pulmonary arteries. The site for access is most commonly either the common femoral vein or the right internal jugular vein. Two access sites and vascular sheaths are usually necessary if bilateral pulmonary artery infusion catheters are planned. If the common femoral vein is selected as the access site, long sheaths (55–70 cm) are required to traverse the pulmonic valve and allow for stability of the infusion catheters for the duration of thrombolysis. Options for infusion catheters include the Cragg-McNamara Valved Infusion Catheter (Covidien, Plymouth, MN), Uni*Fuse Infusion Catheter (Angiodynamics, Latham, NY), and Ultrasound-assisted EkoSonic Endovascular System (EKOS, Bothell, WA). The recommended concentration for t-PA is 0.01 to 0.05 mg/mL and can be infused at rates starting at 0.5 to 2 mg/h.[14] The EkoSonic Endovascular System (EKOS) is an FDA-cleared drug delivery catheter that uses ultrasound delivered through the catheter core. The ultrasound energy is hypothesized to alter the local architecture of the fibrin clot to improve fibrinolytic efficiency and efficacy.

In cases of massive PE, catheter-directed mechanical fragmentation or thromboaspiration may improve pulmonary perfusion and increase left heart filling pressures. When performing fragmentation, the most commonly employed technique is the rotating pigtail.[1] However, clot fragmentation can lead to distal embolization of clot fragments that can cause acute changes in pulmonary pressures and hemodynamics. Preparation for thromboaspiration in conjunction with this technique may be beneficial. The Angio-Jet Rheolytic Thrombectomy (ART) System (Boston Scientific, Marlborough, MA) has been associated with complications of bradycardia, arrhythmia, heart block, hemoglobinuria, renal insufficiency, major hemoptysis, and procedure-related death.[1] As a result, the FDA has issued a black box warning for use of this system in the pulmonary arterial system. New clot aspiration/thrombectomy tools such as the Indigo Cat8 (Penumbra, Inc, Alameda, CA), Flowtriever (Inari Medical, Irvine, CA), and AngioVac (Angiodynamics, Latham, NY) are on the horizon, but have not been formally assessed for safety and efficacy.

Therapeutic anticoagulation does not need to be discontinued prior to the procedure. Supine positioning during these procedures can be challenging due to dyspnea induced by lying flat. In these circumstances, it is important to work together with the nurse, anesthesiologist, if present, and technologist to determine the best position for the patient, which may affect the access site chosen. It is critical to understand that sedation and anesthetic agents can reduce preload and lead to cardiovascular collapse. In cases where anesthesia is necessary, involvement of a specialized cardiac anesthesiologist is recommended.

An assessment of bleeding risks and contraindications to thrombolysis is mandatory. The possibility of blood transfusion should be discussed with all patients prior to initiating thrombolysis. The components of the assessment should include the following questions. If the answer is yes to any of the questions, performance of thrombolysis should be reconsidered or not performed.

- History of recent major surgery, cataract surgery, trauma, cardiopulmonary resuscitation, obstetrical delivery, or other invasive procedure within 10 days. Yes or no?
- History of recent active bleeding within 3 months. Yes or no?
- History of stroke, intracranial/intraspinal bleeding, tumor or vascular malformation. Yes or no?
- History of cancer. Yes or no? If yes, appropriate workup for the possibility of intracranial metastases should be performed.
- History of allergy to heparin, t-PA, or contrast. Yes or no?
- History of an arterial puncture in a noncompressible site within 21 days. Yes or no?

5.3.3 Technical Tips and Tricks and Procedural Details

The first step in performing thrombolysis for PE is selecting the location for venous access. If bilateral pulmonary artery catheter insertion is planned, the majority of interventionalists will place two vascular sheaths, which can be introduced via the same vein or different veins (common femoral or internal jugular). A Cobra catheter, Grollman catheter, pigtail catheter, Sos catheter, or Swan-Ganz catheter can be used to advance into the pulmonary artery. It should be recognized that end-hole catheters can pass through the chordae tendineae, and if large devices follow over the wire, these chordae can tear and lead to hemodynamic deterioration. It is important to observe for any signs of catheter constraint to detect this potential complication and correct catheter position.

Recording pressures while advancing catheters from the right atrium to the RV and the pulmonary arteries will document the severity of right heart dysfunction. Severity of pulmonary hypertension can be defined as mild (pulmonary artery systolic pressure [PASP]: 25–49 mm Hg), moderate (PASP: 50–69 mm Hg), and severe (PASP > 70 mm Hg).[15] Following pressure measurements, end-inspiratory pulmonary arteriograms are performed from the right and left pulmonary arteries. Angled catheters and standard guidewires can be used to gain access to the site of greatest clot burden. Caution should be used when advancing a hydrophilic wire into the desired branch, as it can easily cause trauma to the vessel and lead to pseudoaneurysm formation. Infusion catheters can then be inserted over-wire to cover the entire length of thrombus. A bolus of t-PA can be administered at the operator's discretion.

Infusion of t-PA is most commonly performed at a rate 0.5 to 1 mg/h per lung for a duration of 12 to 24 hours. Varying doses and durations are utilized at different centers with an average dose of 28.0 ± 11 mg in the Pulmonary Embolism Response to Fragmentation, Embolectomy, and Catheter Thrombolysis (PERFECT) registry that included six experienced centers.[16] The dosing regimen used in Prospective, Single-arm, Multi-center Trial of EkoSonic® Endovascular System and Activase for Treatment of Acute Pulmonary Embolism (PE) (SEATTLE II) was a fixed dose of 24 mg at 1 mg/h for unilateral PE and 2 mg/h for bilateral PE.[14] During the infusion of t-PA, there have been variable doses of anticoagulation with unfractionated heparin (UFH) used. The most common dose is 5 units/kg/h or 500 units per hour.[16] Full-dose anticoagulation can be resumed immediately at the conclusion of the t-PA infusion.[14] The need and utility of measuring fibrinogen levels is still unclear; however, there is evidence that fibrinogen ≤ 150 mg/dL is associated with an increased risk of major bleeding during t-PA infusion.[17]

At the conclusion of thrombolytic infusion, it is at the discretion of the provider to perform a follow-up pulmonary arteriogram and pressure measurement or to remove the infusion catheters at bedside. During the ULTrasound Accelerated Thrombolysis of PulMonAry Embolism (ULTIMA) and SEATTLE II studies, postthrombolytic infusion pulmonary artery pressure measurements were obtained through the EKOS catheters that were removed at bedside and showed a significant reduction in pulmonary artery pressures from a baseline of 51.17 ± 14.06 to 37.23 ± 15.81 mm Hg.[16]

5.3.4 Potential Complications or Pitfalls

Bleeding during administration of t-PA is the most significant complication of thrombolytic therapy for PE. Intravenous administration of t-PA is associated with increased major bleeding and intracranial bleeding. Studies using t-PA administered through an infusion catheter (ULTIMA and SEATTLE II) had no intracranial bleeding events in 178 patients.[10,14] However, the SEATTLE II study had 17 major bleeds (10% of patients). The PERFECT registry of 101 patients with submassive and massive PE showed no increase in major bleeding or intracranial hemorrhage with catheter-directed t-PA administration. Minor bleeding events occurred in 13 of 101 patients (12.9%).[16] These data are promising, but more robust studies are necessary to truly understand the bleeding risk of CDT for PE. If there is concern for clinically significant bleeding, cessation of thrombolytic infusion should be considered.

An important intraprocedural technical consideration is the appearance of a catheter crossing a patent foramen ovale (PFO) (▶ Fig. 5.5). This incidence occurs in 25 to 30% of patients.[18] In

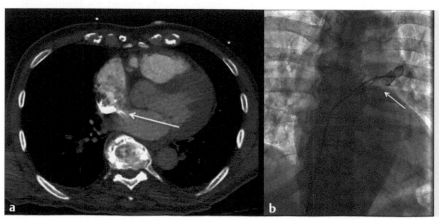

Fig. 5.5 (a) Axial CT imaging showing a contrast jet (*arrows*) through a patent foramen ovale (PFO). (b) Intraprocedural fluoroscopic image demonstrating a modified Grollman catheter traversing the PFO with contrast in the pulmonary vein (*arrow*).

this scenario, the catheter will cross into the left atrium, LV, and potentially the aorta, possibly leading to systemic arterial embolism.

5.3.5 Postprocedural Management and Follow-up

Depending on the duration of tPA infusion and local hospital regulations, the patient will need to be in an intensive care unit or step-down unit for appropriate nursing level of care for the duration of tPA infusion. Once the tPA is discontinued, patients should be transitioned to an anticoagulation regimen, which can be restarted immediately and continued for a minimum of 3 months.[5] The duration of anticoagulation may need to extend longer than 3 months or indefinitely based on the individual patient risk factors for recurrence and bleeding. The risk of recurrent VTE if anticoagulation is continued for 6 to 12 months is similar to the rate with 3 months of anticoagulation.[5] Indefinite anticoagulation reduces the risk for recurrent VTE by 90%, but has an increased risk of major bleeding of 1% per year.[5] Patients with a history of malignancy have an increased risk of recurrent VTE and it is recommended that they remain on indefinite anticoagulation after a PE.[5] Due to improved efficacy for recurrent DVT with low-molecular-weight heparin (LMWH) in cancer patients, LMWH is recommended for at least 3 to 6 months after the index VTE event.[19]

The determination as to which anticoagulant is best should be made in conjunction with the patient and their care team. Direct oral anticoagulants, such as dabigatran, rivaroxaban, apixaban, and edoxaban, have all been compared to standard anticoagulation in noninferiority studies in VTE in both the acute phase and long term. In acute-phase studies, the trials showed noninferiority for recurrent VTE with possibly lower bleeding rates.[20,21,22,23,24,25] The studies of extended treatment of VTE also showed effectiveness in recurrent VTE prevention with similar or slightly lower bleeding rates than traditional anticoagulation therapy.[22,26,27]

There is no clear consensus on the outpatient follow-up regimen for these patients, but it is important to monitor for both recurrent VTE in the short term and pulmonary hypertension in the long term. One sample regimen may include a 1-month, 3-month, 6-month, and annual follow-up. Between 1 and 3 months, a repeat echocardiogram is performed to assess for residual changes in heart function or strain. Additional tests such as exercise testing (e.g. 6-minute walk distance, cardiopulmonary exercise testing) and ventilation perfusion scanning may be necessary in patients who appear to be developing pulmonary hypertension.[28]

5.3.6 Outcomes

The ULTIMA trial studied 59 patients with submassive PE between 2010 and 2013 in Germany and Switzerland who received ultrasound-assisted catheter-directed thrombolysis (USAT) using 10-mg tPA per lung for 15-hour infusion lengths in the USAT arm and UFH in the control arm. Patients who received USAT had a statistically significant reduction in RV:LV ratio from 1.28 to 0.99 ($p < 0.001$) at 24 hours, while there was no change in the UFH group. There was also a statistically

Table 5.1 CDT trial results

	ULTIMA	SEATTLE II	PERFECT
Number of patients	59	150	73
Treatment	USAT	USAT	USAT/CDT
t-PA dose	10 mg per lung	24 mg total	28.0 ± 11.0 mg total
RV:LA ratio reduction	1.28–0.99 (p <0.001)	1.55–1.13 (p <0.0001)	Not reported
Pulmonary artery systolic pressure reduction (mm Hg)	52.0 + 11.5 to 39.7 ± 10.3 (p <0.001)	51.4 ± 16 to 37.5 ± 11.9 (p <0.0001)	51.17 + 14.06 to 37.23 ± 15.81 (p <0.0001)
Major bleeding	None	17 patients (10%)	None
Intracranial hemorrhage	None	None	None

significant reduction in pulmonary artery and right atrial pressure measurements post USAT.[10]

The SEATTLE II studied 150 patients at 22 centers in the United States between 2012 and 2013. The dose of tPA was regimented at 24 mg infused at 1 mg per hour. If the patient had bilateral catheters inserted, the infusion was 1 mg per hour per catheter for a total of 12 hours. There was a statistically significant reduction in RV:LV ratio from 1.55 to 1.13 ($p < 0.0001$), decrease in pulmonary artery systolic pressure of 51.4 to 37.5 mm Hg ($p < 0.0001$), and decrease in Miller index from 22.5 to 15.8 ($p < 0.0001$) 48 hours postprocedure.[14]

The PERFECT registry included 73 patients with submassive PE and 28 patients with massive PE who had CDT for submassive and massive PE between 2011 and 2014. Patients received a variety of doses of tPA and urokinase for a spectrum of durations, using both USAT and standard CDT. The initial results showed clinical success (defined as hemodynamic stabilization, improved pulmonary hypertension or right heart strain, and survival to discharge) in 97.3% of submassive PE patients and 85.7% of massive PE patients. A total of 89.1% demonstrated improved echocardiographic RV function, and 84.8% had a reduction in pulmonary artery pressures. In a subanalysis of USAT versus standard CDT, there was no difference between the pressure changes in the two groups.[16]

It should be noted that both SEATTLE II and PERFECT did not have a control arm, so the observed improvements cannot be attributed to CDT. Results of these studies are summarized in ▶ Table 5.1.

5.4 Pearls of Wisdom

- Assess PE patients with a multidisciplinary team and involve local physicians with expertise and interest in the disease process.
- Identify risk factors and contraindications to thrombolysis to avoid bleeding complications.
- Be cautious with the use of sedation and anesthesia in patients with submassive and massive PE. If anesthesia is absolutely necessary, involve a cardiac anesthesiologist.

- Use the minimum necessary dose of thrombolytics to improve right heart function. The goal is not complete clot dissolution.
- Follow your patients over time to assess for long-term consequences of PE, such as CTEPH.

5.5 Unanswered Questions

- The role of CDT in patients with submassive PE is unclear at this time. While preliminary data are promising, CDT will only be used routinely in this population if rigorous, randomized studies demonstrate that it improves clinically relevant short- and long-term outcomes compared with anticoagulation alone.
- The optimum dose and duration of thrombolytic infusion during CDT has yet to be determined.
- The role of novel mechanical and aspiration devices in the setting of PE is not yet known, and prospective safety, efficacy, and effectiveness trials are necessary to elucidate their value.
- It is unknown whether ultrasound-assisted infusion catheter can shorten the duration of infusion and/or reduce the dose of a thrombolytic drug compared with a standard catheter.
- Methods of assessing the degree of RV distress are underdeveloped; thus, it is currently unknown which submassive PE patients are at risk for poor outcomes and which are most likely to derive benefit from aggressive therapy.

References

[1] Kuo WT. Endovascular therapy for acute pulmonary embolism. J Vasc Interv Radiol. 2012; 23(2):167-79.e4, quiz 179

[2] Rathbun S. Cardiology patient pages. The Surgeon General's call to action to prevent deep vein thrombosis and pulmonary embolism. Circulation. 2009; 119(15):e480-e482

[3] Kearon C, Akl EA, Ornelas J, et al. Antithrombotic therapy for VTE disease: CHEST guideline and expert panel report. Chest. 2016; 149(2):315-352

[4] Vedantham S, Piazza G, Sista AK, Goldenberg NA. Guidance for the use of thrombolytic therapy for the treatment of venous thromboembolism. J Thromb Thrombolysis. 2016; 41(1):68-80

[5] Konstantinides SV, Torbicki A, Agnelli G, et al. Task Force for the Diagnosis and Management of Acute Pulmonary Embolism of the European Society of Cardiology (ESC). 2014 ESC guidelines on the diagnosis and management of acute pulmonary embolism. Eur Heart J. 2014; 35(43):3033-3069, 3069a-3069k

[6] Søgaard KK, Schmidt M, Pedersen L, Horváth-Puhó E, Sørensen HT. 30-year mortality after venous thromboembolism: a population-based cohort study. Circulation. 2014; 130(10):829-836

[7] Kabrhel C, Rosovsky R, Channick R, et al. A multidisciplinary Pulmonary Embolism Response Team: initial 30-month experience with a novel approach to delivery of care to patients with submassive and massive pulmonary embolism. Chest. 2016; 150(2):384-393

[8] Jaff MR, McMurtry MS, Archer SL, et al. American Heart Association Council on Cardiopulmonary, Critical Care, Perioperative and Resuscitation, American Heart Association Council on Peripheral Vascular Disease, American Heart Association Council on Arteriosclerosis, Thrombosis and Vascular Biology. Management of massive and submassive pulmonary embolism, iliofemoral deep vein thrombosis, and chronic thromboembolic pulmonary hypertension: a scientific statement from the American Heart Association. Circulation. 2011; 123(16):1788-1830

[9] Schoepf UJ, Kucher N, Kipfmueller F, Quiroz R, Costello P, Goldhaber SZ. Right ventricular enlargement on chest computed tomography: a predictor of early death in acute pulmonary embolism. Circulation. 2004; 110(20):3276-3280

[10] Kucher N, Boekstegers P, Müller OJ, et al. Randomized, controlled trial of ultrasound-assisted catheter-directed thrombolysis for acute intermediate-risk pulmonary embolism. Circulation. 2014; 129(4):479-486

[11] Lankeit M, Gómez V, Wagner C, et al. Instituto Ramón y Cajal de Investigación Sanitaria Pulmonary Embolism Study Group. A strategy combining imaging and laboratory biomarkers in comparison with a simplified clinical score for risk stratification of patients with acute pulmonary embolism. Chest. 2012; 141(4):916-922

[12] Aujesky D, Obrosky DS, Stone RA, et al. Derivation and validation of a prognostic model for pulmonary embolism. Am J Respir Crit Care Med. 2005; 172 (8):1041-1046

[13] Jiménez D, Aujesky D, Moores L, et al. RIETE Investigators. Simplification of the pulmonary embolism severity index for prognostication in patients with acute symptomatic pulmonary embolism. Arch Intern Med. 2010; 170(15): 1383-1389

[14] Piazza G, Hohlfelder B, Jaff MR, et al. SEATTLE II Investigators. A Prospective, Single-Arm, Multicenter Trial of Ultrasound-Facilitated, Catheter-Directed, Low-Dose Fibrinolysis for Acute Massive and Submassive Pulmonary Embolism: The SEATTLE II Study. JACC Cardiovasc Interv. 2015; 8(10):1382-1392

[15] Pillai MV, Killam J, Legasto AC, Eden E, Tartell L, Minkin R. Prediction and grading of pulmonary hypertension severity with computerized tomography. Am J Respir Crit Care Med. 2013; 187:A4697

[16] Kuo WT, Banerjee A, Kim PS, et al. Pulmonary Embolism Response to Fragmentation, Embolectomy, and Catheter Thrombolysis (PERFECT): initial results from a prospective multicenter registry. Chest. 2015; 148(3):667-673

[17] Skeik N, Gits CC, Ehrenwald E, Cragg AH. Fibrinogen level as a surrogate for the outcome of thrombolytic therapy using tissue plasminogen activator for acute lower extremity intravascular thrombosis. Vasc Endovascular Surg. 2013; 47(7):519-523

[18] Hagen PT, Scholz DG, Edwards WD. Incidence and size of patent foramen ovale during the first 10 decades of life: an autopsy study of 965 normal hearts. Mayo Clin Proc. 1984; 59(1):17-20

[19] Lee AY, Levine MN, Baker RI, et al. Randomized Comparison of Low-Molecular-Weight Heparin versus Oral Anticoagulant Therapy for the Prevention of Recurrent Venous Thromboembolism in Patients with Cancer (CLOT) Investigators. Low-molecular-weight heparin versus a coumarin for the prevention of recurrent venous thromboembolism in patients with cancer. N Engl J Med. 2003; 349(2):146-153

[20] Agnelli G, Buller HR, Cohen A, et al. AMPLIFY Investigators. Oral apixaban for the treatment of acute venous thromboembolism. N Engl J Med. 2013; 369 (9):799-808

[21] Büller HR, Décousus H, Grosso MA, et al. Hokusai-VTE Investigators. Edoxaban versus warfarin for the treatment of symptomatic venous thromboembolism. N Engl J Med. 2013; 369(15):1406-1415

[22] Bauersachs R, Berkowitz SD, Brenner B, et al. EINSTEIN Investigators. Oral rivaroxaban for symptomatic venous thromboembolism. N Engl J Med. 2010; 363(26):2499-2510

[23] Büller HR, Prins MH, Lensin AW, et al. EINSTEIN-PE Investigators. Oral rivaroxaban for the treatment of symptomatic pulmonary embolism. N Engl J Med. 2012; 366(14):1287-1297

[24] Schulman S, Kakkar AK, Goldhaber SZ, et al. RE-COVER II Trial Investigators. Treatment of acute venous thromboembolism with dabigatran or warfarin and pooled analysis. Circulation. 2014; 129(7):764-772

[25] Schulman S, Kearon C, Kakkar AK, et al. RE-COVER Study Group. Dabigatran versus warfarin in the treatment of acute venous thromboembolism. N Engl J Med. 2009; 361(24):2342-2352

[26] Agnelli G, Buller HR, Cohen A, et al. AMPLIFY-EXT Investigators. Apixaban for extended treatment of venous thromboembolism. N Engl J Med. 2013; 368 (8):699-708

[27] Schulman S, Kearon C, Kakkar AK, et al. RE-MEDY Trial Investigators, RE-SONATE Trial Investigators. Extended use of dabigatran, warfarin, or placebo in venous thromboembolism. N Engl J Med. 2013; 368(8):709-718

[28] Bernstein EJ, Mandl LA, Gordon JK, Spiera RF, Horn EM. Submaximal heart and pulmonary evaluation: a novel noninvasive test to identify pulmonary hypertension in patients with systemic sclerosis. Arthritis Care Res (Hoboken). 2013; 65(10):1713-1718

6 Inferior Vena Cava Filters

Robert King and Matthew Johnson

Summary

Inferior vena cava (IVC) filters are commonly employed in contemporary medical practice in the management of patients with deep venous thrombosis (DVT), often in the setting of pulmonary embolism (PE). There is increasing controversy regarding the appropriateness, safety, and efficacy of IVC filters, and there is a great deal of attention currently on determining what specific patient populations benefit from their use. This chapter outlines the historical data for IVC filters and discusses details of patient evaluation for appropriateness. The chapter is accompanied by a detailed discussion of a complex patient presentation, and the decision-making and management inherent in caring for complex DVT patients are discussed.

Keywords: DVT, IVC, IVC filter, retrievable filter, PRESERVE, PE, PREPIC

6.1 Introduction

Venous interruption has been employed as a means to prevent fatal pulmonary embolism (PE) since the late 18th century when John Hunter performed the first femoral vein ligation.[1,2] Bottini reported the first successful interruption of the inferior vena cava (IVC) for prevention of fatal PE in 1893.[1,3] Over the next 60 years, open surgical ligation was the preferred method of IVC interruption, despite an overall mortality rate of 14%, recurrent PE rate of 6%, and a fatal recurrent PE rate of 2%.[1]

In an effort to reduce the mortality rate associated with surgical ligation, as well as improve upon the morbidity of IVC interruption, IVC plication using various staples and clips was developed. This technique improved patient morbidity outcomes modestly, but still carried an overall mortality rate of 12%. Given the persistently high mortality rate, early innovators in the late 1960s began to explore complete and partial IVC-interrupting intraluminal techniques as means to prevent fatal PE. Many intraluminal devices, including detachable occlusion balloons, temporary sieve catheters, and intraluminal clips, were developed.

The most popular device to arise from that early intraluminal experience was the Mobin-Uddin umbrella (▶ Fig. 6.1). The Mobin-Uddin umbrella was intended as a permanent endovascular plication device that would gradually interrupt the IVC via occlusion. Two drawbacks to the design were: (1) because the original umbrella was 23 mm in diameter, it was too small to prevent occasional cranial migration, including embolization to the heart, and (2) development of thrombus within and above the device often caused caval thrombosis and allowed recurrent PE.

The Greenfield filter, introduced in 1973, was designed for operative insertion from either the internal jugular or common femoral vein approach.[1] It was not until a decade later that the first endovascular placement of a Greenfield filter was described, using a 28-French sheath via a transjugular approach.[4]

The Greenfield filter ameliorated the problems inherent in earlier intraluminal devices in that its conical shape allowed continued patency of the IVC and decreased the incidence of cranial migration.

Over the past 40 years, many filters have been introduced. To date, there is no published comparative study to demonstrate superiority between them.[4] The FDA approved retrievable filters in the early 2000s. Although the number of IVC filters placed in the United States has dramatically increased over the past 10 years,[5] only two randomized control trials have been conducted to parse out whether IVC filtration in fact does what it is intended to do: prevent clinically significant pulmonary emboli.[6,7] It should be noted that even a randomized control trial despite careful planning and protocol may be fraught with bias and lead to erroneous conclusions. For instance, the clinical trials by Decousus et al and Mismetti lacked groups consisting of patients with acute deep venous thrombosis (DVT) or PE who received only IVC filters. Hence, patients who did not have a contraindication to anticoagulation received caval filtration. Thus, patients without an accepted indication for caval filtration received filters under the study protocol. That all subjects in both groups in both studies received anticoagulation compromised demonstration of any benefit of IVC filtration, limiting the real-world application of their findings.

Although no randomized control trial has been conducted for the purpose of evaluating retrievable filters, multiple prospective clinical studies evaluating the safety and efficacy of individual retrievable filters have been published.[8] Because currently published data are inadequate to demonstrate safety and efficacy of the filters currently available in the United States, the PRESERVE study, a prospective, multicenter trial of the majority of filters in current use in the United States, was begun in late 2015 (preservetrial.com, ClinicalTrials.gov identifier NCT02381509). Enrollment of 1,430 subjects in that trial was completed on March 31, 2019. Until a more definitive scientific statement can be made regarding the efficacy of filter placement, it is up to the interventionalist to screen patients appropriately and place filters according to guidelines such as those

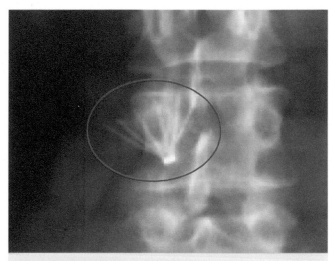

Fig. 6.1 The Mobin-Uddin umbrella filter.

set forth by the Society of Interventional Radiology (SIR) Multi-disciplinary Consensus Conference.[9] This chapter was written with those guidelines in mind and can be used as a best practice guide when considering a patient for IVC filter placement.

6.2 Case Vignette

6.2.1 Patient Presentation

A 29-year-old woman returned to longitudinal interventional radiology clinic for evaluation for IVC filter removal, 3 months following placement of the filter.

She had undergone catheter-directed thrombolysis for symptomatic left iliofemoral DVT as a result of May–Thurner syndrome (discussed elsewhere in this volume), with concurrent left common iliac vein angioplasty and stenting. Due to rethrombosis 3 days following her procedure, while therapeutically anticoagulated with enoxaparin, repeat thrombolysis was performed. After a discussion of risks, benefits, indications, and alternatives to IVC filters, an IVC filter was also placed. Risks specific to the IVC filters that were discussed prior to placement included migration, fracture caval wall penetration, embolization of all or a portion of the filter, recurrent DVT, IVC thrombosis, and PE. The indication for IVC placement was recurrent DVT while on anticoagulation (▶ Table 6.1).

Past medical history was significant for multiple miscarriages, and her DVT event, her first, had followed a recent miscarriage. During evaluation of her DVT, a thrombophilia panel was performed, and was positive for antiphospholipid antibodies.

Since her repeat thrombolysis and placement of the IVC filter, she had been therapeutically anticoagulated with warfarin. She had returned to the office for 1-month follow-up and at that time complained of intermittent left lower extremity pain, but denied swelling. She was tolerating exercise, but had not yet returned to work because of pain with prolonged standing. At the time of the 1-month office visit, duplex ultrasound of the left lower extremity demonstrated patent deep venous system with small residual, nonocclusive thrombus within the common femoral vein. It was determined at that stage to continue filtration, with a return for reevaluation in 2 months.

At the time of 3-month follow-up, she reported improved symptoms and increased activity. A duplex ultrasound of the left lower extremity was unchanged from the prior. Given her stability on warfarin, it was decided to schedule her for venography to include evaluation of the iliac stent and IVC filter retrieval.

6.2.2 Physical Exam

No left lower extremity edema or tenderness to palpation, no erythema. Distal pulses are equal and intact bilaterally.

6.2.3 Labs

Complete blood count and comprehensive metabolic panel are within normal limits; international normalized ratio (INR) is 2.5.

6.2.4 Imaging

Prior CT was reviewed to evaluate for any issues pertaining to the filter. It was noted that the apex of the filter was tilted posteriorly and likely abutting the posterior cava wall (▶ Fig. 6.2).

6.2.5 Specifics of Consent

Prior to the attempt to retrieve the filter, a thorough conversation with the patient included the risks and benefits of both maintenance and retrieval of the IVC filter. She was advised of the absence of data supporting long-term filtration, but of the theoretical risk that removal of the filter could permit PE should she develop unstable DVT in the future. She was also advised of the risks of long-term presence of IVC filters, including IVC thrombosis, filter fragmentation, and migration of the filter or

Table 6.1 Indications for ICV filter placement

Therapeutic (VTE present)	Prophylactic (no current VTE)

1. PE or DVT (caval, iliac, or fem-pop) present plus
  a) high risk or complications from anticoagulation or
  b) absolute or relative contraindication to anticoagulation or
  c) failure of anticoagulation
2. Perioperative anticoagulation interruption
3. Massive PE post-CDT or postsurgical with residual DVT
4. Severe cardiopulmonary disease with DVT
	1. High risk of DVT/PE who cannot receive prophylactic anticoagulation secondary to underlying risk of bleeding related to clinical disease:
	  a) cirrhosis
	  b) acute GI ulcer
	  c) coagulopathy
	  d) severe craniospinal or pelvic/long bone injury resulting in prolonged immobilization
	  e) intra-abdominal mass/hemorrhage compressing the IVC or pelvic veins

Source: Adapted from ACR-SIE-SPR Practice Parameter for the Performance of IVC Filter Placement for the Prevention of Pulmonary Embolism (2016).

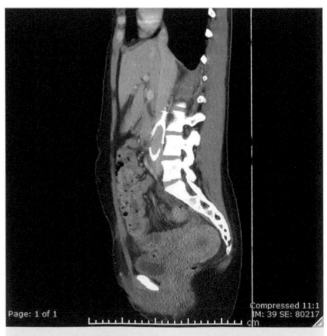

Fig. 6.2 CT of the abdomen demonstrating IVC filter within the lumen of the IVC. Apex of the filter is shown tilted posteriorly, abutting the caval wall.

fragments, as well as strut penetration with vascular injury, bowel injury, or pain. She was also advised that the incidence of these complications was unknown. With respect to risks of the retrieval procedure, the risks of sedation were reviewed, as well as the risks of vascular access, contrast use, and prolonged fluoroscopy. Finally, the risks of failure of retrieval, of caval injury including life-threatening extravasation, and of inadvertent damage to the filter with periprocedural embolization of the filter or fragments were reviewed. Various techniques and tools that might be used during the procedure were also reviewed, with the likelihood of use of devices off-label should the need arise.

6.2.6 Details of Procedure

Access was achieved via ultrasound-guided right internal jugular vein puncture and a 5-French pigtail catheter was advanced to the left common iliac vein for angiographic evaluation of the stented left common iliac vein and the IVC. The external and common iliac veins (including the stent) were widely patent without evidence of thrombus. Caval venography demonstrated no abnormality. A 14-French braided sheath was advanced to the superior IVC, through which a 2.5-cm loop snare was placed for retrieval of the filter.

Despite multiple attempts using different snares, the apex could not be snared, as it was likely embedded in the posterior wall of the IVC. A reverse-curve catheter was advanced over a wire into the caudal IVC. A hydrophilic wire was advanced through the catheter, then back up through the legs of the filter so that the wire could be snared above the filter (▶ Fig. 6.3a). Once the wire was snared, it was pulled through the sheath so that both ends of the wire were accessible at the neck. The reverse-curve catheter was removed and the wire was clamped with a hemostat such that the wire was one cohesive unit, allowing application of back tension during the oversheathing of the filter. With tension on the wire, the retrieval sheath was advanced to the apex of the filter. The apex was partially dislodged from the caval wall but not enough to pull the apex into the sheath (▶ Fig. 6.3b). To fully align the apex with the sheath, the loop snare was readvanced through the sheath, alongside the looped wire, and the retrieval hook was snared in the

conventional fashion. Tension was maintained on the wire during this maneuver to keep the apex in a reasonable position for snaring. The apex was snared, and the retrieval sheath was advanced to the apex, which was over-sheathed (▶ Fig. 6.3c) beyond the filter legs to free the filter and allow for complete removal. The legs of the filter readily released and the filter was removed in its entirety. A pigtail catheter was advanced over a wire into the caudal IVC and postretrieval venography was performed. There was no evidence of injury to the IVC. The catheter and sheath were removed and hemostasis was obtained with manual compression. She was monitored for 2 hours and was subsequently discharged from the department.

Follow-up

The patient was seen at 1, 3, 6, and 12 months in clinic and was doing well and instructed to follow up as needed with interventional radiology. She will undergo lifelong anticoagulation managed by the hematology service.

6.3 Epidemiology and Scope of the Problem

Venous thromboembolism (VTE) accounts for 250,000 hospitalizations annually in the United States. VTE is a major contributor to in-hospital mortality, with rates as high as 30%. Mortality rates are lower among patients with idiopathic venous thrombosis and highest in the setting of cancer. With the arrival of anticoagulants, VTE can be effectively treated. Given the high mortality rate and readily available treatment, anticoagulation is the standard of care in patients without contraindications.[10] In the United States, it is estimated that first-time VTE occurs in approximately 1 per 1,000 persons per year with approximately one-third of cases PE and two-thirds of cases DVT. Rates increase markedly after the age of 45. In patients over 80, incidence increases to 5 cases per 1,000. Risk factors thought to coincide with increasing incidence with age include venous valve incompetence with increased venous stasis, sedentary lifestyle, and acquired comorbidities.[10,11] Rates are slightly higher in men than women. Outcomes of VTE include death,

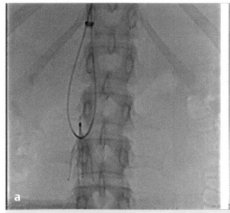 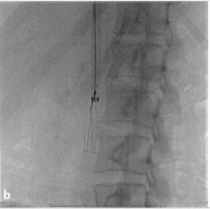 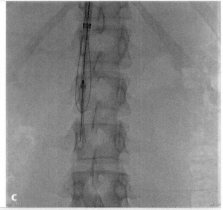

Fig. 6.3 (a) Fluoroscopic image demonstrating a hydrophilic wire passed through a reverse-curve catheter and looped through the struts at the apex of the IVC filter, snared, and passed cephalad through the access sheath, to optimize the orientation of the filter apex for retrieval. (b) Attempted retrieval of filter into sheath, with inability to oversheath the filter due to angulation. (c) Use of both wire loop and hook snare techniques to retrieve angulated filter, with apex successfully passed into sheath.

Table 6.2 Major risk factors for DVT

Age	Cancer
Surgery	Obesity/overweight
Hospitalization	Inherited coagulopathy
Immobility	Acquired coagulopathy
Trauma	
Pregnancy	
Oral contraception	

recurrence, postthrombotic syndrome, and bleeding secondary to anticoagulation.

Given the increasing trend of placing prophylactic filters in patients who are deemed high risk for PE, an understanding of the risk factors for venous thrombosis is necessary. Major risk factors for DVT are shown in ▶ Table 6.2. To mitigate risk of VTE, patients should be risk stratified and modifiable risk factors should be addressed. Thromboprophylaxis should be initiated when deemed appropriate. Half of all VTE in a longitudinal study looking at 21,680 people over a 7-year period were considered secondary to triggering risk factors. Important triggering risk factors that may prompt an IVC filter consultation include hospitalization, cancer, surgery, and trauma.

Prophylactic filter consults for surgical and trauma-related indications have significantly contributed to the sharp increase in IVC filter placements in the United States.[12] It is unclear whether a filter in that population is of any benefit. There is evidence suggesting prophylactic filter placement has no effect on reducing trauma patient mortality, while increasing the incidence of DVT.[13]

IVC filter placement has increased 25-fold in the United States in the past 20 years and 3-fold from 2001 to 2006.[14] Whether increased filter usage has, on the whole, been of benefit to patients is unclear. Guidelines from two societies, the SIR[8] and the ACCP,[15] differ in their recommendations, both with little level 1 data to support their positions. Further, multiple studies have shown poor compliance with both guidelines, with up 50% of filters placed without a clear indication.[16] Inappropriately placed IVC filters put undue risk on patients, and the cost to society can be tremendous. Therefore, strict adherence to the SIR or ACCP guidelines should be the standard of care until better level 1 data are available. Broadly accepted indications include lower extremity DVT in the setting of an absolute contraindication to, or documented failure of, anticoagulation therapy.[16] The SIR has added prophylactic filter placement guidelines to their recommendations. However, these cases should be limited as much as possible as a true benefit has not been shown to date. If a filter is placed for prophylactic reasons, diligence must be taken to ensure that 100% of these filters are removed once the "at-risk" period has passed.

6.3.1 Patient Presentation and Evaluation

When considering a patient for IVC filter placement, one should adhere to the accepted absolute indications as recommended in the SIR guidelines including: (1) failure of anticoagulation, (2) complication while on anticoagulation, or (3) contraindication to anticoagulation.

The other common reason IVC filtration is requested is for short-term prophylaxis against potential PE in high-risk patients for VTE undergoing surgery. This indication, and filter placement status post trauma, are thought to be in large part responsible for the large increase in IVC filter utilization. Although there has been no proven benefit in placing filters for that reason, it has become an acceptable indication in most institutions by proxy rather than by data. The risks and benefits of filter placement should be discussed in detail with the patient prior to the procedure. A retrieval follow-up plan, and the infrastructure to execute that plan, should be in place to ensure retrieval is carried out once the at-risk period ends.

The next consideration is the location and extent of the thrombus. Is it uni- or bilateral? Does the thrombus extend into the popliteal vein? Is there iliofemoral thrombus? Iliocaval? Is there thrombus free floating in the IVC?

In general, if the DVT involves only the veins below the knee, an IVC filter is not recommended. Although there is very little risk for below-knee thrombus to propagate to the pulmonary arteries, close observation for cranial extension within the deep venous system in these cases may be warranted. This risk increases as the thrombus extends cranially within the deep venous system of the leg. If the location or extent of the thrombus is within the popliteal vein or higher and there is an absolute indication for filter placement, the patient may benefit from IVC filtration to protect against clinically significant PE.

Consultations for IVC filter placement for prophylactic reasons are a bit more nuanced. These patients will present with a future contraindication to anticoagulation: impending surgery. However, these patients have yet to develop any DVT and mostly likely never will even despite their high-risk status. IVC filters can be placed safely in this population with little risk.[10] The majority of complications arise when the patients are lost to follow-up and the filters are never retrieved. The 8-year follow-up data from the PREPIC trial demonstrated that although the incidence of PE was significantly lower in the filter group, there was a 37% increased risk of developing DVT in those patients who received IVC filters versus those who did not. It is of utmost importance that these patients are followed up and their filters are retrieved promptly, thereby mitigating the long-term risks of IVC filtration.

6.3.2 Preparation for Procedure

Of those filters placed by radiologists, the majority of IVC filters are placed in an interventional suite. More recently, bedside filter placement via intravascular ultrasound (IVUS) guidance has been described. The latter method should only be attempted if the operator is very experienced in filter deployment and an expert in IVUS imaging techniques. Alternatively, a portable C-arm can be used bedside, but the ICU bed must be able to accommodate the C-arm. In everyday practice, even in a busy academic tertiary medical center, this should be an extremely rare situation. In almost every instance, even the sickest ICU patient should be able to travel to the interventional suite. In an instance in which request is for filter placement via IVUS because of the patient's clinical status, one should evaluate whether the patient will truly benefit from IVC filtration.

Prior to the procedure, review the pertinent imaging again to confirm your procedural plan. Cross-sectional imaging is not mandatory prior to IVC filter placement, but can be helpful in detecting variant venous anatomy and extent of thrombosis. If infrarenal thrombus is present, a suprarenal IVC filter can be placed.

Lab workup should include coagulation panel including INR, partial thromboplastin time, and prothrombin time. For patients at risk for renal insufficiency, creatinine and blood urea nitrogen should also be obtained. The procedure is classified as a "clean" procedure. As such, no prophylactic antibiotics are recommended.

Moderate sedation can be given prior to placement to facilitate patient comfort. However, if urgent IVC filtration is necessary, contraindications to sedation such as NPO status should not delay the procedure. IVC filter placement can be performed safely, quickly, and effectively without sedation if needed.

The interventional suite setup should include an interventional tray including (example from our institution): micropuncture set, 1% lidocaine, 11 blade, two 10-mL and two 20-mL syringes, saline flush, contrast in a bowl, a 0.035-inch wire, 4- or 5-French pigtail catheter if filter sheath is not power-injectable. The injector should be loaded with at least 50 mL of contrast for pre- and postplacement venography. The filter of choice should be readily available for table handoff when you have confirmed that filter placement is safe.

6.3.3 Technical Tips and Tricks and Procedural Details

Position the patient supine on the table. The majority of filter placements will be via right internal jugular or right common femoral vein approach. The operator should also be familiar with left internal jugular and left common femoral vein approach in case there are contraindications to deployment from the right side.

Access is obtained for placement of a flush catheter, which is then advanced over the wire into the caudal IVC. If the status of the iliac veins is not known, the flush catheter can be advanced into each vein and venography may be performed to evaluate for thrombus extension. With the flush catheter at the level of the iliocaval junction, digital subtraction venography is performed with an injection rate of 10 to 20 mL/s for a total volume of 20 to 30 mL. Injection rates can vary, but the above rates and volumes are good starting points.

When evaluating the IVC venogram, the following should be identified: inflow from the right and left common iliac veins, location of the renal veins, presence of an accessory renal vein (▶ Fig. 6.4a), presence of a circumaortic renal vein (▶ Fig. 6.4b), and a duplicated IVC (▶ Fig. 6.4c). A note is made of the level of the most inferior renal vein, as that is often considered, again without supporting data, to be the optimum location for placement of the filter apex. For purposes of measurement of caval diameter, venography can be performed with a radiopaque ruler taped underneath the table, by using the overlying vertebral body as a landmark at the level of the lowest renal vein, or with a marker flush catheter.

A reference image of the caval venogram can be displayed on the reference monitor to help with placement. The flush catheter is removed, if used, and the filter delivery sheath is advanced into the caudal IVC. The filter is then placed within the introducer sheath and advanced until the end of the filter is at the distal tip of the sheath. Meticulous technique should be used to ensure that the legs or apex (depending on site of access) of the filter do not go beyond the tip of the sheath. The introducer sheath is then retracted so the apex of the filter is positioned at the desired level (at the lower of the two renal veins). The filter is now in position to deploy. Under constant fluoroscopic guidance, the filter is unsheathed by retracting the introducer sheath with one hand, while the other hand holds the filter in place. It is important that the hand stabilize the filter and does not move during the unsheathing maneuver. This can be accomplished by stabilizing this hand against your body or on the sterile equipment table. The introducer sheath should

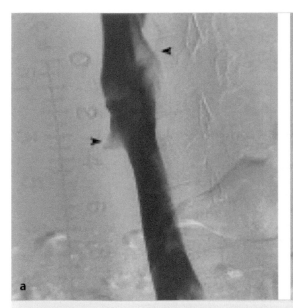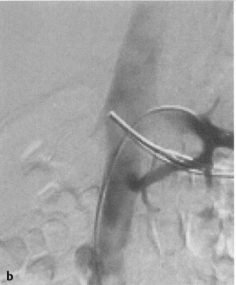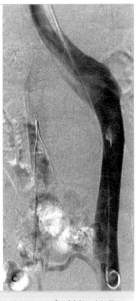

Fig. 6.4 Anatomic variants relevant to IVC filter placement. **(a)** Accessory right renal vein inferior to the location of bilateral unopacified blood inflow (*arrowheads*) that indicates the locations of the left and right renal veins; **(b)** venography of left renal vein demonstrating opacification of a circumaortic left renal vein; **(c)** venography of the left-sided trunk of a duplicated IVC.

be retracted so the apex is completely free of it. The filter is now deployed.

Note that this method applies to most, but not all filters. For example, the bird's nest filter placement is more complicated. If completion venography is desired, a flush catheter or the introducer sheath can be advanced through the filter into the caudal IVC over a wire. If the filter were deployed from the groin, it is not necessary to traverse the filter. Care should be taken when advancing the catheter or sheath through the filter as the filter can be dislodged. Completion venography is performed with contrast injection at a rate and volume similar to those used for preplacement venography; however, less contrast may be used for this injection, as the purpose of the completion venogram is to evaluate for complications and filter position vis-à-vis the cava rather than looking for anatomic variants. Immediate complications include: migration, tilting of filter, filter fracture with embolization of fracture fragment, thrombus formation, deployment of leg or the filter apex into renal vein, filter leg entanglement, and failure to deploy at desired level.

If the completion venogram is negative for complication, the sheath or catheter may be removed. Hemostasis is obtained by manual compression and a small dressing can be placed at the access site. The patient can be transferred back to the floor or to the appropriate holding area for postprocedural monitoring.

6.3.4 Potential Complications or Pitfalls

Complications can be categorized as early or late. Early complications include malposition, excessive tilting, or failure of the filter to deploy completely. Late complications include recurrent or de novo PE or DVT, filter migration, filter fracture with embolization, filter leg penetration, or IVC thrombosis.

Early Complications

The filter can be considered malpositioned if it is deployed in an unintended position. This complication is almost always attributable to operator error. If the malposition is determined to be clinically significant, e.g., legs deployed into a renal vein or filter deployed into the aorta, the filter should be retrieved and appropriately repositioned. If it is determined that the malposition has no clinical consequences, it may be left in place.

A filter is considered excessively tilted if the apex is greater than 15 degrees off-center relative to the axis of the IVC. If the filter is determined to be excessively tilted, filter retrieval or repositioning could be considered. If left in place, an excessively tilted filter may be difficult or impossible to retrieve once its legs become embedded.

Rarely, the filter legs will cross on deployment and become entangled. The filter should be retrieved and redeployment attempted, as that entanglement puts the patient at risk of inadequate filtration and filter migration.[13] If the legs cannot be uncrossed, the filter should be removed and a new filter placed.

Late Complications

The most devastating complication is migration with embolization to the heart or lungs. Occasionally, migration may be asymptomatic. When symptomatic, these patients will present with arrhythmias, myocardial infarction, valve insufficiency, or heart failure. This rare but potentially deadly complication occurs in 0.1 to 1.2% of cases depending on filter type.[10,11,12] If embolization to the heart occurs, an immediate cardiothoracic surgical consult should be made. If the filter embolizes during or shortly after the placement procedure, its percutaneous retrieval could be considered. Groin and neck access should be obtained to allow for more percutaneous options. Site of primary access will be determined by the location of the filter. This procedure should be performed under general anesthesia for patient comfort as well as real-time monitoring of the valves via transesophageal ultrasound. Cardiothoracic surgery should be on call for emergent surgery, if percutaneous retrieval ends in valve tear or fails altogether. If the filter is found to have migrated late, surgical approach is recommended, as a filter that has been in the heart for longer periods of time should not be retrieved by percutaneous techniques, since the perforation risk is high.

Filter penetration through the wall of the cava can be found incidentally on CT. Filter penetration is very common, with the incidence reported as high as 40 to 95%.[13,14] Although it can be a rare cause of abdominal pain, filter penetration is usually asymptomatic. The penetrating leg can cause problems for the patient if it erodes into surrounding structures such as a blood vessel, adjacent bowel, or ureter. (▶ Fig. 6.5). Penetration is diagnosed if the filter strut extends 5 mm beyond the wall of the IVC. If invasion of a surrounding structure is noted, filter retrieval should be considered. A penetrated filter may be difficult to retrieve in that the feet may not be easily retracted back through the caval wall. Occasionally, advanced retrieval techniques, such as use of forceps, must be employed. Because of the difficulties that can arise from this procedure, general anesthesia may be considered for patient comfort. If the filter cannot be retrieved via endovascular techniques, a surgical consult should be considered if the clinical impact of the penetration is high.[16]

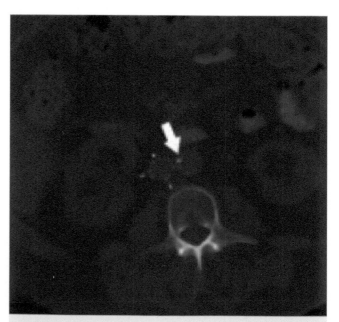

Fig. 6.5 CT of the abdomen with contrast, showing caval penetration by struts of the IVC filter. The strut at the 3 o'clock orientation appears to have penetrated the wall of the aorta, projecting into its lumen (*white arrow*).

Risk of caval thrombosis increases over time with an overall risk of 2.7%.[11] Symptoms include bilateral lower extremity swelling and pain. These symptoms warrant further workup, first with noninvasive imaging and then with venography. Catheter-directed thrombolysis may be indicated. This technique is discussed in other chapters.

Filter fracture incidence has been reported at 2 to 10%. Fracture puts the patient at risk for fragment embolization. Fracture may change the structural integrity of the filter, which may change the flow dynamics and increase the risk of caval thrombosis. This also puts the patient at an increased risk of recurrent PE. Thus, when filter fracture is encountered, the filter, and optimally the lesser fragments, should be retrieved. If the patient needs ongoing IVC filtration, a new filter may be placed at the time of retrieval.

Permanent filters decrease the risk of recurrent PE. The exact incidence of recurrent PE is unknown, but it is thought to be close to 3%. Because risks likely increase with length of filtration,[17] in patients in whom permanent filtration is not required, retrievable filters should be placed, and retrieved when possible. High filter retrieval rates can be achieved with high clinical success.[8] The PRESERVE trial will shed more light on whether placement of retrievable filters improves the incidence of late complications.

6.3.5 Postprocedural Management and Follow-up

After the procedure, the patient should be placed on bedrest and observed for a period of time appropriate for the site and caliber of venous access. If sedation was used, vital signs should be monitored every 15 minutes and the patient should be discharged according to institutional sedation recovery policy. Follow-up clinic visit can be set up according to preplacement discussion with the patient and referring service. If IVC filtration duration is not known at the time of the procedure, a 1-month follow-up clinic visit should be scheduled and filter retrieval assessment should be made at that time. Once the filter has been removed, the patient may be discharged from the interventional radiology clinic.

6.3.6 Outcomes

The PREPIC trial demonstrated the efficacy of permanent IVC filters with decreased recurrent PE rates in both short- and long-term follow-up compared to the group receiving anticoagulation alone. The tradeoff with permanent filtration lies with the increased risk of DVT. Over the 8-year period, 37% of patients with filters experienced DVT compared to 26% in the anticoagulation-only group. Surprisingly, there was no difference in postthrombotic syndrome rates. Furthermore, there was no difference in mortality. Also of importance was an IVC thrombosis rate of 13%. It has been extrapolated from those data that patients with retrievable filters would experience better outcomes as the long-term increased DVT and caval thrombosis risk would be eliminated once the filter was removed. The data are lacking in that regard. A study comparing the clinical effectiveness of permanent versus retrievable filters over a 12-month follow-up period demonstrated an incidence of symptomatic PE in 4% versus 4.7% in the permanent and retrievable filter patients, respectively. Symptomatic DVT occurred in 11.3% versus 12.6% in the permanent versus retrievable filter patients, respectively. Symptomatic IVC thrombosis occurred in 1.1 and 0.5% in the permanent versus retrievable filter patients, respectively.[18]

6.4 Pearls of Wisdom

- Place IVC filter only if patient meets accepted indications.
- Review all relevant imaging, including cross-sectional imaging, to evaluate for anomalous vasculature.
- Know the venographic appearance of all known caval anomalies and know where to place the filter if a vascular anomaly is encountered.
- Know how to deploy the filter from the neck or groin.
- Be familiar with snare techniques and have a snare readily available in case of postdeployment migration or embolization.
- Follow-up with patients who receive a retrievable filter is a must.
- Retrieve filter as early as possible. The longer it remains in situ, the more difficult the retrieval.
- Retrieve all filters that should be retrieved. 100%.

6.5 Unanswered Questions

The rationale for retrievable IVC filter use is extrapolated from PREPIC trial data. To date, there are no randomized control trials looking at the safety and efficacy of retrievable filters. The PRESERVE trial, a large prospective, open-labeled, multicenter trial, is currently underway with full patient enrollment expected in 2018. These results may change the IVC filter paradigm by answering simple but pertinent questions: Are retrievable filters safe and do they work? The answer may be "no" in some or most clinical scenarios. The interventional community should be prepared to deal with the ramifications of that very real possibility. If the answer is "yes," as would seem to be likely for patients with, e.g., recurrent PE despite adequate anticoagulation, we will be armed with high-level data. In that event, guidelines might become more robust, and hopefully a standard of care for IVC filter placement will emerge. Until such data are available, interventionalists should use best practices based on the guidelines such as those set forth in this chapter.

References

[1] Greenfield LJ. Evolution of venous interruption for pulmonary thromboembolism. Arch Surg. 1992; 127(5):622–626

[2] Hunter J. Observations on the inflammation of the internal coats of veins. Trans Soc Improvement Med Chir Knowledge.. 1793; 1:18

[3] Bottini. Cited by: Dale WA. Ligation of the inferior vena cava for thromboembolism. Surgery 1958;43:22–44

[4] Molvar C. Inferior vena cava filtration in the management of venous thromboembolism: filtering the data. Semin Intervent Radiol. 2012; 29(3):204–217

[5] Kuy S, Dua A, Lee CJ, et al. National trends in utilization of inferior vena cava filters in the United States, 2000–2009. J Vasc Surg Venous Lymphat Disord. 2014; 2(1):15–20

[6] Mismetti P. Randomized trial assessing the efficacy of the partial interruption of the inferior vena cava by an optional vena caval filter in the prevention of the recurrence of pulmonary embolism. PREPIC 2 trial: prevention of embolic

recurrences by caval interruption (prospective, multicentric, randomised, open trial) [in French]. Rev Pneumol Clin. 2008; 64(6):328–331

[7] Decousus H, Leizorovicz A, Parent F, et al. A clinical trial of vena caval filters in the prevention of pulmonary embolism in patients with proximal deep-vein thrombosis. Prévention du Risque d'Embolie Pulmonaire par Interruption Cave Study Group. N Engl J Med. 1998; 338(7):409–415

[8] Kaufman JA, Kinney TB, Streiff MB, et al. Guidelines for the use of retrievable and convertible vena cava filters: report from the Society of Interventional Radiology multidisciplinary consensus conference. J Vasc Interv Radiol. 2006; 17(3):449–459

[9] Johnson MS, Nemcek AA, Jr, Benenati JF, et al. The safety and effectiveness of the retrievable option inferior vena cava filter: a United States prospective multicenter clinical study. J Vasc Interv Radiol. 2010; 21(8):1173–1184

[10] Fields JM, Goyal M. Venothromboembolism. Emerg Med Clin North Am. 2008; 26(3):649–683, viii

[11] Cushman M. Epidemiology and risk factors for venous thrombosis. Semin Hematol. 2007; 44(2):62–69

[12] Cushman M, Tsai AW, White RH, et al. Deep vein thrombosis and pulmonary embolism in two cohorts: the longitudinal investigation of thromboembolism etiology. Am J Med. 2004; 117(1):19–25

[13] Hemmila MR, Osborne NH, Henke PK, et al. Prophylactic inferior vena cava filter placement does not result in a survival benefit for trauma patients. Ann Surg. 2015; 262(4):577–585

[14] Stein PD, Kayali F, Olson RE. Twenty-one-year trends in the use of inferior vena cava filters. Arch Intern Med. 2004; 164(14):1541–1545

[15] American College of Chest Physicians Evidence-Based Clinical Practice Guidelines. Available at: http://journal.publications.chestnet.org/issue.aspx?journalid=99&issueid=23443&direction=P#tocHeading_26198

[16] Joels CS, Sing RF, Heniford BT. Complications of inferior vena cava filters. Am Surg. 2003; 69(8):654–659

[17] Morales JP, Li X, Irony TZ, Ibrahim NG, Moynahan M, Cavanaugh KJ, Jr. Decision analysis of retrievable inferior vena cava filters in patients without pulmonary embolism. J Vasc Surg Venous Lymphat Disord. 2013; 1(4):376–384

[18] Kim HS, Young MJ, Narayan AK, Hong K, Liddell RP, Streiff MB. A comparison of clinical outcomes with retrievable and permanent inferior vena cava filters. J Vasc Interv Radiol. 2008; 19(3):393–399

7 Chronic Venous Occlusive Disease

Deepak Sudheendra

Summary

Chronic venous occlusive disease (CVOD) is commonly treated conservatively by the medical community at large. Most patients with symptomatic CVOD are managed with long-term extremity compression garments, and often with chronic anticoagulation. Many patients suffer from lifestyle-limiting symptoms, and sequelae can include signs and symptoms of chronic venous stasis, with soft tissue changes or ulceration. This chapter familiarizes the reader with standards for evaluation and management of patients with symptomatic CVOD, including review of techniques for recanalization of occluded venous segments with tips for postprocedural longitudinal management of these patients.

Keywords: deep vein thrombosis, stents, postthrombotic syndrome, angioplasty, caval thrombosis, venous thrombosis, IVC filter, May–Thurner syndrome

7.1 Introduction

Chronic venous occlusive disease (CVOD) resulting from deep vein thrombosis (DVT) is characterized by a constellation of symptoms collectively known as postthrombotic syndrome (PTS). The characteristic chronic leg swelling, pain, skin changes, varicose veins, and venous stasis ulcers affect nearly 50% of patients with proximal iliofemoral DVT within the first 1 to 2 years of presentation.[1] CVOD results in significant morbidity as well as personal, emotional, and economic costs to the individual and society.[2] The vast majority of patients with CVOD never undergo treatment and most are never referred to a vascular specialist for management.

Most commonly, CVOD can broadly be categorized into those cases resulting from inferior vena cava (IVC) filter complication and those due to proximal DVT. The technical approach and medical management of these conditions are discussed herein.

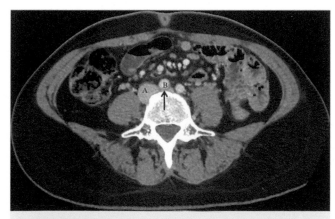

Fig. 7.1 CT venogram showing bifurcation of the IVC into the right common iliac vein **(a)** and the left common iliac vein (*arrow*) that is compressed by the overlying right common iliac artery **(b)**.

7.2 Case Vignette 1

7.2.1 Patient Presentation

A 35-year-old woman developed acute left iliofemoral DVT 2 days postpartum, presenting with chronic left leg swelling, muscle fatigue, cramping, and intermittent left buttock pain. Warfarin therapy was prescribed for 6 months, followed by treatment with rivaroxaban (Janssen Pharmaceuticals, Rariton, NJ) for 3 months. Nine months following her initial presentation, due to ongoing symptoms of CVOD, a CT venogram was obtained and demonstrated significant left common iliac vein compression and thrombotic occlusion of the left external iliac vein. At that time, she underwent an unsuccessful attempt at recanalization of her left external iliac vein. It was recommended that she continue anticoagulation indefinitely and wear thigh-high compression stockings. Two years later, she presented for reevaluation. At that time, she reported significant swelling in the left lower extremity with failure to use compression. She was an avid runner and unable to run long distances or do prolonged physical activity due to pain and swelling.

7.2.2 Physical Exam

On physical examination, the patient was a slender woman with mild asymmetric enlargement of the left lower extremity, relative to the right. She had no obvious skin manifestations, varicosities, or ulcers.

7.2.3 Noninvasive Testing

Review of the initial preoperative CT venogram from 2 years prior showed significant compression of the left common iliac vein by the overlying right common iliac artery, suggestive of May–Thurner syndrome (▶ Fig. 7.1a; ▶ Fig. 7.1b). A duplex ultrasound (US) performed contemporaneous to the consult revealed occlusion of the left external iliac vein with patent common femoral, femoral, and popliteal veins (▶ Fig. 7.2).

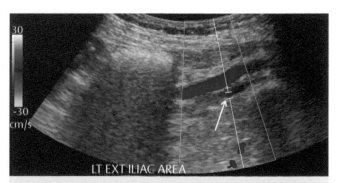

Fig. 7.2 Duplex US showing no venous flow in the left external iliac vein (*arrow*).

7.2.4 Invasive Testing

The catheter venogram from the prior recanalization procedure showed a left common femoral vein access with occluded left external iliac vein and mature pelvic collaterals draining to the right external iliac vein.

7.2.5 Specifics of Consent

The risks and benefits of reattempting recanalization of the patient's chronically occluded left external iliac vein were discussed in detail. Specifically, the expectation of getting through a chronic occlusion that had been previously attempted was put into perspective. Potential complications such as vascular injury and bleeding were discussed. Complications such as iliac vein thrombosis or stent occlusion that could necessitate additional procedures in the future were also described. Self-limited side effects, including access site pain and back pain, that may accompany iliac vein stenting were discussed. Although the likelihood of using thrombolytics was low due to the chronicity of the occlusion, the risks of bleeding from thrombolytics was discussed if acute or subacute thrombus was found during the procedure requiring pharmacomechanical thrombectomy. Finally, a tentative plan for postprocedural anticoagulation was outlined, including the type and length of anticoagulation.

Details of Procedure

A preprocedural plan was formulated to ensure the best possible outcome. The plan was to gain access to the left femoral vein in the midthigh or the left great saphenous vein with an 8F, 10-cm sheath and perform a venogram. Attempts would be made to cross the occluded left external iliac vein with a hydrophilic guidewire, 5F Bern catheter (Boston Scientific, Marlborough, MA), followed by angioplasty and Wallstent placement (Boston Scientific, Marlborough, MA). Intravascular US (IVUS) (Volcano Corporation, San Diego, CA) would also be used for sizing and stent positioning and to determine the extent of compression of the left common iliac vein.

The patient was placed in the supine position, general anesthesia induced, a bladder catheter placed, and US evaluation performed to determine the optimum access site. The right neck and left groin down to the knee were prepped. Initially access was gained in the left greater saphenous vein should stenting be required into the femoral vein. Venography was performed which showed occlusion of the left common iliac vein with patent left internal iliac draining to the iliac confluence and cross-pelvic collaterals draining to the right external iliac vein (▶ Fig. 7.3a). Second access was obtained in the right internal jugular vein and a long 6F braided sheath was placed to the level of the left common iliac occlusion (▶ Fig. 7.3b). Several

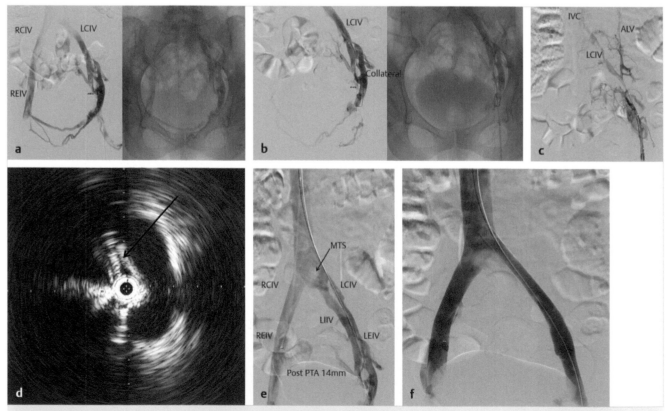

Fig. 7.3 (a) Venogram showing complete occlusion of the *supposed* left external iliac vein with prominent collateral draining to right external iliac vein (REIV). The right common iliac vein (RCIV) is patent. The *supposed* left common iliac vein is patent. (b) Sheath is shown in what appears to be the left common iliac vein (LCIV) and catheter tip is in large pelvic collateral vein. (c) Venogram illustrating ascending lumbar vein (ALV) joining a severely stenotic left common iliac vein (LCIV). A trace amount of contrast is seen draining into the IVC. (d) Compression of the left common iliac vein (*arrow*) as seen by IVUS. (e) Venogram after angioplasty of the stenotic LCIV shows two venous channels. The vein that was thought to be the patent LCIV is actually the left internal iliac vein (LIIV) that has a high bifurcation directly from the IVC. The area where no contrast is seen is characteristic of May–Thurner syndrome (MTS). (f) Completion venogram after Wallstent placement that extends slightly into the IVC to minimize rethrombosis as the weakest parts of the stent are proximal and distal ends.

attempts were made with a 5F Bern catheter and stiff hydrophilic wire to cross the occluded left common iliac vein without success.

Venography was performed in different obliquities in an attempt to find a channel that resembled the occluded left external iliac vein. Oblique femoral venography showed a very diminutive venous collateral representing the ascending lumbar vein, a branch of the left common iliac vein (▶ Fig. 7.3c). Accessing the channel to this venous branch, a 5F Quick-cross catheter (Spectranetics, Colorado Springs, CO) was used with a hydrophilic wire to traverse the occluded left common iliac vein. Angioplasty was performed with a 6-mm balloon after which IVUS was used to determine the extent of compression and facilitate stent sizing (▶ Fig. 7.3d). Serial angioplasty was performed up to 16 mm (▶ Fig. 7.3e).

The length of the common iliac and external iliac vein requiring stenting was approximately 16 cm. An 18 mm × 9 cm Wallstent was placed in the left common iliac vein with 1 cm extending into the IVC and was balloon dilated to 16 mm, resulting in a total stent length of 10 cm. A second 16 mm × 9 cm Wallstent with 1 cm of overlap into the left common iliac stent was placed in the left external iliac vein down to but not past the inguinal ligament and ballooned to 16 mm (▶ Fig. 7.3f). IVUS was repeated and showed significant improvement in iliac vein diameter, completion venography was performed, and hemostasis was achieved with manual pressure.

There were no postprocedure complications. The patient was extubated, the bladder catheter removed, and the patient transferred to recovery. The patient was admitted to ensure that there were no postprocedure complications; pain was adequately controlled, and anticoagulation was appropriately administered.

7.2.6 Follow-up

At a 3-week postprocedure clinic visit, symptoms of CVOD had resolved and she had returned to her normal activity including long-distance running.

7.3 Case Vignette 2

7.3.1 Patient Presentation

A 61-year-old male was referred 3 days after undergoing coronary artery bypass grafting complicated by acute IVC and bilateral iliac vein thrombosis. The patient had been on warfarin for a right lower extremity DVT and, in preparation for surgery, had a Trapease IVC filter (Cardinal Health, Dublin, OH) placed 3 weeks prior to surgery. After examination of the patient and extensive discussions with the cardiac surgery team at our institution, the decision was made to discharge the patient on anticoagulation and compression stocking therapy with follow-up evaluation in interventional radiology (IR) clinic in 4 to 6 weeks, as it was determined that thrombolytic therapy would not be safe in the immediate post–cardiac surgery setting.

One month later, the patient presented to IR outpatient clinic for evaluation. The symptoms of bilateral lower extremity swelling had minimally improved with anticoagulation and stockings. He continued to have significant lower extremity pain and swelling and was unable to stand or ambulate for long periods of time. He had gained nearly 25 lbs from lower extremity

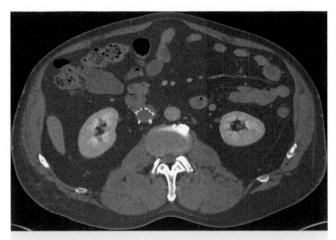

Fig. 7.4 Complete thrombosis of the IVC with permanent Trapease filter in place.

edema. The patient felt that his cardiac rehabilitation was compromised due to his symptoms resulting from extensive lower extremity clot burden.

7.3.2 Physical Exam

On physical examination, the patient had significant bilateral lower extremity swelling. His calves were tender to palpation and he was unable to stand for more than a few minutes without developing lower extremity pain and fatigue. He had no obvious skin manifestations, varicosities, or ulcers.

7.3.3 Imaging

A CT venogram demonstrated the permanent IVC filter with occlusive thrombosis of the infrarenal IVC and bilateral iliac veins (▶ Fig. 7.4).

7.3.4 Specifics of Consent

Of particular importance in this case were the risks of stenting across the permanent IVC filter, which included vascular injury, bleeding, and filter fracture or migration. All other benefits and risks as outlined in the first case were also discussed.

7.3.5 Details of Procedure

A preprocedural plan was formulated to ensure the best possible outcome. The plan was to gain bilateral common femoral vein access, perform bilateral iliofemoral venography, and traverse the bilateral iliac and IVC occlusions. This would be followed by pharmacomechanical thrombectomy up to the level of the filter. The IVC and iliac veins would then be reconstructed with Wallstents that would involve "crushing" the filter against the caval wall.

General anesthesia was induced, a bladder catheter placed, and the patient placed in the supine position. Initial access with 10F vascular sheaths was obtained in the bilateral common femoral veins using US guidance. Bilateral lower extremity venograms were performed (▶ Fig. 7.5a). A 5F Bern directional

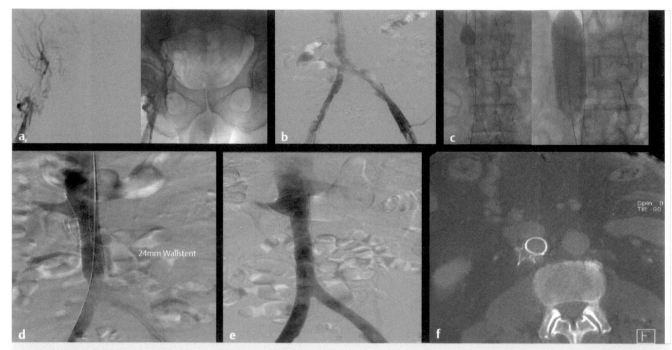

Fig. 7.5 **(a)** Right lower extremity venogram showing multiple pelvic collaterals due to chronic occlusion of the right iliac veins. The left lower extremity venogram (not pictured) looks the same. **(b)** Reestablishment of flow into the iliac veins and IVC after pharmacomechanical thrombectomy and angioplasty. **(c)** Trapease filter is crushed with 24-mm balloon again IVC wall. **(d)** Recanalized IVC after placement of 24 mm × 7 cm Wallstent. Note that the stent does cover the renal veins. **(e)** Final venogram showing reconstruction of the IVC and iliac veins. **(f)** Cone-beam CT shows compression of the IVC filter against the caval wall by the Wallstent with no evidence of vascular injury or hematoma.

catheter, stiff hydrophilic wire, and 5F Quick-cross catheter were used to traverse the occlusions in the bilateral common femoral and iliac veins and distal IVC. The right internal jugular vein was then accessed and a long 12F braided sheath was placed. A stiff hydrophilic wire was used to cross the chronically occluded IVC filter. From the left common femoral vein access, the wire was snared and through and through wire access was established.

Pharmacomechanical thrombectomy with the Angiojet thrombectomy device (Boston Scientific, Marlborough, MA), using pulse spray, was performed in both iliac veins and IVC through the filter. To minimize hemoglobinuria and potential renal injury, thrombectomy of the iliac veins and IVC was limited to a total volume of 300 mL. Repeat venography was performed that showed a moderate thrombus reduction, reestablishment of flow, and significant long-segment stenoses in the bilateral common and external iliac veins, treated with 14- and 16-mm angioplasty balloons (► Fig. 7.5b). Through the 12F sheath, a 24-mm balloon was used to "crush" the IVC filter against the caval wall (► Fig. 7.5c). This was then followed by placement of a 24 mm × 7 cm Wallstent in the IVC spanning the length of the IVC filter and crossing the renal veins. The stent was deployed and ballooned to 24 mm. Repeat venography showed reestablishment of flow in the IVC (► Fig. 7.5d). The bilateral common iliac veins were stented with 14 mm × 9 cm Wallstents and the external iliac veins were stented with 14 mm × 6 cm Wallstents. Repeat venography showed brisk flow through both lower extremities and the IVC with no evidence of contrast extravasation (► Fig. 7.5e). In addition, cone-beam CT was performed and showed exclusion of the IVC

filter and no evidence of hematoma or filter fracture (► Fig. 7.5f). Hemostasis was achieved with manual pressure.

There were no postprocedure complications. The patient was extubated, the bladder catheter was removed, and the patient was transferred to recovery. Due to the complexity of the procedure, he was admitted for 2 days to ensure that there were no postprocedure complications; pain was adequately controlled, and anticoagulation was appropriately administered.

7.3.6 Follow-up

One-month postprocedure, the patient was doing extremely well with minimal lower extremity swelling. His exercise tolerance had significantly increased and he had lost 45 lbs of fluid weight. CT venogram showed that his IVC and iliac stents were patent. One-year postprocedure, the patient continued to do well and remained on anticoagulation. He is currently being evaluated for superficial venous insufficiency in his right lower extremity due to ongoing symptoms of leg fatigue, cramps, and heaviness.

7.4 Epidemiology and Scope of the Problem

PTS affects nearly half of all patients with acute proximal DVT within the first 2 years. About 5 to 10% of patients with symptomatic proximal DVT will develop severe PTS, including venous ulceration, which results in significant disability and impaired quality of life (QOL).[1] Iliofemoral DVT confers a greater risk of recurrent DVT and thereby a higher risk of PTS compared to femoral-popliteal DVT due to the lack of collateral outflow from the deep femoral.[3,4] Calf DVT, not a completely benign process in its own right, can extend to involve more proximal veins in 10 to 20% of patients and lead to PTS in nearly 20% of those patients.[5] QOL studies have shown that severe PTS has a QOL similar to that of cancer or congestive heart failure.[6] While few studies have examined the costs differentiating acute DVT from its complications, the estimated medical cost of treating VTE and its complications in the United States is $6.7 to $9.8 billion per year.[7]

7.4.1 Patient Presentation and Evaluation

Patients who present with CVOD demonstrate PTS of varying severity. During the initial office consultation, the natural history of DVT and PTS is discussed. Patients are evaluated according to both CEAP classification and VCSS scoring to determine baseline presentation and severity of symptoms. Other factors that are considered are the overall health of the patient and coexisting medical conditions that would complicate a procedure, such as renal insufficiency, heart failure, and morbid obesity. A thorough physical examination is performed and preprocedural photographs of the affected extremities are taken for the medical record. If diagnostic imaging has not been previously performed, duplex US or, most commonly, cross-sectional imaging with either MR/CT venography is performed.

Patient suitability for moderate sedation is assessed. Factors that may require general anesthesia include a plan for extensive recanalization of the deep venous system (i.e., IVC and bilateral iliac vein occlusion vs. single common femoral vein occlusion), the need for assisted ventilation (i.e., CPAP or BIPAP), and pain tolerance and anxiety level.

A critical factor in determining whether a patient is suitable for treatment is likelihood of compliance with anticoagulation, as this is paramount to a successful outcome. Those patients who are noncompliant with medications, including history of compliance with anticoagulation, or who are not suitable candidates for deep vein recanalization may be treated with conservative therapy, including referrals as needed to hematology or lymphedema specialists.

7.4.2 Preparation for Procedure

Low-molecular-weight heparin (LMWH; enoxaparin) is started 48 hours prior to the procedure and continued through the day of the procedure. This move away from using unfractionated heparin has anecdotally led to decreased on-table thrombosis, improved efficiency for the IR and floor nursing staff due to the lack of monitoring activated clotting times (ACTs) or partial thromboplastin time (PTT), and fewer subtherapeutic blood levels in the 1 month postprocedural period, which is the most susceptible rethrombosis period. In cases in which the patient will also be undergoing a complex IVC filter retrieval, unfractionated heparin may be preferable, should quick reversal be needed with protamine for caval injury.

On the day of the procedure, patients are kept NPO. Depending on the proposed length of the procedure, which can range from 2 to 6 hours, a decision is made for bladder catheterization. The patient is placed in either the supine or prone position and US evaluation is performed to determine the ideal access point. Commonly used equipment includes:

- Sheaths (6–16F) including long braided support sheaths.
- Hydrophilic and stiff 0.018- and 0.035-inch guidewires.
- Angioplasty balloons ranging from 4 mm for a tibial vein to 25 mm for an IVC. Balloons (120-cm working length) are often needed when working from a calf vein access.
- Angled catheters (4–5F) and chronic total occlusion catheters.
- Mechanical thrombectomy devices:
  - Angiojet (Boston Scientific, Marlborough, MA).
  - Arrow Trerotola thrombectomy device (Teleflex, Wayne, PA).

In addition to preprocedural antibiotics and moderate sedation medications, nursing staff are advised to keep atropine, protamine, heparin, and nitroglycerin readily available.

7.4.3 Technical Tips and Tricks and Procedural Details

Preprocedural planning to determine the ideal access point and the major steps in the procedure is one of the most important components of performing a deep venous recanalization procedure. Common access points such as the popliteal vein, common femoral vein, and internal jugular veins are evaluated. US is used to determine the most peripheral part of the extremity in which a patent deep vein is visualized. For example, if a patient has chronic thrombus involving the popliteal vein, access is achieved in a patent deep vein segment peripheral to the level of the occlusion, such as the posterior tibial or peroneal vein, to maximize venous inflow and recanalize the full length of the popliteal vein. Occasionally, the small saphenous vein may be used if it joins a patent popliteal vein segment.

7.4.4 Potential Complications or Pitfalls

The complications from deep venous recanalizations are few and generally not life-threatening. Venous rupture is a common and easily managed complication treated with prolonged balloon tamponade and, in rare cases, a stent. More challenging technical complications include stent undersizing that can lead to rethrombosis, or oversizing that can result in intractable back pain, especially in left common iliac vein stenting in May–Thurner syndrome. While IVUS can be beneficial for stent sizing and for evaluating major and subclinical areas of venous stenosis, its use is not an absolute requirement in our experience if good quality multiplanar venography is performed.

7.4.5 Postprocedural Management and Follow-up

Having a well-defined management plan that deals with anticoagulation issues, rethrombosis, pain, and ongoing postthrombotic symptoms is key to a successful outcome in the eyes of the patient. Shortly before the end of the procedure, the heparin infusion is stopped and an ACT is checked before removal of the sheaths (sheaths removed if ACT < 200 sec). If the patient is on LMWH, the sheaths are removed without checking any parameters. Once hemostasis is achieved, the patient is transferred to and observed in the recovery room.

Depending on the complexity of deep vein recanalization, the patient is either discharged the same day or admitted for overnight observation. In some cases, patients are admitted for 1 to 2 days if they have other comorbidities such as renal insufficiency or congestive heart failure that may require further monitoring. All patients are admitted to the IR service.

If patients are admitted, nursing staff are instructed to monitor the patient for access site complications and pain control and to ensure that anticoagulation is maintained.

Anticoagulation with LMWH is restarted the same day if the patient is on heparin during the procedure. Compression garments should be fitted and obtained prior to the day of the procedure. If the patient does not have appropriate compression stockings, a lymphedema team, if available, should be consulted for compression garments to be fitted within 24 hours of the procedure.

Prior to discharge, the patient is examined for access site complications and pain control, and relevant bloodwork is reviewed. Thigh-high compression stockings, 20 to 30 mm Hg, should be worn daily for 1 month until first office follow-up. Office visits are performed at 1, 6, and 12 months postprocedure. Imaging, consisting of duplex US or CT venography, is performed at 1-month postprocedure for patients with infrainguinal disease and IVC/iliac thrombosis, respectively. Additional imaging is generally not needed at subsequent follow-up unless there is a concern for rethrombosis or PTS symptoms recur that may necessitate a repeat intervention. Patients are generally discharged with a 1-month supply of twice-daily dosing of LMWH and a narcotic for pain. Since the degree of initial venous occlusion correlates with the likelihood of developing reflux, patients are followed yearly for signs and symptoms of superficial venous insufficiency and, if clinically indicated, are treated with saphenous vein ablation.[8]

If available, it is beneficial to work with a multidisciplinary thrombosis service on all patients presenting with acute and chronic DVT. Hematologists should be familiar with relevant procedures, and protocols for managing patients with CVOD may be developed collaboratively. In the process of building this relationship, all parties have an opportunity to learn about thrombosis and its complications. It can be useful for patients to have a follow-up appointment with a hematologist, who will monitor and make recommendations regarding anticoagulation after the 1 month of LMWH.

The American College of Chest Physician guidelines are a useful guide regarding the duration and type of anticoagulation. Use of an antiplatelet agent in conjunction with anticoagulation may confer higher risk of bleeding than do anticoagulants, alone, and there is lack of evidence for an antiplatelet/anticoagulation regimen in venous disease. However, once patients have completed their course of anticoagulation, aspirin 81 mg daily may be useful as secondary prevention against recurrent thrombosis.

7.4.6 Outcomes

With the advent of endovascular techniques, the options available for patients with severe CVOD have expanded. Nearly two

decades ago, Nazarian et al described their experience in stenting IVC and iliofemoral occlusions with primary and secondary 1-year patency rates of 50 and 81% and 4-year patency rates of 50 and 75%, respectively.[9] More recently, in patients with iliofemoral CVOD, Razavi et al performed a meta-analysis of 37 studies including 2,869 patients (nonthrombotic, 1,122; acute thrombotic, 629; chronic postthrombotic, 1,118) that underwent stenting and found a high rate of stent patency and minimal complication rate. At 1 year, primary and secondary patency rates were 96 and 99% for nonthrombotic, 87 and 89% for acute thrombotic, and 79 and 94% for chronic postthrombotic.[10] While limited retrospective series have shown promising outcomes in the management of CVOD, presently there are no prospective randomized studies comparing these procedures to conservative measures. However, many patients who seek medical attention for severe PTS have been unable to receive adequate, if any, medical attention for CVOD and thereby have been suffering for years with more conservative therapies (i.e., compression stockings) that are often difficult to maintain long term.

7.5 Pearls of Wisdom

- Be persistent. These cases can be very long and challenging. Sometimes you will need to bring the patient back another day and try again.
- Make sure the patient is adequately anticoagulated during the procedure; otherwise, rethrombosis will occur on the table or shortly thereafter.
- Have a low threshold for using a crossing catheter to traverse an occlusion. It can mean the difference between minutes and hours.
- Patients may complain of back pain after stenting in May–Thurner syndrome. If back pain continues for more than a week, a short, tapering course of steroids is often helpful to decrease pain and inflammation.
- Maximize inflow by obtaining access at a location peripheral to the occluded vein segment.
- Avoid telling the patient that their swelling and other postthrombotic symptoms will resolve within a few days of venous recanalization. Often, it can take 4 to 6 weeks for patients to notice a significant improvement.
- If unsuccessful in recanalization attempt, consider sending patient to a more experienced center.

7.6 Unanswered Questions

CVOD is a non-life-threatening condition that is often inadequately treated from a patient QOL perspective. Patients with PTS are often not referred to an appropriate vascular specialist because there is a widespread lack of understanding about venous disease and available treatments. The care of patients with PTS often requires a multidisciplinary approach including but not limited to IR, hematology, surgery, podiatry, lymphedema specialists, and physical therapy.

Areas that require further research include:

- Investigating the natural history of PTS in those with calf or isolated popliteal DVT.

- Examining the role of venous inflow and its effect on recurrent thrombosis rates.
- Identifying the optimal anticoagulation/antiplatelet regimen after venous recanalization.
- Appropriate timing for thrombolysis/recanalization in the setting of recent surgery.
- Stent sizing optimization.

References

[1] Baldwin MJ, Moore HM, Rudarakanchana N, Gohel M, Davies AH. Post-thrombotic syndrome: a clinical review. J Thromb Haemost. 2013; 11(5):795–805

[2] Guanella R, Ducruet T, Johri M, et al. Economic burden and cost determinants of deep vein thrombosis during 2 years following diagnosis: a prospective evaluation. J Thromb Haemost. 2011; 9(12):2397–2405

[3] Tick LW, Kramer MH, Rosendaal FR, Faber WR, Doggen CJ. Risk factors for post-thrombotic syndrome in patients with a first deep venous thrombosis. J Thromb Haemost. 2008; 6(12):2075–2081

[4] Douketis JD, Crowther MA, Foster GA, Ginsberg JS. Does the location of thrombosis determine the risk of disease recurrence in patients with proximal deep vein thrombosis? Am J Med. 2001; 110(7):515–519

[5] Meissner MH, Caps MT, Bergelin RO, Manzo RA, Strandness DE, Jr. Early outcome after isolated calf vein thrombosis. J Vasc Surg. 1997; 26(5):749–756

[6] Kahn SR, Ducruet T, Lamping DL, et al. Prospective evaluation of health-related quality of life in patients with deep venous thrombosis. Arch Intern Med. 2005; 165(10):1173–1178

[7] Grosse SD, Nelson RE, Nyarko KA, Richardson LC, Raskob GE. The economic burden of incident venous thromboembolism in the United States: A review of estimated attributable healthcare costs. Thromb Res. 2016; 137:3–10

[8] Markel A, Manzo RA, Bergelin RO, Strandness DE, Jr. Valvular reflux after deep vein thrombosis: incidence and time of occurrence. J Vasc Surg. 1992; 15(2): 377–382, discussion 383–384

[9] Nazarian GK, Bjarnason H, Dietz CA, Jr, Bernadas CA, Hunter DW. Iliofemoral venous stenoses: effectiveness of treatment with metallic endovascular stents. Radiology. 1996; 200(1):193–199

[10] Razavi MK, Jaff MR, Miller LE. Safety and effectiveness of stent placement for iliofemoral venous outflow obstruction: systematic review and meta-analysis. Circ Cardiovasc Interv. 2015; 8(10):e002772

8 Peripheral Venous Insufficiency

Mary Costantino

Summary

This chapter provides guidelines for the evaluation, management, and treatment of patients with chronic venous insufficiency, with two comprehensive case discussions, demonstrating the range and complexity of patient presentations. The chapter presents a useful algorithm for clinical evaluation, ultrasound interrogation, and treatment selection. There is a comprehensive overview of management approaches, as well as presentation of the technical details of procedural management.

Keywords: CEAP, venous stasis, venous insufficiency, sclerotherapy, vein ablation, varicose veins, perforator, reflux

8.1 Introduction

Peripheral venous insufficiency is underdiagnosed and is often unrecognized. It affects an estimated 25 million U.S. adults, with 20% of those progressing to end-stage disease. Evaluation and management of a patient with peripheral venous insufficiency follows a straightforward algorithm using both clinical and radiological expertise.

No one clinical specialty treats venous disease. Podiatrists, dermatologists, vascular surgeons, and interventional radiologists, among others, all are involved in the evaluation and treatment of peripheral venous insufficiency. Given the multidisciplinary nature of treatment, many societies have published guidelines and criteria for evaluation and treatment. This can be a source of confusion to the beginning practitioner who must sort through multiple societal guidelines. The American College of Phlebology (ACP), Society for Interventional Radiology (SIR), American Venous Forum (AVF) and Intersocietal Commission for the Accreditation of Vascular Laboratories (ICAVL) are recommended resources.

8.2 Case Vignette 1

8.2.1 Patient Presentation

A 52-year-old man presented with a large painful left calf and pretibial varicosity. The varicosity initially developed in his late 20 s, and it has been slowly progressive. When the patient first noticed the varicosity, he was completely asymptomatic. In his late 40 s, the patient developed increasing discomfort related to the varicosity, starting as a tingling and aching sensation before progressing to a burning pain. The varicosity became increasingly symptomatic, eventually becoming disruptive to his daily activities. The patient is required to stand for prolonged periods of time at work, which became increasingly limiting to his required activities. He had worn compression socks for 2 years prior to presentation, usually the calf-high athletic type. The symptoms improved significantly with elevation, leading him to seek to elevate his legs at every opportunity.

8.2.2 Physical Exam

A 4- to 5-mm bulging varicosity extended over the left medial calf and pretibial region, extending from the level of the patella to the distal calf, with multiple reticular veins and telangiectasias within the anterior lower calf. Small aneurysmal dilatations were seen, presumably representing dilated, incompetent venous valves. Physical exam findings were highly suggestive of great saphenous vein (GSV) reflux supplying this enlarged branching varicose tributary.

8.2.3 Noninvasive Testing

An upright duplex ultrasound exam was performed, demonstrating a dilated GSV measuring 11 mm at the saphenofemoral junction (SFJ), with greater than 500 ms of reflux documented. A large varicose tributary measuring 6 mm in diameter was demonstrated, correlating to the visible and painful varicosity evident on physical exam. At the midcalf, there was a 2-mm incompetent perforating vein, which supplied an overlying 3-mm varicosity. A second 5-mm varicosity within the lower calf was identified with origin not determined. The small saphenous vein (SSV) was normal in caliber without retrograde flow. There was no deep vein thrombosis (DVT).

8.2.4 Initial Management

The patient was prescribed medical grade thigh-high compression stockings providing 20 to 30 mm Hg of compression. In the absence of venous ulceration or recurrent superficial thrombophlebitis, the majority of third-party payers require a minimum 3-month trial of conservative therapy consisting of medical grade (20–30 mm Hg) compression stocking use, exercise program including walking, periodic leg elevation, and the use of over-the-counter pain medications. A past history of compression stocking use often does not contribute toward the patient's insurance approval, as many insurance carriers require a supervised conservative therapy program under the care of the treating physician. However, if the patient notes symptoms have responded favorably to prior compression stocking use, the treating clinician can reasonably conclude the patient's symptoms are related to venous congestion and may improve with future therapy.

Following 3 months, the patient returned for follow-up evaluation. Although the compression stockings provided him some relief, symptoms of leg pain, throbbing, burning, and pruritis quickly returned when compression was removed.

After documenting failure of symptom resolution with conservative measures, treatment options were discussed with the patient, including continued daily compression stocking use as well as endovenous ablation. The patient elected to proceed with GSV ablation.

8.2.5 Specifics of Consent

The key concerns to discuss with the patient prior to endovenous ablation are DVT, nerve injury, pain, swelling, bruising, and treatment failure. Endovenous saphenous vein ablation carries a small (1–2%) risk of DVT, which is discussed at length with the patient. Saphenous vein thermal ablation is associated with a slight risk of nerve injury, usually transient if access is performed at the level of the midcalf or above. Patients are counseled to expect varying degrees of tenderness, bruising, and swelling. Patients are also informed that a small percentage of patients may not experience relief of their symptoms following treatment.

8.2.6 Details of Procedure

GSV thermal ablation was performed as described in detail in this chapter. A follow-up postprocedure ultrasound was done to exclude DVT and extension of heat-induced thrombus (EHIT) as well as to assess for adequate vein closure.

Following ablation and while still supine on the procedural table, thigh-high 20 to 30 mm Hg compression stockings were applied. If the patient is unable to wear stockings, various methods are used to provide postprocedure compression including elastic bandages, gauze wraps, self-adherent inelastic dressings, and knee-high compression socks.

8.2.7 Follow-up

Thigh-high compression was prescribed for 7 to 10 days postablation. The patient returned to clinic 1 month following GSV ablation and demonstrated regression of the bulging varicosity previously supplied by the GSV. Small residual symptomatic varicosities present in the lower leg were managed with ultrasound-guided foam sclerotherapy. Three months following treatment, the patient returned to clinic and noted complete resolution of his symptoms.

8.2.8 Periprocedural Troubleshooting and Decision Points

In this patient, the dominant decision points were regarding whether to proceed with ablation alone, ablation plus phlebectomy, or ablation plus phlebectomy with ultrasound-guided foam sclerotherapy. There is a variable approach to these types of vessels. Although there is literature support for performing phlebectomy with ablation in the same visit, many patients can experience excellent clinical results with endovenous ablation alone, obviating the need for phlebectomy. The benefits of ablation alone are a shorter procedure time and fewer incisions and scars. The benefits of performing phlebectomy concurrently with ablation are the elimination of all residual varicosities in one visit and the prevention of the pain and hyperpigmentation of superficial thrombophlebitis, which may occur if there is delay in performing phlebectomy after GSV ablation.

8.3 Epidemiology and Scope of the Problem

Peripheral venous insufficiency affects an estimated 25 million U.S. adults, with 25% of those progressing to chronic venous disease with skin changes and healed or active venous ulcers.

Six percent of adults in the United States have more advanced chronic venous disease consisting of skin changes including hyperpigmentation and/or lipodermatosclerosis with active or healed ulcers. Eighty percent of lower extremity ulcers are venous in nature. Peripheral venous insufficiency is underdiagnosed and is often unrecognized. Evaluation and management of a patient with peripheral venous insufficiency follows a straightforward algorithm using both clinical and imaging expertise.

Endovenous thermal ablation was FDA approved in 1999. Due to the ease of the procedure, favorable outcomes, low complication rates, and ability to perform thermal ablation in an office setting, venous stripping fell out of favor rapidly and thermal ablation was adopted across specialties. There are two thermal ablation modalities available in the United States for endovenous ablation; radiofrequency (RF) and laser energy. RF and 1,480-nm laser are comparable in terms of outcomes and complications, with improvements in outcomes seen with transition from a laser frequency of 810 nm, which was associated with a higher reported rate of bruising and postprocedure pain.

Because there are so many involved societies and a wide variety of practitioners, there are large gaps in data which can be somewhat confusing for the beginning practitioner, such as: How long does the patient wear compression stockings following treatment? How quickly will symptoms subside? What are expected outcomes? Most practices differ, with the more advanced practitioner tailoring his/her practice based on past experiences.

8.3.1 Patient Presentation and Evaluation

Patient presentations may be extremely variable. Prior to a discussion of the detailed evaluation of the individual patient, a review of the lower extremity venous anatomy is provided in order to form a basis for discussion.

Anatomy

A detailed understanding of the lower extremity venous anatomy is of critical importance to any practitioner wishing to intervene on the venous system.

The venous system in the lower extremity is divided into the superficial and deep systems. The superficial system is comprised of the GSV and the SSV. The GSV courses from the inguinal crease along medial leg to a point posterior to the medial malleolus. The GSV is found within the saphenous compartment, between the superficial fascia and the deep fascia. Any vein seen outside of this compartment is a GSV tributary, and if the "GSV" extends outside of this compartment it is no longer called the GSV. If the compartment is empty, the GSV is considered atretic in that segment. The saphenous compartment demonstrates a classic "Egyptian eye" appearance. The GSV is most easily located at the SFJ; it then can be followed peripherally down the leg with focus on the saphenous compartment.

Two common accessory veins are the anterior accessory great saphenous vein (AAGSV) and posterior accessory great saphenous vein (PAGSV). The AAGSV and the PAGSV parallel the saphenous vein originating near the SFJ and course toward the anteromedial (AAGSV) or posteromedial (PAGSV) thigh. The

AAGSV can be seen on physical exam in a typical location running across the anterior thigh. The PAGSV is typically seen running across the posterior thigh. The PAGSV is any venous segment that extends parallel to the GSV and is posterior; the AAGSV is any venous segment being parallel with the GSV and is located anteriorly. Both the AAGSV and PAGSV are by definition found within the saphenous compartment. The AASV and PPSV may demonstrate reflux, and may develop varicosities, and if so should be treated in the same manner as the GSV. There may be clinical failure despite technical success in treating the GSV in the setting of an untreated incompetent accessory GSV. The accessory GSVs usually have a proximal straight segment supplying tortuous varicosities distally.

The deep system of the leg is comprised of the common femoral vein, femoral vein, popliteal vein, posterior tibial vein, peroneal vein, and anterior tibial veins. Reflux can be found within this deep system due to primary valve failure or often due to prior DVT leading to damaged and scarred venous valves.

Perforators are small short veins that connect the deep system to the superficial system, and these are named according to location. Huntington's perforators are found in the proximal thigh, Dodd's perforators are found in the distal thigh, Boyd's perforators are found around the knee, and Cockett's perforators are found within the posterior calf. Perforators physiologically flow from superficial to deep, but can reflux. This is of particular importance in cases of venous ulcers. When perforators are visualized, the direction of flow should be determined. If the direction of flow is going from a refluxing superficial system into the deep system, then this is called a reentry perforator, where the perforator is serving to decompress the superficial system by emptying blood into the deep system. However, if flow is from the deep system to the superficial system, this indicates that a point of abnormality is actually within a refluxing perforator and is the source of the physiologic abnormality. These refluxing perforators should be treated.

The vein of Giacomini is a variant important to the treatment of venous insufficiency. Also called the intersaphenous vein, the vein of Giacomini connects the GSV to the SSV, coursing along the medial posterior thigh. Reflux within this segment must be identified and treated.

The superficial system normally connects to the deep system in the following locations: (1) in the inguinal region where the GSV connects with the femoral vein, forming the SFJ; (2) in the posterior knee where the SSV connects with the popliteal vein at the saphenopopliteal junction; (3) perforating veins in the thigh and lower leg. An understanding of each patient's anatomy is imperative in forming a successful treatment plan.

It is recommended that new practitioner perform diagnostic and mapping ultrasound until he/she fully understands the anatomy and complexity of the lower extremity venous pathways.

8.3.2 Decision Making

Once the anatomy is understood, an algorithmic approach to the patient may be applied. First, start with the clinical status. With the information provided during the history, evaluate the symptoms: duration, quality, severity, location, and exacerbating and ameliorating factors.

Obtain a thorough patient history including family history of venous disease, personal history of DVT, compression use, superficial venous thrombus, coagulation disorder, and detailed description of lifestyle limitations. Symptoms of venous insufficiency include lower extremity heaviness, fatigue, pain, cramping, pressure sensation, burning and itching, swelling, and restless leg symptoms. Symptoms usually occur when standing and worsen throughout the day. Symptoms are exacerbated by warm weather and are relieved by leg elevation and exercise that included calf muscle-pump activity. Symptoms of venous insufficiency must be differentiated from other disease processes causing leg pain or discomfort including peripheral arterial disease, arthritis, and neurogenic conditions.

The traditional textbook notion of arterial disease being worse at night, when the legs are elevated on the bed, and venous disease being worse during the day, while the patient is upright, is not reliable. Patients with venous insufficiency can describe symptoms worse at night, even preventing sleep. Although the legs are elevated, the symptoms of aching and throbbing will persist. Venous insufficiency is often misdiagnosed as "restless leg syndrome" as the patient complains of itchy, burning legs at night resulting in constant leg movement. This is thought to represent the typical symptoms of venous disease exacerbated by the heat of sheets or blankets. Patients will often describe kicking the blankets off of their legs. Any patient with restless leg syndrome and signs of venous insufficiency should be evaluated for reflux.

8.3.3 Physical Exam

Patients with venous insufficiency often demonstrate characteristic physical exam findings. These include lower extremity swelling and typical cutaneous manifestations of tissue congestion and damage. Cutaneous manifestations of chronic venous insufficiency are edema, hyperpigmentation, venous eczema (stasis dermatitis), lipodermatosclerosis, atrophie blanche, and venous ulceration. Cutaneous manifestations are progressive and graded according to the CEAP classification (▶ Table 8.1). The pathophysiology of cutaneous manifestations relates to tissue level venous hypertension resulting in microcirculatory changes and inflammation.

With venous congestion, capillary dilatation occurs and recruited white blood cells release inflammatory mediators. Edema demonstrates a typical pattern in the perimalleolar region and ascending up the leg. The edema does not extend into the foot. This is an important physical exam finding which helps to differentiate venous edema from lymphedema. Continued swelling then leads to a cycle of increased permeability and capillary damage. Symptoms are often worse in hotter climates due to increased capillary dilatation.

Inflammatory changes are thought to occur because white blood cells are trapped due to increasing blood flow; these white blood cells accumulate and release toxic oxygen metabolites and proteolytic enzymes, which lead to further capillary damage, increased permeability, microlymphatic damage, and ultimately fibrin formation. At the microcirculatory level, increased capillary diameters, decreased capillary number, and endothelial damage are seen. The increased capillary permeability also leads to accumulation of extravasated red blood cells within the interstitial space.

Table 8.1 CEAP classification

- C0: No visible or palpable signs of venous disease
- C1: Telangiectasias, reticular veins, malleolar flares
- C2: Varicose veins
- C3: Edema without skin changes
- C4: Skin changes ascribed to venous disease (pigmentation, venous eczema, lipodermatosclerosis)
- C4a: Pigmentation or eczema
- C4b: Lipodermatosclerosis or atrophie blanche
- C5: Skin changes as above with healed ulceration
- C6: Skin changes as above with active ulceration

Symptoms

- S: Symptomatic
- A: Asymptomatic

Etiologic classification

- Ec: Congenital
- Ep: Primary
- Es: Secondary (postthrombotic)
- En: No venous cause identified

Anatomic classification

- As: Superficial veins
- Ap: Perforator veins
- Ad: Deep veins
- An: No venous location identified

Pathophysiologic classification

- Pr: Reflux
- Po: Obstruction
- Pr,o: Reflux and obstruction
- Pn: No venous pathophysiology identifiable

Score: C _, S/A, E_, A_, P_

In patients with lipodermatosclerosis, in addition to increased white blood cell accumulation, proinflammatory cytokines such as IL-1A and IL-IB are present. Lipodermatosclerosis is characterized by hyperpigmentation and fibrosis of the dermal and subcutaneous tissues and demonstrates a high association to chronic venous insufficiency. Chronic congestion leads to pericapillary fibrin formation, which leads to decreased oxygen diffusion. These changes inhibit new collagen formation, which impairs healing, and hence, nonhealing ulcers.

Dry skin and pruritus are often associated and can lead to venous eczema, which is a pruritic process usually beginning at the level of the ankle and again rising cephalad.

Superficial telangiectasias and spider veins are often present. On ultrasound, these rarely demonstrate a visible connection to the deep system and are not specifically indicative of reflux, except in cases of corona phlebectatica. Corona phlebectatica is a cluster of normally visible cutaneous vessels within the medial ankle. Corona phlebectatica has been found to correlate with the clinical severity and hemodynamic abnormalities of chronic venous insufficiency. Although it is not included in the CEAP classification, there is a strong correlation with underlying hemodynamic venous disturbances.

Venous ulceration is the end stage of chronic venous insufficiency. An estimated 20% of chronic venous insufficiency patients will develop venous ulcers; 1 to 4% of the U.S. adult population has had an active or healed ulcer, and 80% of lower extremity ulcers are venous in nature. Many physicians and care providers do not recognize venous ulcers for what they are; 40% of patients with venous lower extremity ulcers have an open ulcer for over 1 year. Many practitioners will recognize these as "stasis ulcers," yet be unaware that these are *venous* stasis ulcers. Many patients spend months and months undergoing painful debridement and wound care appointments, without the ulcers being recognized as venous in etiology. Venous ulcers occur within the medial malleolar region and this location is nearly pathognomonic for venous stasis.

Understanding the patient's symptom complex and based on physical exam, some conclusions may be drawn. The next step is obtaining a thorough lower extremity venous duplex. Duplex sonography evaluating a patient for superficial venous insufficiency is distinct from an examination to evaluate for DVT. The overwhelming majority of patients who have a previous venous duplex will report a normal ultrasound examination. Lower extremity duplex sonography performed at hospitals and imaging centers will examine the deep system in order to exclude DVT. Rarely is the superficial system or the presence or absence of deep venous reflux evaluated. Do not let the history of a "normal ultrasound" deter from pursuing a specialized ultrasound to evaluate for GSV reflux.

8.3.4 Venous Ultrasound

Ultrasound for the diagnosis and characterization of lower extremity venous insufficiency requires venous mapping, which is complex and requires time and attention to detail. A complete exam usually requires 45 to 60 minutes.

The examination of the deep system can be performed supine. Ideally, the superficial system is evaluated in the standing position with the patient's weight on the leg not being interrogated. The leg being examined should be placed with the foot flat on the ground (the heel should not be raised; this is a natural tendency and must be avoided as this position activates the calf pump) and the leg externally rotated. If the patient is unable to stand for the duplex ultrasound, a tilt table should be utilized with at least 15 degrees of reverse Trendelenburg. The calf or SSV may be scanned with the patient seated on the exam table with the leg hanging over the side of the table.

Ultrasound should: (1) determine the venous anatomy with mapping of the superficial system and all connections to the deep system; (2) evaluate for DVT and superficial venous thrombosis; (3) evaluate for reflux in the superficial and deep systems; and (4) note any perforators and communications to visible tributaries or varicosities.

The initial focus should be on the GSV, and reflux is evaluated throughout the length of the GSV, with size and reflux measurements taken at the junction, proximal thigh, midthigh, knee, and calf, and size and presence of reflux noted. The origin of reflux determines treatment options and can be found anywhere along the lower extremity venous system. Reflux can start peripherally and ascend to the SFJ (the ascending theory), or can start centrally and progress peripherally (descending or waterfall reflux). Reflux is assessed by placing Doppler on the vessel of interest and applying pressure to the vein cephalad to the area of interest. Doppler will demonstrate blood refluxing toward the foot. Reflux is defined by the American Venous

77

Forum as reversed flow within the femoropopliteal junction > 1,000 ms, superficial veins > 500 ms, or perforators > 350 ms.

To assess for reflux, augmentation of the vessel of interest is used. There are many ways to perform augmentation; several are covered here. However, finding the method that works best for each practitioner will give the most reproducible results. Venous ultrasound is complex and initially difficult; when starting a practice, one should work closely with one or two appointed specialized ultrasound technologists, to ensure complete and accurate exams. Venous ultrasound is a specialized skill, and if using a technologist, he/she should have additional training in the diagnosis of venous reflux.

To elicit reflux at the SFJ, Valsalva is used to produce increased intra-abdominal pressures. Within the more peripheral saphenous system, Valsalva is not as effective and manual hand compression can be used over the muscles within the calf. Activation of the calf pump can be used with active dorsi- and plantar flexion of the foot while evaluating the flow with Doppler. The piranha maneuver uses the muscle pump, the patient rocking back and forth to engage the calf muscles or to shift from one leg to the other. Automatic cuff devices inflated to 80 to 120 mm Hg can also be used. Proximal augmentation in which pressure is applied central to the vessel of interest is often used; however, there is debate over whether this method is valid and accurate within the superficial system, as this is a forced reflux rather than applying a physiologic situation such as Valsalva or muscle pump techniques.

Each clinic should develop a form that the sonographer uses to communicate data to the operator. It is helpful to include on the form a basic diagram of the venous structures for each leg, to provide a location for notations and a visual overview of the extent of disease. Ultrasound reports are usually standardized, as this meets the requirements of insurance companies and requires the least amount of time for physician interpretation. However, venous disease is often complex and descriptive verbiage is encouraged so that the reader can really understand what is occurring within the venous system.

In summary, for reporting purposes the diameter of each GSV and SSV is documented in the upper, mid, and lower thigh as well as below the knee. Visible anterior or posterior accessory saphenous veins are also evaluated. The presence and duration of reflux are documented at each location. The location, diameter, and severity of reflux are also documented for each major varicose tributary. The sonographer should provide a detailed diagram documenting the location and extent of bulging and nonbulging varicose tributaries. All incompetent perforating veins are also documented noting their diameter and severity of reflux as well as proximity to active or healed ulcers or focal symptomatic lipodermatosclerosis. In practice, what is most important is defining the levels of reflux and characterizing the anatomy to determine a treatment strategy.

When the patient's clinical symptoms are highly suspicious for venous congestion and ultrasound is negative, it is worth repeating an ultrasound at a different time of the day (ideally as late as possible) with the patient fully hydrated, and in a warm room. With an adequate clinical history, the diagnosis of venous congestion should be confidently made and the purpose of the ultrasound is to find the underlying etiology.

Should the clinical and radiographic evaluations conclude that venous insufficiency is present, deciding on the best treatment is next. There are three treatment options: thermal ablation (RF or laser), ultrasound-guided sclerotherapy (USGS), and microphlebectomy (i.e., ambulatory phlebectomy)

8.3.5 Preparation for Procedure

The ultrasound report, with diagrams of the patient's anatomy and points of reflux, as well as the summary history for understanding of the patient's dominant symptoms, should be available and reviewed in advance of the procedure. Staff should be well oriented to the use of the ablation equipment, and tumescent anesthetic should be prepared and in the room.

The tumescent solution is 50 mg of lidocaine in 1,000 mL of normal saline, and should be prepared in advance. If a pump is used for delivery of tumescent, this should be in place and set up in a convenient location for the operator. If sclerotherapy is planned, sclerosant should be available in the room, with appropriate syringes and access needles on the table.

It is recommended that the room be warm and the patient be advised to fully hydrated. It can be helpful to mark the patient's leg in advance, with the patient standing, to demonstrate the locations of visible varicosities. Topical anesthetic is often used, applied in advance of the procedure to improve patient tolerance.

8.3.6 Technical Tips and Tricks and Details of Procedure

Ablation

The patient is placed in a supine position in reverse Trendelenburg. The leg is placed in external rotation with the knee slightly bent. Ultrasound is performed to identify the SFJ and the diseased vessel; GSV will be used for illustration.

Prior to prepping the patient, the diagnostic ultrasound is reviewed and ultrasound is again used to confirm findings. Based on factors such as patient's hydration status, anxiety level, and the temperature in the room, the veins may be smaller or larger than seen on the original diagnostic study. If they are smaller, this can lead to access issues.

The procedure is often performed with an ultrasound technologist as well as the operator. Different practitioners approach the site of access in various manners, but the goal should be treatment of the entirety of the diseased, refluxing vein. A peripheral access will ensure complete closure of the vein being treated, with a plan to ablate as much as the diseased vein as possible, and to cross over any perforators or varicosities that could become pathologic in the future. However, with GSV ablation there is a higher risk of thermal injury to the sural nerve as access moves more peripherally, below the belly of the gastrocnemius muscle. Nerve damage is caused by inadvertent heat translocation during ablation, which can be prevented by adequate perivenous tumescent around the venous fascia. Damage results in anesthesia in the medial malleolar region which resolves by 6 months to 1 year, usually within the first several months. Every patient with low access should be informed that they may experience numbness of the medial lower and midcalf, and if properly prepared, patients are not bothered by this transient side effect of the treatment.

The point of access is marked. The leg is then prepped using betadine or chlorhexidine, with a sterile towel at the groin, and a sterile drape over the remainder of the leg. The operator is in a sterile gown and gloves, and a sterile cover is placed over the ultrasound probe. Following identification of the point of access, 0.1 to 0.2 mL of lidocaine 1% is used to numb the access site. Using ultrasound guidance, a 21-gauge needle is advanced into the vein. Typically, this is done in a longitudinal direction; however, if the vein is small, this may be easier to perform in the transverse direction. It is important to try and access the vessel in a single stick, as veins can be quite spasmodic. If multiple sticks are made, the vein can clamp down, rendering it inaccessible. If this happens, it is best to place a warm blanket on the patient and remove the needle for a period of time. One may consider applying 1 inch of nitropaste and wait 20 to 30 minutes prior to reaccessing; however, there is some risk of profound hypotension with use of nitropaste, so this should be used with some caution. If access still cannot be obtained, and the initial site was low enough, follow the vein 2 to 3 cm cephalad to a patent lumen. Overinjecting lidocaine will compress the vein. It is notable that patents have a variable degree of venous spasm. Anecdotally, younger women have the most spasmodic veins, and particular attention is given to this subgroup (incidentally, they are also more likely to feel the catheter thread through their vein).

Once access is obtained, there should be brisk return of blood. A 0.018-inch microwire is placed through the access needle. When accessing the vein, care should be taken to prevent partial access, with the needle bevel partially within the lumen and partially within the wall of the vein. If this happens, flow through the back end of the needle will be present but not brisk. If a microwire is inserted through the needle and advanced in this scenario, the microwire will actually advance with ease about 6 to 7 cm. The operator will think the wire is intraluminal when indeed the wire is dissecting the vein wall. This will result in spasm of 8 to 10 cm of vein, and render the vein inaccessible.

Avoid advancing the microwire unless one is sure an intraluminal position is obtained. In difficult access cases (usually accessing a 1–3-mm vein, or a vein with a thick wall), ultrasound guidance can be used to make slight adjustments in position, direction, and tip orientation of the bevel of the needle and to observe the advancing wire within the lumen.

Once access is obtained, the table should be flattened to help empty the venous system and decompress the vein around the catheter.

Following placement of the microwire, if using RF, a small dermatotomy is made and the 7-French sheath is advanced into the vein. The wire and inner dilator are removed. The RF catheter is then advanced through the vein bare, to terminate 2 to 3 cm from the SFJ. If using laser, a transitional dilator is placed over the microwire, the microwire is removed, and a 0.038-inch wire is advanced to the SFJ. The catheter and sheath are advanced over the wire to terminate at the SFJ, the wire is removed, and the laser is advanced through the sheath to the final position 2 to 3 cm from the SFJ, at which point the sheath is pulled back to uncover the fiber. The laser fiber should not be advanced bare through the venous segment.

Whether using laser or RF, there should be no resistance to advancing the catheter cephalad. The catheter should be advanced slowly and with ease. A small number of patients have spasmodic vessels and may feel the catheter advance centrally. As long as the catheter advances with ease, continue to advance the catheter to the SFJ and reassure the patient. If there is resistance, ultrasound is then used to visualize the catheter tip as it advances through the vein. Resistance is caused by spasm, a slight bend in the vein, or placement of the catheter or sheath into a side branch.

If the vein of interest is anything less than perfectly straight, advancement of the RF catheter may be difficult. If there is any tortuosity or a serpiginous area within the treated vein, the catheter will not advance centrally and will need to be advanced over a 0.025-inch wire to the SFJ. Wire advancement through tortuous segments can be performed fairly readily with ultrasound guidance. Care should be given to estimating how far the wire needs to go to advance to the SFJ, as there is no need for the wire to be central. With the wire just distal to the SFJ, the thermal ablation catheter can be safely advanced over the wire to bypass the stenotic or serpiginous segment.

Once the device is 2 cm from the SFJ, tumescent is applied. The tumescent solution is 50 mg of lidocaine in 1,000 mL of normal saline; the volume of tumescent is limited by the maximum daily lidocaine dose of 5 mg/kg. The purpose of the tumescent is to anesthetize the vein, provide a heat sink to protect surrounding tissues, and to compress the vein around the catheter. Using ultrasound guidance, any micropuncture needle, usually a 21 gauge, is advanced to the vein sheath and tumescent is infused within the sheath and surrounding the vein. The tumescent may be delivered with use of a commercial pump designed for this purpose, or may be delivered by hand using 20-mL syringes. It is important to bathe the vein circumferentially with tumescent, in contact with the vein, particularly in the calf where the sural nerve runs parallel to the vein. In the lower leg, the vein should be at least 1 cm deep at the time of ablation; therefore, in the distal leg, more tumescent is applied to the superficial aspect of the vein than to the deep aspect.

Following delivery of tumescent, the distance from the catheter tip to the SFJ is reconfirmed to be 2 to 3 cm from the SFJ. Ultrasound should also be used at this point to visualize the entire length of the catheter, to confirm that tumescent completely surrounds the catheter. Once this final ultrasound survey is performed and considered to be satisfactory, treatment can begin.

In the case of laser ablation, protection goggles are applied and the activated laser, along with its sheath, is slowly withdrawn at a rate of 7 s/cm to a point just central to the level of the access site. The laser must be deactivated prior to exiting the vein lumen. The wattage applied to the vein varies greatly in practice; however, a treatment range 80 to 100 J/cm is a reasonable target.

RF ablation is performed using 20-second RF cycles, during which the catheter will heat to greater than 120 watts and the impedance should drop to < 20 ohms. Typically, two cycles are used at the most cephalad treatment point. The catheter is then withdrawn segmentally in 5 cm increments based on the calibrated markings on the catheter, applying RF cycles at intervals along the length of the vein to treat the entire saphenous vein.

Care should be taken to ensure that the thermal device is turned off far from the skin insertion site. Skin burns will occur if the subcutaneous tissue or dermis is accidently treated. At the completion of the case, the catheter is completely removed. The coagulated blood within the vein can be expressed from the vein through the incision, the leg is cleaned, and a Steri-Strip is applied.

Large varicosities can be painful and unsightly. If varicosities are problematic, the practitioner should determine whether the vein needs focal treatment. Following ablation of the GSV, often a bulging pain will regress over several months, especially if the varicosity arises from the treated GSV and has no collateral supply. If the vein is large, receives supply from multiple sources, or is very symptomatic, targeted treatment of the varicosity can be performed at the time of the GSV ablation.

Ultrasound-Guided Sclerotherapy versus Phlebectomy

Use of various techniques for management of varicosities, specifically, will vary clinic to clinic; some clinics perform ablation and USGS or phlebectomy in the same setting as ablation, while others perform ablation with watchful waiting for 1 to 3 months to determine whether the varicosities decompress once the refluxing GSV is treated. One argument in favor of staged treatment is that, once tumescent is applied, and in particular with an anxious patient with spasm, the varicosities may actually be quite small and nonaccessible. However, in patients in whom this does not occur, concurrent treatment may allow for earlier relief and reduce the chance a second procedural session is required. In the event of inability to complete the phlebectomy or sclerotherapy at the time of ablation, USGS can be planned for performance at the time of the follow-up ultrasound to rule out DVT, done 3 to 5 days following the procedure.

It is important to describe both the phlebectomy and sclerotherapy techniques to each patient with large dilated varicosities and, based on the relative acceptance of the cosmetic outcomes expected and the desired results, a treatment can be chosen. When a varicosity is long and solitary and/or large and protruding, a singular phlebectomy provides the most immediate cosmetic result, but leaves behind small scars. USGS is ideal when the patient is less concerned about a residual blue vein and there is a large network of veins, since foam used for sclerotherapy can percolate through multiple side branches, easily eliminating a network of varicosities. Careful discussion should be had with patients with the AAGSV coursing across the thigh from the inguinal crease to the lateral knee if sclerotherapy is considered. The location of this vein is highly visible, so realistic outcomes should be described. Inform patients that following USGS they will still see the blue vein; however, the bulging will disappear.

Ultrasound-Guided Sclerotherapy

Using ultrasound guidance, a 23-gauge butterfly needle is inserted into the vein of interest. A clean syringe is attached to the back of the butterfly needle and blood is aspirated to the syringe. A solution of 0.25% foam sodium tetradecyl sulfate (STS), consisting of 1% STS 1 mL: air 3 mL, is then made using a three-way stopcock; the treatment syringe is then attached to the butterfly needle and foam Sotradecol is infused into the vein under ultrasound guidance. The foam can be visualized coursing through the vein with an immediate result. When the syringe is empty, the needle is removed, the area is compressed, and the sclerosant is massaged through the veins. In this manner, any individual varicosities and smaller side branches can be treated. Note is made of varicosities that empty into the deep system or communicate with a large refluxing perforator and, for these, phlebectomy should be considered to prevent STS from coursing centrally. Should foam STS enter into the deep system, DVT is rare due to the high flow within the deep system. However, it should be avoided as much as possible. When USGS is used in veins with communication to the deep system, manual compression or compression with the transducer can be performed at the communication, and a less aggressive amount of STS can be used. These veins may require multiple treatments.

STS may be purchased in concentrations of 1 or 3%. Most clinics purchase 3% and dilute to 0.25%. Occasionally, 0.5% is used for larger veins (5–6 mm).

Phlebectomy

Microphlebectomy (or ambulatory phlebectomy) is typically done at the time of ablation. With the patient in the standing position prior to the beginning of the ablation procedure, the veins of interest are marked using an indelible marker. Following ablation, using the tumescent solution, a 25-gauge needle is used to apply tumescent around the vein and subcutaneous tissues for anesthesia. A small skin incision, approximately 4 mm, is made over the vein. A phlebectomy hook expressly designed for this purpose is inserted through the skin incision to hook the vein. Hemostats are used to capture the vein and continued gentle traction is applied to free the vein from the subcutaneous tissue. Occasionally, the vein will not come out in long segments and only small pieces of vein are removed. Any residual, visible vein that presents in follow-up can be treated with USGS.

8.3.7 Potential Complications or Pitfalls

Complications in saphenous vein ablation are few, with EHIT with or without DVT, thrombophlebitis, pain, localized nerve injury, and ulceration being potential complications. EHIT is a complication of thermal ablation occurring in approximately 5% of cases.[1] The endothelium is damaged and a local inflammatory reaction occurs with resultant, therapeutic thrombotic occlusion of the treated venous segment. In cases of EHIT, thrombus propagates toward the SFJ and potentially into the deep system. EHIT is thought to behave differently from true DVT, with a rate of nonfatal pulmonary embolism occurring at a rate of 0.03%.[2] Risk factors for EHIT include male gender, large vein diameter, and multiple phlebectomies. There are four grades of EHIT and treatment includes recurrent monitoring with ultrasound, nonsteroidal anti-inflammatory medication, antiplatelet therapy, or anticoagulation. Because EHIT is asymptomatic, routine follow-up ultrasounds 2 to 7 days following ablation should be performed. Each clinic should develop a protocol for EHIT treatment.

Thrombophlebitis is painful and debilitating, without significant long-term sequelae. If the patient develops thrombophlebitis, focal pain can be quite severe, and management consists of symptom control. A recommended regimen is aspirin daily for 5 days, compression stocking use, and warm compresses as first-line treatment. In severe cases, a small incision may be made over the thrombosed segment and the clot can be expressed from the vein to provide immediate relief.

The most dangerous potential complications are the result of inadequate operator knowledge of the venous anatomy and the complexities of venous insufficiency. It is imperative to ensure a thorough knowledge of each patient's anatomy and flow patterns. In understanding the landscape, one can ensure that there is no access obtained to the deep venous system during venous ablation procedures. Irreversible limb-threating injury will be the result of mistakenly accessing and ablating or sclerosing the deep system.

8.3.8 Postprocedural Management and Follow-up

Following ablation, compression should be applied before the patient stands. An assistant or the patient may place the compression stocking. A variety of devices can be used to aid with placement, such as a simple silk bootie that allows the stocking to roll over the ankle. A 20 to 30 mm Hg thigh-high compression stocking is the most common option, with an open-toe version being most comfortable for many patients. Alternatively, a gauze wrap with overlying elastic bandage followed by a compression stocking is occasionally used. Caution should be used when using self-adherent, inelastic wraps, such as Coban (3 M, Maplewood, MI), due to the risk of tourniquet effect, and even elastic bandages should be used with care as it is common to inadvertently wrap the leg more tightly than is recognized with resultant neurovascular compromise.

Immediately following ablation, the patient is encouraged to ambulate to decrease the risk of clot extension. Clot can propagate centrally from ablation site toward the SFJ, causing EHIT, and ambulation is thought to assist in prevention of DVT.

8.4 Case Vignette 2

8.4.1 Patient Presentation

A 65-year-old male with nonhealing right medial malleolar ulcer for 6 months is undergoing regular debridement under the direction of his family physician. Despite twice a week debridement, the ulcer has decreased in size by only 10%.

8.4.2 Physical Exam

The ulcer measures 5 × 3 cm and is wet, oozing serosanguineous fluid from its base.

8.4.3 Noninvasive Testing

Ultrasound demonstrated GSV reflux bilaterally, right SSV reflux, and a refluxing perforator subjacent to the ulcer.

8.4.4 Decision Making

This patient had CEAP-6, EP, SP disease and treatment is indicated. In venous ulceration, compression is the primary form of

treatment, with ablation serving to hasten healing and prevent reoccurrence. In the setting of ulceration, a refluxing perforator underlying the ulcer must be ablated as well. The order of ablation should be GSV, SSV, and then the perforator. Some centers do each ablation on separate days, while others combine the GSV and SSV.

8.4.5 Specifics of Consent

Specifics discussed with a patient undergoing vein ablation for venous ulceration relate largely to setting expectations for outcome, and for the likelihood of multiple procedures to complete treatment. Additionally, when treating the SSV, a specific consideration is injury to the posterior tibial nerve with the result of foot drop.

When treating multiple veins, whether to extend over multiple sessions is largely dependent on limitations around volume of tumescent anesthesia, with a maximum daily lidocaine dose of 4 mg/kg. Though both GSVs can be ablated in the same session, or certainly a GSV and SSV, care should be taken to accurately deliver the tumescent in the perivenous tissues to maximize the length of vein treated. Another limiting factor may be that some insurance companies may not approve same-day, multisite ablations. Patients should be prepared for multiple treatments, each performed 2 to 3 days apart. This means multiple visits to the clinic. If the patients are forewarned, most are happy to comply.

8.4.6 Details of Procedures

The initial ablation was performed on the ipsilateral GSV. Two days later, the SSV was ablated and this was followed by ablation of the perforator 1 week following the SSV procedure. For SSV ablation, the patient is positioned prone, and the SSV is accessed from the posterior calf just above the Achilles tendon. The catheter is advanced to 2 to 3 cm from the saphenopopliteal junction.

8.4.7 Follow-up

The patient was instructed to wear compression socks around the clock for 1 week, followed by 2 weeks of daytime-only wear, for a total time of 3 weeks. The patient returned in 3 to 5 days for a follow-up ultrasound to rule out EHIT/DVT. Postprocedure compression varies widely, with no consensus on how long stockings need to be worn. The purpose of the stockings is to apply continuous compression to the vein to prevent recanalization, decrease pain, and increase physical function following ablation.

8.5 Venous Ulceration

8.5.1 Epidemiology and Scope of the Problem

Venous ulceration is the end stage of chronic venous insufficiency. An estimated 20% of chronic venous insufficiency patients will develop venous ulcers, 1 to 4% of the U.S. adult population has had an active or healed ulcer, and 80% of lower extremity ulcers are venous in nature. Many physicians and care providers do not recognize venous ulcers for what they are; 40% of patients with venous lower extremity ulcers have an open ulcer for over 1 year.

8.5.2 Patient Presentation and Evaluation

When presented with an extremity ulcer, the differential diagnosis of arterial, neuropathic, or dermatologic ulceration must be considered and, if necessary, the patient referred for the more appropriate evaluation. Venous insufficiency ulcers have a classic pattern, with ulceration occurring in the medial malleolar region or occasionally within the posterior lower calf, and this location of a wet ulcer should always prompt evaluation for venous stasis as the etiology. This pattern is distinct from ulcers resulting from peripheral arterial disease, which occur within the digits/distally in arterial watershed distributions, or those secondary to neuropathy and diabetes, which occur more frequently on the plantar aspect of foot. Venous ulcers are traditionally shallow, wet ulcers from 1 to 10 cm, with apparent granulation tissue and fibrin formation. The utility of ultrasound is to discover the underlying pathologic venous physiology.

8.5.3 Conservative Management

In venous ulceration, compression is the primary form of treatment, with ablation serving to hasten healing and prevent recurrence. Currently, all insurance companies require 3 months of compression stockings 20 to 30 mm Hg prior to approving invasive treatment. However, in the case of active ulceration or active hemorrhage from a small aneurysm, this waiting period is waived. Most vein practitioners use thigh-high 20 to 30 mm Hg stockings, with advanced adjustable compression devices recommended for patients who are unable to don the compression stockings.

8.5.4 Technical Tips and Tricks and Details of Procedure

When compression is combined with venous ablation therapy, there is a 12-month ulcer recurrence rate of 5%, versus 67% with compression alone. In a second study, there are similar findings with a 12-month ulcer recurrence rate of 12%, versus 28% with compression alone.

In patients with complex, multilevel venous insufficiency with ulceration, the order of ablation should be GSV first, and then SSV. In the setting of ulceration, a refluxing perforator underlying the ulcer must be ablated as well. Ulceration and symptomatic focal lipodermatosclerosis are two of the clinical situations in which ablation of perforators is indicated.

The SSV is treated in a fashion similar to that for treatment of the GSV; however, the patient is placed prone on the table and the SSV is accessed from the posterior calf just above the Achilles tendon. The catheter is advanced to 2 to 3 cm from the saphenopopliteal junction for initiation of ablation. A special consideration in the case of the SSV is the posterior tibial nerve, which can be avoided by ablating only the superficial component of the SSV, peripheral to the point at which it dives deep to the fascia.

For perforator ablation, ultrasound is used to access the perforator percutaneously. The catheter is advanced into the perforator, 1 cm from the deep system and, following delivery of tumescent anesthesia, the perforator is ablated. Using the RF system there is a unique perforator stylet that is used. The stylet has an inner needle, allowing for a single puncture technique. The needle/catheter combination is used to directly puncture the perforator; the needle is removed with the ablation catheter left behind. The perforator stylet has a heating component 3 cm in length (vs. 7 cm for the regular RF catheter.) Perforator treatment is comprised of one or two 4-minute treatment cycles in the case of RF, or a short ablation in the case of laser. Perforator treatment is distinct from routine ablation and proper catheter selection should be reviewed with the vendor.

8.5.5 Potential Complications or Pitfalls

Damage to the posterior tibial nerve is a specific concern when performing SSV ablation. If the SSV drops deep to the deep fascia, the posterior tibial nerve is at risk. This is a motor nerve and damage can result in foot drop, which can be permanent. This is a much more serious complication than is transient diminished sensation. To avoid this, if the SSV dives deep to the fascia, the ablation is started just peripheral to this, even if this point is > 3 cm from the saphenopopliteal junction.

Ablation of perforators should be performed with care, and only after the practitioner is highly competent in performance of standard ablation procedures. Familiarity with devices and excellent understanding of the anatomy are critical, as extension of ablation into the deep venous system is a risk, as is cutaneous ulceration from performance of ablation within the tissue tract.

8.5.6 Postprocedure Management and Follow-up

In patients with multilevel venous insufficiency and ulceration, it is common to find a component of lymphedema as an underlying factor. In patients with lymphedema, obese patients, complex venous pathology, or extensive deep vein reflux, it behooves the vein specialist to find a local physical therapist specializing in compression and treatment of lymphedema. These patients will likely need lifelong compression therapy. Lymphedema specialists will properly fit patients with the correct device, teach and perform lymphatic massage, and stay current in techniques to manage edema. Conservative management can be optimized in patients who find standard thigh-high 20 to 30 mm Hg compression stockings difficult to don due to mobility, thigh or leg shape, or debilitating conditions such as arthritis.

Patients with ulcers should have high-quality wound care. When embarking on the management of patients with venous ulcers, referral to a wound care clinic is advised, with mastery of wound care reserved for a mature practice.

8.6 Pearls of Wisdom

Interventional radiologists have a distinct advantage over other specialists when starting a vein practice because of a unique skill set in image-guided access. The biggest challenge is proper patient selection and predicting patient outcome.

- Venous disease is complex and very poorly understood. Insurance companies have limited understanding of this disease and equate clinical venous congestion simplistically with junctional reflux.
- In the current environment, reimbursement for vein ablation is based on the size of the vein, although there are no data to support the concept that degree of clinical symptoms correlates to size of the saphenous vein. Therefore, in spite of payer paradigms, this notion should be disregarded by the clinician.
- Large dilated varicosities do not necessarily equate to symptomatic patients and vice versa. A patient can have extensive dilated visible veins and be asymptomatic. Likewise, a patient can have a normal exam yet be quite symptomatic with achy, burning legs. Do not judge a book by its cover.
- Use of compression can help determine if symptoms are due to venous congestion in equivocal patients.
- Women who are 30 to 40 years old with edema have less predictable results following treatment. The degree of lymphedema versus venous edema is difficult to predict. In the case of a positive ultrasound, under-promise and treat one leg first to see how the patient responds.
- As a corollary, where there is venous edema, there is lymphedema.
- "Screening ultrasounds" with the probe placed only at the SFJ are discouraged. Venous congestion is a clinical diagnosis, and once it is determined that it is present, the goal of the ultrasound is to find the level of the disease.
- Once a venous patient, always a venous patient.
- About 50% of patients are "complex," meaning simple GSV reflux without the addition of refluxing AAGSV, perforators, complex anatomy, etc. Treatment can be a journey, and you and the patient should be prepared for follow-up ultrasounds, clinic visits, and additional treatments.
- Every patient scheduled for bilateral GSV reflux should be warned that the GSV is used for cardiac bypass, and these veins will not be available for grafting in the future. If patients

are high risk, contact their cardiologist to discuss prior to bilateral ablation.

- Never touch the deep system. If there is any question that one is in the deep system, terminate the procedure. Irreversible limb-threating damage will be done if one is mistakenly within the deep system.

8.7 Unanswered Questions

Venous disease is much more complex than many appreciate. Young (20–40-year-old) women present a unique subset of patients with symptoms of venous congestion, seemingly out of proportion to junctional reflux. Estrogen receptors are known to modulate vascular dilatation in arteries, with a known link to arterial disease such as cardiovascular disease and migraines. There is a known association with estrogens and DVT, and interestingly, many women describe the onset of venous disease with pregnancy. Though certainly the gravid uterus applies pressure to the central venous system, the question of a peripheral process occurring at the capillary level should be raised. Venous congestion is oversimplified to meet insurance criteria. However, the severity of symptoms and edema in younger women with mild junctional reflux suggests a more peripheral process. This is similar to a central neuropathy versus a peripheral neuropathy.

How long must a patient wear compression prior to an ablation? Insurance companies mandate an arbitrary 3-month trial of conservative therapy. This is implemented in vein clinics across the United States and is based on an attempt to prevent coverage. A multicenter study should be performed to debunk this arbitrary wait time.

References

[1] Kane K, Fisher T, Bennett M, et al. The incidence and outcome of endothermal heat-induced thrombosis after endovenous laser ablation. Ann Vasc Surg. 2014; 28(7):1744–1750

[2] Sufian S, Arnez A, Labropoulos N, Lakhanpal S. Incidence, progression, and risk factors for endovenous heat-induced thrombosis after radiofrequency ablation. J Vasc Surg Venous Lymphat Disord. 201 3; 1(2):159–164

9 Venous Access

Todd Hoffman, Laura K. Findeiss, and Gordon McLennan

Summary

Central venous access procedures are frequently performed by interventional radiologists, and are most commonly considered straightforward. However, knowledge of the nuances of placement, management, and troubleshooting of central venous catheters is necessary for an effective and successful venous access practice. In particular, management of patients with limited access options is nearly completely within the purview of interventional radiology. This chapter will review guidelines relevant to the management of central venous access, and will present techniques for achieving access in patients with venous occlusions.

Keywords: central venous catheter, port, SVC syndrome, TIVAD, recanalization, vascular access

9.1 Introduction

Central venous access is a cornerstone procedure in the modern interventional radiology (IR) practice. Technical mastery of routine catheter placement is straightforward. The expertise provided by the interventional radiologist in both basic and advanced catheter management helps patients and referring physicians navigate the complexities of long-term central venous access such as optimizing catheter choice, managing catheter-related complications, and achieving optimal venous access. The aim of this chapter is to provide a construct for managing central venous access using evidence-based strategies and state-of-the-art techniques.

9.2 Case Vignette

9.2.1 Patient Presentation

A 54-year-old woman with a history of recurrent pancreatic cancer status post Whipple procedure presented 2 months after placement of a left subclavian vein dual-lumen port with neck, facial, and bilateral upper extremity edema. Computed axial tomography (CT) of the chest was performed with contrast, revealing thrombus within the superior vena cava (SVC) surrounding the catheter tip (▶ Fig. 9.1). Incidental note was made of small pulmonary emboli, from which she was asymptomatic. The patient was treated with a heparin drip as a bridge to oral anticoagulation. Facial and neck edema resolved completely, and at discharge there was minimal symmetric bilateral upper extremity edema.

A few months later the patient was referred to the IR department for evaluation of a malfunctioning port, with documentation of unsuccessful aspiration through both lumens and resistance to injection resulting in prolonged infusion times.

9.2.2 Physical Exam

Vital signs were within normal limits and the patient was in no acute distress. There was trace residual pitting edema noted in the bilateral forearms, right slightly greater than left. Small anterior chest wall collateral venous structures were noted. No head and neck swelling was present, her neck exhibited normal range of motion, and there was no respiratory distress suggesting airway compromise. Mallampati score was 2. Positive S1/S2 heart sounds were auscultated with normal cardiac rate and rhythm. Lungs were clear bilaterally.

9.2.3 Noninvasive Testing Imaging

At the initial presentation at the time of acute symptoms, the patient had bilateral upper extremity duplex ultrasound interrogation revealing thrombus in her bilateral axillary and subclavian veins. A chest CT performed at the same time demonstrated thrombus throughout the SVC as well.

For evaluation of the etiology of port dysfunction, a venogram was performed via port access. This revealed restriction of contrast flow from the tip of the catheter, indicative of a fibrin sheath (▶ Fig. 9.2), with palpable resistance to injection of contrast through both lumens.

A follow-up chest CT was obtained prior to intervention for procedural planning. This demonstrated narrowing of the SVC with resolution of the previously visualized thrombus. In addition, asymmetric right chest wall venous collateral channels had formed (▶ Fig. 9.3).

9.2.4 Specifics of Consent

The spectrum of options were discussed, including attempted snaring/stripping of the original access versus complete removal of the left subclavian port, with new port placement through right internal jugular vein access, and techniques for managing SVC stenosis. Standard procedural risks were discussed, including those relative to moderate sedation, risk of bleeding, pneumothorax, and infection. In addition, the likely need for SVC venoplasty and attendant possibility of stent placement were reviewed, including risk of SVC perforation and

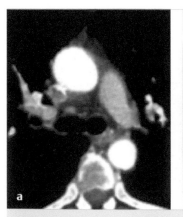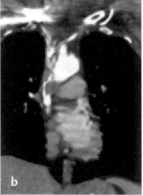

Fig. 9.1 Axial (**a**) and coronal (**b**) reformatted CT reveals extensive thrombus burden throughout the superior vena cava below the tip of the port catheter.

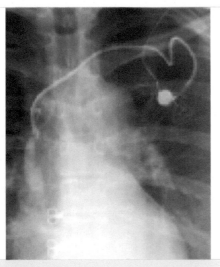

Fig. 9.2 Contrast injection through the medial lumen of the catheter reveals a fibrin sheath distorting the contrast column through the tip of the catheter with slight reflux of contrast along the distal catheter tip. Also note the tortuous course of the catheter from the chest wall insertion site to point of entry within the left subclavian vein.

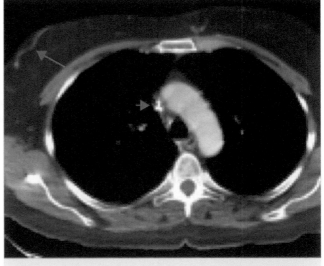

Fig. 9.3 Note early development of anterior chest wall collaterals (blue arrow) and narrowed superior vena cava surrounding the port catheter (blue arrowhead).

hemopericardium from SVC balloon dilatation, leading to surgical intervention or death. The patient elected for attempted stripping of her preexisting port with subsequent new port placement if this was unsuccessful, and consented to balloon dilation with possible stent placement in the SVC.

9.2.5 Details of Procedure

After obtaining informed consent, the patient was placed on the fluoroscopy table in supine position. Patency of the right common femoral vein was confirmed with a brief ultrasound exam. The right groin was prepped and draped in the usual sterile fashion. The skin and subcutaneous soft tissues were anesthetized using 1% lidocaine. A small incision was made with a #11 scalpel. Access to the right common femoral vein was obtained with ultrasound guidance using micropuncture technique and a 25-cm 6-French vascular sheath was positioned with its tip in the inferior vena cava (IVC). The sidearm of the sheath was flushed and connected to an infusion of heparinized saline solution.

Over a 0.035-inch, 180-cm-length Glidewire Advantage guidewire (Terumo Medical Corporation, Somerset, NJ), a 4-French 100-cm hydrophilic angled catheter was advanced across the SVC stenosis into the right brachiocephalic vein and venography was performed (▶ Fig. 9.4a). There was retrograde flow of contrast from the right brachiocephalic vein into the azygous vein without opacification of the SVC or right atrium.

The diagnostic catheter was exchanged for an 8 mm by 4 cm Ultraverse balloon (BARD Peripheral Vascular, Tempe, AZ). Balloon dilation of the SVC was performed, with a significant waist identified at the level of the catheter tip (▶ Fig. 9.4b; ▶ Fig. 9.4c; ▶ Fig. 9.4d). Subsequently, a 10 mm by 4 cm balloon was easily inflated at the same level without residual waist or patient discomfort. Final central venography confirmed restored antegrade flow of contrast from the right brachiocephalic vein through the SVC (▶ Fig. 9.4e). Due to presentation with port

dysfunction without symptoms of SVC syndrome, stenting of the SVC was not pursued.

Due to persistent adherence of the catheter to the vein wall/fibrin sheath, with inability to snare the catheter to strip the sheath, decision was made to place a new catheter in the reestablished lumen. A new 9.5-French dual-lumen port was placed without difficulty via right internal jugular vein access (▶ Fig. 9.5), with removal of the left subclavian port. The catheter tip was positioned significantly deeper than the original port, with the tip terminating at the junction of the upper and mid-thirds of the right atrium. The patient's cardiac rhythm was observed for several minutes to ensure no evidence of ectopy incited by the catheter. The patient was discharged home the same day.

9.2.6 Follow-up

The new port served the patient well up to 6 months after the intervention. Unfortunately, the patient's metastatic disease burden continued to progress despite therapy. She declined further therapy and pursued hospice care.

9.3 Epidemiology and Scope of the Problem

The spectrum of disease processes treated for which long-term central venous catheter access is required is vast, including but not limited to end-stage renal disease, cancer, infection, malnutrition, and pulmonary hypertension. Any patient requiring chronic, recurrent peripheral infusion therapy may also require central venous catheter access as peripheral veins thrombose.

Over 5 million central venous catheters are placed in the United States each year.[1,2] From 1992 to 2011, placement of long-term central venous access devices in the Medicare patient population increased by an astounding 303% nationally, from

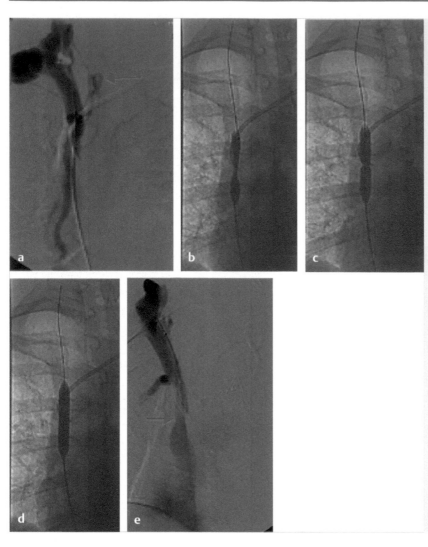

Fig. 9.4 (a) Central venogram demonstrating retrograde contrast flow from the right brachiocephalic vein into a prominent azygous vein and mediastinal venous collaterals (*arrow*). Note lack of inline anterograde flow along the diagnostic catheter. (b–d) Inflation of the balloon at the level of the port tip resulted in a significant waist that persisted through subsequent inflation and was eventually overcome at burst pressure. (e) Central venogram performed above the left subclavian port catheter tip demonstrates improved inline flow from the right brachiocephalic vein through superior vena cava with robust right atrial and early pulmonary artery enhancement. A small residual waist of the mid SVC was noted (*arrow*) but not pursued with stent placement at this time due to the appearance of brisk flow past the stenosis.

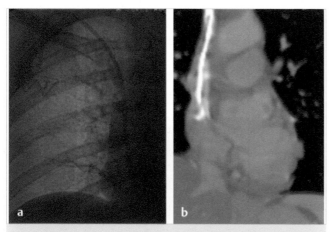

Fig. 9.5 New dual-lumen 9.5-French port catheter placed via right internal jugular vein approach. When compared to Fig. 9.1, note deeper positioning of the catheter (a). Depth of the catheter somewhat exaggerated by low inspiratory lung volumes on this image. Note with arms over head on a chest CT, the catheter pulls back to the superior cavoatrial junction (b).

76,444 to 307,838.[3] Per the U.S. Renal Data System, 80.2% of patients with end-stage renal disease were using dialysis catheters for initiation of hemodialysis by the end of 2013, translating to approximately 376,900 patients.[4]

As the clinical indications for and number of patients requiring central venous access increase, the demand for expertise in those managing venous access also increases. The interventional radiologist is in a unique position as both procedural and clinical content expert in the entire range of central venous access challenges and considerations. While many medical providers are able to place central venous catheters into a patent subclavian, internal jugular, or basilic vein, it is incumbent upon the interventional radiologist to uphold National Kidney Foundation Kidney Disease Outcomes Quality Initiative (NKF KDOQI) guidelines (www.kidney.org) for correct vein choice and preserve arm veins for possible future dialysis fistula/graft creation. Any clinician can remove a catheter in a bacteremic patient; the interventional radiologist should remind the clinical team of current Centers for Disease Control (CDC) guidelines and provide strategies that potentially preserve access for these patients.

Any clinician can manage a patient with a stenosed or occluded SVC by placement of a femoral catheter; the interventional radiologist can reconstruct, preserve, or obtain central venous access through a wide variety of techniques.

As the number and duration of long-term central venous catheters increases, managing complex vascular access will become a greater need. The interventional radiologist, as a steward of central venous access, should work to ensure excellent outcomes for patients from initial catheter placement and beyond.

9.3.1 Patient Presentation and Evaluation

There are numerous factors to be considered in the evaluation of a patient for central venous access, and the evaluation should allow selection of the most appropriate catheter for the patient's needs. In simplest terms, the interventional radiologist needs to determine what the catheter will be used for, how many lumens are necessary, how long the catheter will dwell within the patient, and how frequently it will be accessed. It is unreasonable to expect the referring provider to understand the nuances associated with the current breadth of central venous catheter choices, and the interventional radiologist should be prepared to make recommendations regarding appropriate access choice, rather than simply provide a technical service. A cursory understanding of how the catheter will be used will rapidly narrow down the choices for the correct catheter. ▶ Table 9.1 provides a basic framework for catheter selection and procedural planning.

Table 9.1 Framework for venous access patient evaluation

Catheter choice	• Type of therapy—continuous vs. intermittent • Duration of therapy—long term vs. short term

Previous access	• Reason for removal:
	  ○ Vessel thrombosis
	  ○ Infection
	  ○ Catheter migration or malposition
	• Patient experience:
	  ○ Issues with sedation at the time of or prior to catheter insertion
	  ○ Catheter's impact on quality of life

Preprocedure workup	• Consents
	• Labs:
	  ○ Platelet level—ensure > 30,000/mL
	  ○ Coagulation panel
	• Appropriate medications withheld
	• Allergies reviewed
	• Assessed for moderate sedation

Anatomy	• Jugular vein patency • Potential candidate for dialysis fistula graft • History of physical exam signs of central venous occlusion

Technique	• Conventional ultrasound/fluoroscopic approach
	• Central venous recanalization
	  ○ Central venous stent
	  ○ Crossing technique
	  ○ *Standard wire/catheter technique*
	  ○ *Sharp recanalization*
	  ○ *Radiofrequency wire*

9.3.2 Duration of Access Requirement

Short-term access can generally be achieved with a peripheral IV (PIV). PIVs are appropriate for nonsclerosant and nonvesicant agents that need to be administered intravenously for short durations. The most common indication for a PIV would be for intravenous crystalloid infusions during hospitalization or for rapid resuscitation. Saline is isotonic to the blood and can be rapidly infused in a peripheral vein with few adverse consequences. Many hospitals require that PIVs be changed every few days to avoid thrombophlebitis or local infection. With ever shortening lengths of stay, most patients will likely only need one PIV during a hospitalization. For this reason, the CDC recommends peripherally inserted central catheters (PICCs) and midline catheters only be placed when the duration of IV access will be more than 6 days.[5]

When access is needed for a longer duration, for example, 6 weeks of IV antibiotics for treatment of osteomyelitis, a PICC is a suitable peripherally inserted line that can be maintained for a long duration with limited risk of infection. When treatment is needed for several months or longer, then a tunneled catheter may be better than a PICC because the use of a tunneled cuffed catheter can further reduce the risk of infection. Finally, ports represent long-term access devices that are appropriate when accessed only intermittently.

9.3.3 Sclerosants and Vesicants

Sclerosants and vesicants are drugs that have a direct caustic effect on the endothelium, related to the pH and the osmolality of the medication. Vesicants are defined as drugs that can cause tissue destruction or skin blistering, while irritants are any drug with a pH of less than 5 or greater than 9. Examples of drugs and infusions that are vesicants are 10% dextrose, dopamine, midazolam, lorazepam, nitroprusside, potassium chloride in > 40 mEq, total parenteral nutrition (TPN), and vancomycin. Irritants include drugs such as ciprofloxacin, ceftriaxone, fluconazole, morphine, octreotide, and propofol.

It is very important to restrict the use of vesicants and irritants to central veins where adequate mixing can occur. This is important for the prevention of thrombophlebitis and venous occlusion. It has been demonstrated that extremes of pH and osmolarity increase venous thrombosis rate.[6,7]

9.3.4 Lumens Required

The more lumens a catheter has, the larger the device and the more manipulation it will undergo. This leads to an increase in the risk of infection and venous thrombosis. Ideally, when requested to provide venous access, systems should be in place to ensure that each lumen of the access device is justified on the basis of either continuous simultaneous infusion or incompatibility of medications. When there are more lumens, each will be frequently manipulated during changes of medications and the risk of infection goes up. For this reason, CDC guidelines recommend limiting the number of lumens to the minimum needed for infusions.[8]

Another consideration with respect to lumens is that the size of the catheter increases with increasing number of lumens. As a consequence, in a study of triple-lumen PICCs, the trial was terminated early due to an unacceptable thrombosis rate associated with three-lumen 7-French PICC lines.[8]

9.3.5 Frequency of Use: Intermittent or Continuous Access

The frequency of administration is a factor when considering placing a port. In general, the advantage of a port over an externalized tunneled catheter is a lower rate of infection because the port does not need to be continuously accessed. For example, typical chemotherapy regimens involve several days of chemotherapy every 3 to 4 weeks. In this situation, the port makes sense because between treatments the port is completely subcutaneous and at very low risk of infection. However, if a port were used for TPN, daily access would raise the infection rate to one approaching that of a tunneled catheter. The consequences of an infected port are greater, in that an infected port would require an incision and dissection to remove the device. For this reason, daily infusions or continuous infusions should be given through tunneled catheters rather than ports.

9.3.6 Flow Rates

Flow rates should be considered for specific situations such as dialysis and plasmapheresis. Flow rates are directly proportionate to catheter inner diameter (ID), and inversely proportionate to catheter length. Therefore, for volume resuscitation, short large catheters are best, whether peripheral or central, and resuscitation through a PICC should be avoided. In general, the highest flow rates are required for dialysis treatments (generally between 400 and 500 mL/min), and for this purpose a large ID is desired. It is reasonable to attempt to place the smallest outer diameter (OD) catheter that will accomplish necessary flow rates, due to the higher risk of vascular thrombosis or stenosis with larger catheters. Minimizing catheter length may allow for placement of a smaller diameter catheter for improved long-term outcomes. Plasmapheresis is generally run at flow rates of 250 mL/min and some of the older dialysis catheters designs can achieve this with a slightly smaller profile than current dialysis catheters (12.5 vs. 14.5 French). The 9.6-French Hickman catheter (Bard Peripheral Vascular, Tempe, AZ), which is 90 cm in length and has a 1.6-mm ID, can sustain a flow rate of 80 mL/min. This is typically adequate for most infusion therapy.

9.4 Considerations for Specific Indications

9.4.1 Hemodialysis

Understanding the pathogenesis of the patient's renal insufficiency and close communication with the nephrology service is vital. In cases of acute renal insufficiency, determine whether a temporary, nontunneled catheter will suffice until there has been appropriate treatment and recovery of the patient's native renal function. If more long-term or permanent dialysis needs are anticipated, determine where along the arc of decision making the patient may be for upper extremity fistula/graft creation allowing avoidance of ipsilateral catheter placement if possible.

9.4.2 Infection

For most patients, a PICC will suffice for long-term intravenous antibiotic therapy. A key consideration is the patient's underlying renal function. The AV Fistula First Breakthrough Initiative National Coalition recommends against using PICCs in patients at risk for or with known midstage 3 chronic kidney disease or higher renal disease. In this instance, it is prudent to use a low-profile tunneled central venous catheter placed via an internal jugular vein approach, rather than peripherally inserting a catheter, due to the long-term consequences of endothelial damage in this patient population. While many larger health systems have protocols in place to prevent PICC placement in patients with renal insufficiency, this practice is by no means universal. The interventional radiologist can be a key advocate in assuring hospital compliance with this initiative.

An additional consideration in assessing for PICC versus tunneled catheter placement is a patient's mentation. If the patient has an altered mental status potentially placing the PICC at risk of accidental removal, tunneled access may be more suitable and secure. For a patient who may be aggressive enough to remove tunneled catheters, these may be tunneled across the supraclavicular fossa, superficial to the trapezius musculature, to make the catheter harder to reach by the patient.

9.4.3 Total Parenteral Nutrition

TPN is a broad title given to any intravenous supplementation used to bypass the gastrointestinal tract. The initial decision regarding catheter type again comes down to duration, determining whether a PICC is adequate or if a tunneled catheter will be needed. There are a variety of tunneled catheters that differ in their OD, number of lumens, and ID. The type of TPN solution the patient will receive will dictate the caliber of lumen needed. The TPN lumen should only be used for TPN. If there is anticipation for intravenous medication or frequent blood draws, this will require at least one additional lumen.

A complete review of the various catheters and their properties would exhaust the space in this text. Review of the vendor catalogues which provide details of the different catheter characteristics is a useful endeavor to establish a basic knowledge of the pros and cons of different devices for different uses. For example, there are significant differences between a 10-French dual-lumen Leonard catheter (Bard Peripheral Vascular, Tempe, AZ) and a 9-French dual-lumen Hickman catheter. The Leonard catheter lumens are equal in ID (1.3 mm) as compared to the Hickman catheter, with a 1.3-mm red lumen ID and a 0.7-mm white lumen ID. Careful consideration as to the viscosity of the solution for which each lumen is utilized will help optimize infusion rates, minimize catheter size, and decrease possibility of luminal occlusion. An active dialogue with the TPN service can help determine which catheters meet the needs of the majority of the patient population. Maintaining and regularly reviewing practice level quality data, including catheter-related infections and frequency of need for catheter repair/exchange, can help guide quality improvement efforts to optimize patient care in this arena.

9.4.4 Chemotherapy

The most common catheter choice for administration of chemotherapy is the subcutaneous port. Choice between single- and dual-lumen port catheter placement should be predicated upon the need for simultaneous infusion. Single-lumen catheters will suffice for the majority of cancer patients and are anecdotally better tolerated by patients due to smaller profile of the reservoir. Reservoirs come in a variety of compositions from various manufactures and will not be comprehensively reviewed here.

Determining a patient preference for side of placement may help improve the patient's functionality and quality of life. One patient disclosed that he preferred a left-sided chest port because he was an avid rifle shooter and was concerned how the butt of the rifle would sit against his chest with the subcutaneous reservoir in place. Furthermore, he raised the question about the kick of the gun resulting in disconnection between the catheter and reservoir. Therefore, a left-sided port was placed. Though a regionally common example, this example underlines the importance of the consideration of patient needs, to facilitate improved quality of life.

9.4.5 Previous Vascular Access

When replacement or repeat vascular access is needed, knowledge regarding the circumstances of the prior access is necessary: what, where, when, and why? The answers to these questions should be known before the patient arrives in the IR suite.

What type of catheter did the patient previously have? Something as simple as prior central line placement may be pertinent if there was a documented complication or difficulty at that time. Prior tunneled dialysis catheter placement or prior malpositioned port introduces the possibility of access vein occlusion and central venous stenosis.

Location of the prior catheter is an important consideration. Multiple prior right internal jugular vein tunneled dialysis catheter placements will decrease the probability of right internal jugular vein patency and should prompt a thorough ultrasound assessment prior to the patient being prepped and draped.

When and why the prior access was removed are important questions to answer. If the patient's most recent port or tunneled dialysis catheter was removed for infection, has the patient been appropriately treated? Do they meet criteria for new implanted/tunneled catheter placement or should a temporary catheter be placed until they do? Management of this scenario will be discussed in detail below.

9.5 Technical Tips and Tricks

9.5.1 Basics of Procedure

Most interventional radiologists have a routine, automatic approach to the placement of the uncomplicated central venous access. There is an advantage to establishing a standard approach, the fundamentals of which are outlined here. High variability exists in the approach used and the order of completion of the steps to catheter placement.

1. Ultrasound the anticipated target vein prior to scrubbing and ensure that the ultrasound settings are optimized to see the vein best.
2. Ensure that a complete barrier scrub is performed to minimize the risk of infection from placement. For physician performance measures, standard documentation

of the procedure should include the adherence to "CLIP" (central line insertion practices) bundle criteria mandated by the CDC: chlorhexidine scrub, prep dry prior to insertion, five maximal sterile barriers used, including gloves, gown, cap, mask, and large sterile drape covering patient's entire body.
3. Puncture the vein with direct visualization with ultrasound, directly observing the needle tip puncture the wall of the vein.
4. Advance a wire into the vein. Use of a micropuncture system may reduce the risk of air embolus.
5. Make the tunnel +/– port pocket.
6. Exchange the access catheter for the peel-away sheath.
7. Quickly exchange the wire for the catheter to avoid air embolus.
8. Perform fluoroscopy to ensure the tip is appropriately positioned before removing the peel-away sheath.
9. Remove the peel-away sheath and adjust the catheter to optimize placement of the tip near the junction of the SVC and the right atrium.
10. Obtain an image of the catheter to document appropriate location. Note that this will be supine and that the tip position is likely to change when the patient is moved form a supine to an upright position.

9.5.2 Access Dilation

Passage of dilators and the peel-away sheath reflects one of the most critical moments of central venous access. Kinking of the guidewire causes a sharp point at the bend of the wire, which can penetrate the SVC/right atrium when aggressively advanced as a unit. There are a few technical maneuvers that can significantly reduce the risk of wire kinking and thus reduce the risk of vascular trauma. One technique is to slightly withdraw the wire during advancement of the dilators and peel-away sheath ensuring a smooth coaxial interface between the wire and dilator/sheath. Immediately upon encountering resistance, advancement of the dilator/sheath should stop, and the trajectory of the dilator/sheath evaluated under fluoroscopy. Changing the plane of the dilator/sheath to one more parallel with the patient/vessel will usually allow advancement. Difficult anatomy may require a wire upgrade from that which comes with the catheter kit. In tough cases, a longer wire placed deep into the IVC will ensure enough purchase to perform the withdraw technique while not losing access.

In the event of persistent resistance to dilation, increased guidewire stiffness is helpful. For patients that have a history of multiple prior catheters, anticipate encountering scar tissue and select an appropriately stiff wire for dilation. Another useful approach is the addition of intermediate dilator sizes. Most tunneled dialysis catheter kits come with two dilators and the peel-away sheath. A few intermediary dilatations in addition to what is provided in the kit may facilitate peel-away sheath passage.

9.5.3 Left-Sided Access

Left-sided central venous access is inherently more challenging due to two natural curves the catheter must traverse before taking its final position: (1) curve at the junction of the left internal jugular vein (LIJV) with the left subclavian vein (LSCV); (2) curve at the junction of the left brachiocephalic vein junction with the right, forming the SVC. Therefore, catheter length from left-sided access must take into account both the increased distance of LIJV access compared to right internal jugular vein, and the length "eaten up" by the aforementioned curves as well. On initial placement, the catheter will tend to be stiffer, somewhat straightening the anatomic curves. As the catheter warms to body temperature and becomes more compliant, it will tend to conform more to the curvatures and foreshorten from its original position.

Foreshortening of left-sided access is particularly problematic for several reasons. From a simple malposition perspective, a tunneled dialysis catheter that was in the right atrium upon implantation may not function adequately if the tip is reduced back to the SVC. A unique malposition challenge from left-sided access is the tip terminating in the azygos vein, either acutely or upon delayed foreshortening/repositioning. In the acute setting, this is easily remedied by retracting and repositioning the catheter. If there is any doubt about stability of position, it is reasonable to exchange for a longer catheter in the acute setting to prevent the delayed grief.

9.5.4 The Kinked Peel-Away Sheath

This challenge tends to go hand in hand with left-sided internal jugular vein access as the inherent curves, described above, exert force upon the sheath as the internal dilator is removed. The kink can make it difficult or impossible to advance the catheter. Kinks at the skin level are easily remedied by pinching out the kink or peeling down to/beyond the kink. Internal kinks are more challenging. One initial approach to remedying a kink is to replace the inner dilator to relieve the kink and either advance or slightly retract the sheath/dilator system and reattempt catheter passage. Sometimes the kink will return immediately upon removing the internal dilator. Placing a stiff wire through the sheath, over which to advance the catheter, or placement of a stiff wire into the catheter to give the catheter more body for pushability may allow passage. If still unsuccessful, consider exchange for a new peel-away sheath.

9.6 Potential Complications and Pitfalls

9.6.1 Acute and Intraprocedural Complications

Pneumothorax: The overall pneumothorax rate associated with central venous access placement ranges from 1 to 6% in the literature, with well-established elements that increase the risk including catheters placed in emergent situations, subclavian vein access, increased number of passes, and larger bore catheters.[9] These data do not discriminate between attempts under ultrasound guidance versus anatomical landmarks. Ultrasound guidance has been proven to prevent the number of mechanical complications.[10,11] With impeccable ultrasound-guided technique where there is constant visualization of the needle approaching the jugular vein, the risk of pneumothorax likely approaches 0%.

There are some patients that are inherently more challenging in terms of optimizing visualization of the internal jugular vein. The standard trifecta is the obese tracheostomy patient with a short neck. It may only be possible to get a portion of the ultrasound footprint in a useful position for guidance. If the needle is not aligned perfectly with the probe, there is a chance of overreaching the target and creating a pneumothorax. Use help from all members of the team, such as requesting assistance from the respiratory therapist in turning the patient's head and stabilizing the airway. The other consideration is to allow a slightly higher access above the clavicle than usual for better visualization. Both of these adjustments will decrease the likelihood of complication.

9.6.2 Air Embolism

The true incidence of air embolization during central venous access is likely higher than the reported 0.2 to 1%[12] due to the range of presentations. The clinical manifestations of a significant air embolism can include chest pain, dyspnea, coughing, hypoxemia, and tachyarrhythmia with possibility of fulminant cardiopulmonary collapse.

Air can be introduced into the venous system at multiple points throughout central venous access placement with the underlying commonality of poor seal between the external atmosphere and negative pressure environment of the vein lumen. While not an original concept, it bears repeating that prevention is key. Patients who can comply with commands should be talked through performing a Valsalva maneuver during wire exchanges, advancement of dilators, and advancement of a catheter through the peel-away sheath. For patients unable to follow commands, timing the transitions with exhalation is advised. Several larger bore catheters have valved peel-away sheaths which has been proven to reduce the risk of air embolism.[13]

If suspected, immediately provide a nonrebreather oxygen mask at 100%. This intervention alone has been described as sufficient to resuscitate the patient without additional maneuvers. If the patient does not respond or continues to decompensate, attempt to position the patient in left lateral decubitus position and place the table in Trendelenburg. The goal is to trap the antidependent air in the right atrium. This should be followed by catheter aspiration to remove the trapped air.

9.6.3 Arrhythmia

It is hypothesized that wire/catheter irritation of the myocardial surface instigates arrhythmia. The exact mechanism of this is not fully understood. A study by Stuart et al reviewed arrhythmias presenting during central venous access/exchange procedures in 51 patients and concluded that atrial arrhythmias occurred in 41% of procedures, while ventricular arrhythmias occurred in 25%.[14]

When venous access is performed in the IR suite, patients should receive continuous hemodynamic monitoring, regardless of the type of sedation/anesthesia employed. Electrocardiographic monitoring is key in evaluating for arrhythmias during wire/catheter manipulation, which may otherwise go unnoticed until clinically deleterious.

There is some ability to predict which patients will be at higher risk of arrhythmia during central venous access procedures. A study by Fiaccadori et al looked at 201 guidewire insertions in 171 patients and concluded that acute renal failure was an independent risk factor for developing arrhythmia.[15] Perhaps less risky with fluoroscopic guidance, guidewire overinsertion was also determined as an independent risk factor for inciting arrhythmia. Serum hyperkalemia was not identified as a significant independent risk factor. It is important to note that all cases of arrhythmia were transient without acute cardiopulmonary complication or lasting sequelae.

There is some debate as to whether knowledge of an increased chance of arrhythmia during central venous access should change the procedural plan. For patients in acute renal failure, some will opt to place a femoral catheter until the patient has undergone dialysis to correct serum electrolyte abnormalities, followed by placement of more long-term access when the patient has clinically improved. Others proceed with intended internal jugular access with mental preparedness to deal with periprocedural arrhythmia if needed. There is no study or data to definitely advocate one approach over the other.

Prompt removal of the wire will resolve the arrhythmia a vast majority of the time. If arrhythmia persists, it may be necessary to initiate ACLS (advanced cardiac life support) protocols and, in some instances, activate the institutional code team.

9.6.4 Catheter Malposition

The definition of optimal catheter tip position has evolved over time. In 1989, the Food and Drug Administration (FDA) stated that central venous catheter tips should not be placed in or allowed to migrate into the heart. By 1998, the National Association of Vascular Access Networks released a position statement that the tip of a PICC should be placed in the lower one-third of the SVC close to the junction of the SVC and right atrium. In 2003, the SIR *Reporting Standards for Central Venous Access* stated that the "ideal tip location for central venous access catheters has yet to be determined."[16]

The crux of the controversy is a potential conflict between optimizing patient safety and optimization of catheter performance. The key complications observed, which inform these recommendations, are cardiac perforation and tamponade, arrhythmias, and catheter-induced thrombosis. Currently, efforts to clarify optimal catheter tip position are ongoing. The Society of Interventional Radiology (SIR) promotes use of the American College of Radiology/Society of Interventional Radiology (ACR/SIR) IR Registry and structured reporting for purposes of broad-based data collection on elements of central venous catheter placement. The registry will allow analysis of multiple data elements, including the relevance of catheter tip position to outcomes. Tracking of tip position in the registry is by description of position relative to vertebral body units, based on the observation that cavoatrial junction is reproducibly described using this nomenclature.

Definitive critical analysis of ideal catheter tip position has been hindered by lack of uniformity in nomenclature, investigational methods, and reporting standards. Determination of catheter tip position with chest radiography is often imprecise with significant interobserver variability. A study by Song et al evaluated the position of the cavoatrial junction by correlating CTAs and chest X-rays (CXR) in 560 patients presenting in acute coronary syndrome. These authors discovered the mean cavoa-

trial position was 2.5 vertebral body units below the carina on CTA and 2.4 vertebral body units below on CXR with 95% limits of agreement between –0.6 and +0.3.[17] The initial goal of the Venous Access: National Guideline and Registry Development (VANGuaRD) initiative, launched in 2015 and cosponsored by the SIR, is to develop an "interoperative vocabulary" for reporting to allow for data collection to improve patient-centered outcomes relative to central venous access.

9.6.5 Delayed Complications

Infection

Infections in the setting of existing central venous access are a common clinical challenge. Catheter-related infection is the leading cause of morbidity and subsequent catheter removal in dialysis patients.[18,19] More specifically, infection is cited as the second leading cause of death in patients with end-stage renal disease, with catheter-related bloodstream infection (CRBSI) being the underlying cause in the majority of infections.

A primary consideration in placement of central venous access devices is prevention of infection. The site of catheter insertion should be appropriately prepped and draped. The skin should be prepped with an antiseptic solution. According to a 2002 article in the *Annals of Internal Medicine*, there was a significant reduction of bloodstream infections associated with central venous access insertion when chlorohexidine gluconate was used versus povidone-iodine.[20] Per 2011 Guidelines for the Prevention of Catheter-Related Infections (CDC), the skin should be cleaned with > 0.5% chlorohexidine solution. Most institutions use 2% chlorohexidine. The solution should be applied by a vigorous back-and-forth rubbing for at least 30 seconds. The solution should be allowed to air dry for at least 2 minutes. Elements of maximal sterile barrier precautions are defined by the CDC, and include wearing a sterile gown, sterile gloves, mask, and cap. These recommendations also define that a sterile whole-body drape should be used. Per the 2016 Physician Quality and Reporting System, there must be documentation that all elements of maximal sterile barrier technique (CLIP bundle) were employed during catheter placement.

The next consideration for infection prevention is whether antibiotic administration is appropriate. Regarding routine prophylaxis for central venous access procedures, the SIR Practice Guideline for Adult Antibiotic Prophylaxis during Vascular and Interventional Radiology Procedures concluded "no consensus" with respect to their use, but did note that for immunocompromised patients requiring access for chemotherapy, or those with a history of catheter infection, one could consider use of cefazolin, 1 g intravenously, or vancomycin or clindamycin in patients with penicillin allergy.[21] Similarly, the CDC recommends against using systemic antimicrobial prophylaxis routinely before placement of an intravascular catheter. There is a tendency to routinely use a preprocedure antibiotic with port insertion, with the rationale that these patients are often in an immunocompromised state. Johnson and colleagues recently published a systematic review, evaluating 2,154 patients undergoing placement of totally implantable vascular access devices (TIVADs) to evaluate the benefit of prophylactic antibiotic use. The authors showed no statistically significant effect on development of catheter infection with use of antibiotics, but did demonstrate increased risk of allergic reaction and additional cost in the antibiotic cohort, supporting only selective use of antibiotics in patients undergoing TIVAD placement.[22]

A pertinent consideration is the use of various impregnated catheters. A 2009 meta-analysis by Rabindranath et al evaluated a total of 29 trials including 2,886 patients and 3,005 catheters. This study revealed that antimicrobial lock therapy and exit-site antimicrobial therapies were successful in reducing CRBSI. The challenge becomes potential promotion of antimicrobial resistance with antimicrobial lock therapy; thus, there is no agreed universal recommendation as to when it is appropriate or an optimal regimen. The Rabindranath study revealed no significant reduction in CRBSI when utilizing antimicrobial-coated hemodialysis catheters or perioperative systemic antibiotic administration.[23]

The next consideration is management of the patient that presents with a suspected bloodstream infection. It is important to first validate the diagnosis of CRBSI, ensuring that requirements for making a diagnosis have been met. According to the 2009 Infectious Diseases Society of America (IDSA) guidelines,[24] specimens should be obtained both from the catheter hub and from a peripheral vein, with equal volume in both samples, prior to initiation of antimicrobial therapy. The two specimens should have specific characteristics to meet criteria for CRBSI. These include same organism from both specimens; colony count of microbes from catheter sample should be at least three times greater than that in the peripheral sample; growth of microbes from the catheter sample should precede growth from peripheral blood sample by at least 2 hours (differential time to positivity [DTP] criterion). A sample from the catheter or from peripheral blood, alone, is not sufficient to confirm CRBSI.

The 2009 IDSA guidelines recommend removal of long-term catheters in the following settings:
- Severe clinical sepsis.
- Suppurative thrombophlebitis.
- Confirmed endocarditis.
- Confirmed osteomyelitis.
- Bloodstream infection persisting despite greater than 72 hours of antimicrobial therapy, to which the infecting microbes are susceptible.
- Infections due to confirmed *Staphylococcus aureus*, *Pseudomonas aeruginosa*, fungi, or mycobacteria.

Uncomplicated CRBSI involving long-term catheters (patients in which fever resolves within 72 hours, without intravascular hardware and with no evidence of endocarditis or suppurative thrombophlebitis) due to coagulase-negative *Staphylococcus* species, enterococci, or gram-negative bacilli can initially be treated with attempted catheter salvage using a combination of systemic antimicrobial and antimicrobial lock therapy. When antibiotic lock therapy cannot be used, systemic antibiotics should be administered through the colonized catheter if catheter salvage is desired. In these instances, catheters should be removed if there is persistent or relapsing bacteremia after 72 hours of antibiotic therapy, or clinical deterioration.[24]

Catheter Malfunction

The cause of a catheter malfunction will often be evident combining the details obtained from patient and referring provider interviews, interrogation of a chest radiograph, and inspection of the catheter, itself (▶ Fig. 9.6). Catheter malfunctions can be related to any segment of the catheter or device, including issues with the external connections, the reservoir and its connection to the catheter (in the case of a port), the subcutaneous tract, the catheter lumen, the intravascular course, the tip position, or the status of the terminal vessel. The nature of the dysfunction should be determined (inability to access, inability to aspirate, inability to flush, resistance to flushing, pain with flushing, etc.) to guide the potential approach to remediation.

The most common causes of catheter malfunction are suboptimal tip position and development of catheter tip thrombosis or fibrin sheath (▶ Fig. 9.7). With catheters that fail to aspirate, but continue to have adequate infusion rates, tip position above the SVC should be considered, and this should be evident on a chest radiograph. In this scenario, it is recommended that the catheter be replaced and repositioned, such that the tip is free from the vessel wall at an optimized position in the distal SVC or superior right atrium. Other catheter tip displacements can be seen, secondary to proximal catheter buckling, either within the vessel or, if a tunneled catheter, within the subcutaneous tract. Attempts can be made at preserving the catheter by snaring the tip in order to reduce the kink or buckle, but such catheters often ultimately require replacement due to anatomy or catheter memory reproducing the kink after repositioning.

Catheters that appear to be appropriately positioned that continue to fail on aspiration likely have developed a fibrin sheath surrounding or adjacent to the tip. Such failing catheters can be fluoroscopically evaluated with performance

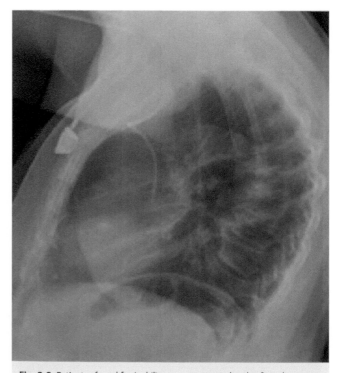

Fig. 9.6 Patient referred for inability to access port shortly after placement. Lateral view of the chest demonstrates a 180-degree flip of the reservoir.

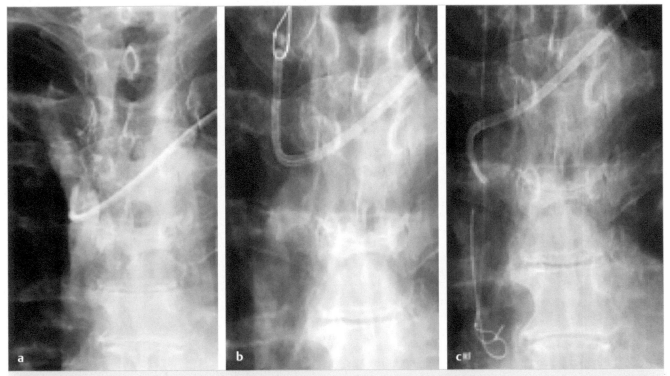

Fig. 9.7 Surgically placed port was sent for a portogram due to inability to aspirate through the catheter. The portogram demonstrated ease of flushing through the catheter (**a**); however, the tip was directed toward the right innominate vein instead of centrally. Through right internal jugular vein access, the catheter tips were secured with a snare and guidewire, then redirected inferiorly (**b, c**). Final portogram demonstrated improved aspiration through the catheter and good central venous opacification. This catheter is too short and, in all likelihood, will again migrate to malposition.

of venography through the catheter to evaluate for contrast retention surrounding the tip. It is advisable to be prepared to fix or replace the catheter in the same setting as the evaluation, as these catheters almost invariably require intervention. Various approaches exist to management. Some operators will place a wire through the catheter, removing it and advancing a balloon over the wire for angioplasty of the fibrin sheath. Such disruption of the fibrin channel should allow for resolution of the issue with placement of a new catheter over the same wire. However, others choose to select a completely new path outside of the formed sheath, placing a new catheter via a fresh stick, such that it is free from the channel, alongside the fibrin sheath, and then removing the malfunctioning catheter. Finally, some choose to attempt to snare the catheter, from either an internal jugular or common femoral approach to "strip" the sheath away from the catheter.

Ports are accompanied with their own set of challenges requiring specific considerations. As these devices tend to have prolonged dwell times, catheter fracture, catheter fixation within mature fibrin sheath, and disconnection of the catheter from the reservoir are all considerations in a longstanding port. Similarly, with poor catheter maintenance, catheter lumens may become chronically occluded and unsalvageable, requiring removal or replacement. In particular, ports can be seen to repeatedly malfunction in patients with higher body mass index (BMI) due to special challenges related to placement. In patients with substantial subcutaneous fat in the upper chest and neck, port access can be a chronic problem and the placement of the port should take into consideration the ability

to access. Larger devices, ideally placed in a relatively superficial position over a bony prominence if possible, will facilitate access, as it is helpful to have a "backstop" to stabilize the reservoir for needle insertion. Reservoirs may rotate or flip when the subcutaneous pocket is capacious, and this concern may warrant placement of anchoring sutures in selected patients even when it is not the usual practice of the operator. To avoid excessive retraction of the catheter tip when in upright position, chest wall soft tissues may be intentionally retracted caudally during tip positioning to reproduce the effects of gravity.

SVC Thrombosis

There are a number of risk factors for SVC thrombosis and stenosis, with longstanding central venous catheters representing the most common cause. With chronic irritation of the vessel wall, thrombosis and stenosis are seen to develop and seem to be accelerated in patients with subsequent placement of upper extremity arteriovenous fistula or graft. This acceleration of stenosis in the central veins is thought to be due to high flow rates seen in dialysis, with increased shear stress impacting remodeling of the veins.

The diagnosis of SVC stenosis can often be made clinically, based on upper extremity and facial edema and development of superficial venous collaterals that can be observed on physical exam. The distribution of edema and collateral formation will typically point to a unilateral central venous stenosis (brachiocephalic or subclavian), versus SVC when the process is bilateral. Symptoms can range from absent, to visible swelling, to functional compromise and pain, to life threatening in the case of SVC syndrome. Specific characteristics of SVC syndrome include facial and upper extremity edema, airway compromise, and headache, and warrant urgent intervention.

Depending on the presentation, SVC thrombosis may warrant intervention. With a chronic picture, many operators will elect for catheter thrombolysis to uncover underlying fixed stenosis, followed by angioplasty and stenting only if needed for symptom improvement. In the acute setting of SVC syndrome with SVC occlusion, it may be warranted to perform some degree of angioplasty up front at the initiation of thrombolysis to establish a lumen.

Upper Extremity Deep Venous Thrombosis

Development of upper extremity deep venous thrombosis (DVT) in the setting of central venous catheters is common. Prospective consideration of the risk of DVT in an individual patient is advisable prior to placement of central venous catheters, to determine best type and position for access. PICC placement exposes the longest segment of vein to endothelial damage, and poses the greatest risk for DVT. In general, it is advisable to avoid placement of catheters via a subclavian approach, since the subclavian access exposes a long segment of vein to catheter irritation, which can lead to stenosis/thrombosis. Catheters placed directly in subclavian veins are typically larger than the small-caliber PICCs leading not only to endothelial irritation, but also to luminal obstruction, adding to the risk of thrombosis. Internal jugular access exposes a shorter segment of central vein to catheter irritation, reducing the risk of clinically significant stenosis and thrombosis.

When patients with central venous catheters develop thrombosis, management should take into account the risk of the thrombosis, the ability to anticoagulate the patient, and the risk of removing versus maintaining the catheter. It is a common practice in some institutions to remove a vascular catheter when DVT is identified and to place a catheter contralaterally. This practice is not recommended, as it then exposes the patient to risk for additional DVT in a second location. Central venous catheter–associated DVT should be managed conservatively, maintaining any clinically useful catheter in place and anticoagulating, if possible, using low-molecular-weight heparin.

9.6.6 Central Venous Recanalization

In general, there are three techniques for venous recanalization, which can facilitate central catheter placement in patients with central venous occlusion. These include conventional wire/catheter navigation, sharp recanalization, and energy-based (radiofrequency, laser) recanalization. This section aims to provide a technical blueprint for each procedure, discuss the individual risks and possible complications of each technique, and provide a current literature review to evaluate their efficacy and safety.

Regardless of technique employed, all patients require a thorough workup. A detailed history and physical examination will help define the location and extent of central venous stenosis/occlusion and help determine what measures must be taken for central venous recanalization, such as whether to stent or not. Review of pertinent imaging is vital to make the patient's time in the IR suite as productive as possible. Venous Doppler

interrogation will help verify patent peripheral access sites and help infer the degree and severity of the central venous lesion. The importance of recognizing a benign from a malignant stenosis or occlusion cannot be overstated, and a quality CT angiogram of the chest can assist in evaluating for extrinsic compressive processes, determining lesion length, and establishing normal venous measurements for angioplasty and stent placement, if necessary. Review of standard laboratory values is important. Knowledge of compromised renal function in patients not yet requiring hemodialysis may lead to consideration of alternatives to iodinated contrast use, such as intravascular ultrasound, or minimization of contrast use.

Initial venous access for lesion characterization and crossing can be obtained from either internal jugular, brachial, femoral, or even subclavian vein if necessary. The right common femoral vein, if patent, provides a mechanical advantage for many lesions. Alternatively, upper extremity access can provide needed "running room" for approaching subclavian lesions. A 6- or 7-French-long sheath, with its tip positioned at the point of contact with the occlusion, will provide stability for the wire/catheter system. Some operators advise connecting the sidearm of the sheath to an infusion line of heparinized saline to avoid thrombus formation at the end of the sheath. Use of a tapered, directional catheter and a hydrophilic wire is recommended, attempting to maintain an intraluminal path. Subintimal recanalization can be difficult in veins. The subintimal space is subject to enlargement with manipulation, more readily that is seen in arterial recanalization, and this makes reentry a challenge. In the chest, the consequences of perforation are potentially life threatening. Therefore, maintenance of an intraluminal path is of greater importance.

For the interventional radiologist lacking experience in peripheral arterial disease interventions, developing familiarity with the current wires and catheters designed specifically to assist crossing chronic total arterial occlusions may be useful as these devices can be translatable to venous occlusions. For example, the Quick-Cross catheters (Spectranetics, Colorado Springs, CO) are support catheters that range in size from 0.035 to 0.014 inch. These catheters have a great deal of axial stiffness, and taper well onto a wire. The additional stiffness prevents catheter buckling when pushing into a tight channel over a guidewire. Additionally, there are specialized crossing wires with various tip stiffness (tip weighting), which provide more body to the wire tip when seeking a channel through the occlusion. This prevents distal wire tip buckling, which ultimately can lead to subintimal or extraluminal transgression. These crossing wires are also highly torqueable, allowing for greater directional control of the tip.

If the central venous occlusion cannot be crossed with the conventional wire/catheter technique from one anatomic approach, additional access is recommended, which may facilitate crossing the lesion from another direction. If unsuccessful, the dual access will still be beneficial for either sharp or radiofrequency wire recanalization.

Sharp recanalization encompasses a broad spectrum of instruments to cross a fibrous occlusion ranging from the back end of a stiff Glidewire (Terumo Medical Corporation, Somerset, NJ) to a modified Colapinto or Rosch-Uchida needle (Cook Medical, Bloomington, IN) (▶ Fig. 9.8). One interesting case report discussed using an Outback-LTD vascular reentry catheter

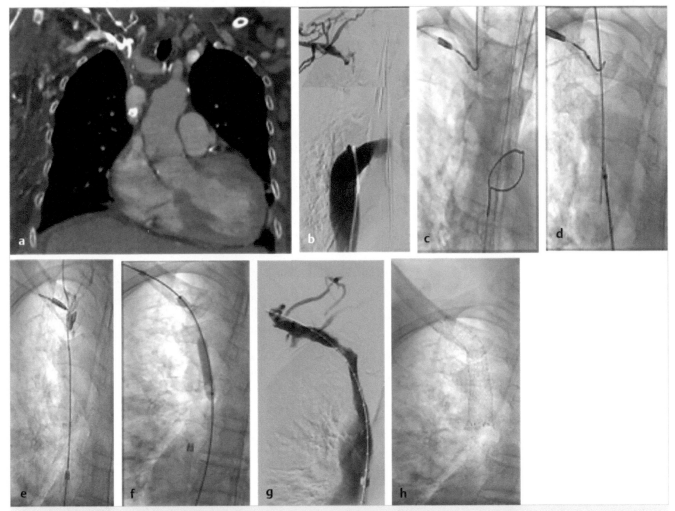

Fig. 9.8 Example of sharp recanalization. Coronal CT image **(a)** demonstrates a fibrous, partially calcified occlusion of a patient that presented with asymmetric right upper extremity edema. Access was gained via the right brachial and right common femoral veins to demonstrate the length of occlusion **(b)**. Snares were positioned on either side of the occlusion **(c)** which provided targets for the sharp needle recanalization. Needle entrapment within both snares **(d)** ensures a true-lumen course. Wire access was secured and angioplasty was performed **(e, f)** followed by venography **(g)** demonstrating establishment of a patent lumen with residual stenosis at the junction of the right subclavian and brachiocephalic veins. A 12-cm S.M.A.R.T. Control self-expanding nitinol stent (Cordis, Cardinal Health, Miami Lakes, FL) was placed across the lesion from the right subclavian vein to the superior vena cava **(h)**.

(Cordis, Cardinal Health, Miami Lakes, FL) resulting in successful right brachiocephalic vein recanalization.[25] The Outback LTD is a reentry catheter intended for chronic arterial occlusions that uses a 22-gauge nitinol cannula as a needle for passage of an 0.014-inch wire across an obstructing tissue plane.

For use of any sharp recanalization device, access on both sides of the lesion is suggested. Access will typically be obtained at the common femoral vein as well as via the internal jugular, brachial, subclavian, or large-enough collateral venous structures.[26,27] Diagnostic venography is performed to determine the extent of the occlusion. A target, such as a snare device, inflated balloon, or pigtail catheter, is placed on one side of the occlusion and the sharp device is carefully advanced toward the target. Advancement should be performed slowly using various obliquities to ensure the device does not deviate into an extraluminal course. Once the lesion has been crossed, a wire is passed through its lumen and snared, creating "through-and-through" secure wire access across the lesion.

No large trials have investigated the safety or efficacy of sharp recanalization. While not a thorough meta-analysis, review of four studies demonstrates a technical success rate approaching 96%.[26,27,28] Of 23 patients included in these series, one episode of mediastinal contrast extravasation was documented and treated with a stent graft; no significant clinical harm was reported as a result of this complication.[25]

Radiofrequency wire recanalization employs the same conceptual steps as described by Ferral et al for sharp recanalization: vein recanalization, creation of through-and-through access, and central catheter placement.[26] Guimaraes et al provide an excellent procedure description using the PowerWire RF Guidewire (Baylis Medical, Montreal, Quebec).[29] The PowerWire is a 0.035-inch wire that comes in a length of 250 cm. The distal tip of this device is short, rounded, radiopaque, and designed to be atraumatic when not active. Upon foot pedal activation from the power generator, a short radiofrequency burst is emitted from the tip. The catheter is advanced with intermittent power application under fluoroscopic guidance, targeting a snare device placed on the opposite side of the occlusion. Once the lesion is completely traversed, the Power-Wire is snared and pulled through the second access sheath to create through-and-through access as described with sharp recanalization technique. The same wire can be used as a support wire to perform subsequent venoplasty and stent placement, if necessary.

There is a limited pool of data currently available for radiofrequency wire central venous recanalization. The Guimaraes paper described successful central venous recanalization in 42 patients, with 100% technical success of this technique.[29] There was one complication reported in this series; a cardiac tamponade attributed to balloon dilatation following stent placement. A series by Sivananthan et al addressed 12 patients with 13 occlusions.[30] In this study, there was a technical success in crossing 9 out of 13 lesions (69%). Higher success rates were correlated with shorter occlusions and right brachiocephalic lesions compared to left. There was no statistical difference in success of crossing more versus less chronic occlusions. Vascular perforation by the radiofrequency wire occurred in four patients (31%) and did prove to be of clinical significance, or require additional intervention, in all four. A major complication, tracheal perforation, was reported in a patient with a long left brachiocephalic vein occlusion resulting in termination of the procedure, intubation, and escalation of care. The patient was extubated 8 days later and subsequently died on the same admission.

Upon successful crossing of the lesion, deciding what to do next depends on the clinical presentation and end goal. If the patient has well-developed collaterals and is relatively asymptomatic, the focus should be on making a channel large enough to accommodate the catheter. Once the lesion is crossed, angioplasty with a relatively small-caliber balloon should be performed to create a channel sufficient for passage of the peel-away sheath and catheter. If the patient has significant symptoms related to central venous stenosis or occlusion, central venous stenting prior to catheter placement will have a clinical benefit. In the case of dialysis patients, if upper extremity grafts/fistulas remain a consideration, central venous stenting should be pursued, as this may allow for sufficient venous flow to allow for optimizing dialysis access, beyond placement of a catheter.

9.7 Alternative Sites for Central Venous Access

9.7.1 Translumbar Approach

The translumbar venous access approach was first described in 1985 by Kenney et al,[31] and is a mainstay of venous access in patients with occlusion of conventional central venous access sites. Viewed as an end-stage vascular access option, translumbar catheter placement should be reserved for patients who have failed attempted recanalization, or are at high risk for complications from recanalization attempts. A series of 31 patients undergoing placement of translumbar IVC ports published by Butros et al revealed a 30-day complication rate of 9.7%, with average catheter use of 14.1 months, and an infection

rate of 0.08 per 1,000 catheter days.[32] A recent series of 33 patients with translumbar hemodialysis catheters by Nadolski et al revealed a major complication rate of 3.3% and median catheter time in situ of 61 days.[33] Interestingly, no significance in durability or complication rate was seen in patients with elevated BMI > 25, suggesting that patients with high BMI should not be excluded from consideration for this technique. Another series of translumbar hemodialysis catheters suggests higher complication rates, with review of 84 catheters in 28 patients over a period of 7 years revealing high catheter failure rates (patency at 3, 6, and 12 months of 43, 25, and 7%, respectively). Poor blood flow was observed in 40% of catheters, and 36% of catheters became infected, leading to 35.9% catheter removal.[34]

The technique has been described in detail elsewhere. The patient should be positioned prone, and translumbar access to the IVC can be achieved directly via right paraspinal approach using CT or fluoroscopic guidance and a standard low-profile access set, such as an AccuStick (Boston Scientific, Natick, MA) or Aprima (Cook Medical, Bloomington, IN). Access to the IVC can be confirmed with aspiration and observation of wire course, or with contrast injection under fluoroscopy. A 45-degree medial and cephalad approach through the soft tissues may facilitate advancement of the catheter, and provide a gentler course of the catheter for tunneling. In most cases, the trajectory should be selected to allow access to the IVC at the L2–L3 level, below the renal veins, although access above the renal veins can be used when circumstances favor such an approach (thrombosed IVC filter, etc.). A long catheter should be available, taking into account the depth from the skin to the IVC, the length of the tunnel, and the expected intravascular length, with termination of the catheter at the inferior cavoatrial junction. It is advisable to tunnel the catheter prior to dilation of the tract, after measurement of the distance from the skin to the desired catheter tip location, which can be performed using the access wire. Once the entire desired length of catheter from tip to cuff is known, the tunnel length can be selected, tunneling may be performed, and then dilation and placement of the peel-away sheath can be carried out. Ideally, a long peel-away should be used, in the range of 18 to 20 cm, for ease of catheter placement. An anterolateral subcostal exit site for a dialysis or other tunneled catheter is best for patient comfort and ease of catheter use. For placement of a port, positioning of the reservoir overlying the iliac crest is preferred to improve ease of reservoir access.

9.7.2 Transhepatic Approach

An alternative to translumbar access is transhepatic access to the hepatic veins as an approach to the IVC. This approach may be desirable in patients with IVC occlusion in addition to thoracic central venous occlusions. First described in a letter to the editor by Crummy and colleagues,[35] then published by Kaufman et al,[36] the technique for access to the hepatic veins should be familiar to the interventional radiologist, as it is similar to that used for percutaneous transhepatic cholangiography and catheter placement. A right midaxillary approach is used to obtain access to a hepatic vein, again with a microintroducer set; once access to a hepatic vein branch is confirmed, the tract may be upsized, and with similar technique as that described for translumbar access, catheter placement can be achieved.

The risk profile for transhepatic catheter placement appears elevated, relative to that for translumbar access and conventional access sites. Smith and colleagues published a series of 16 patients undergoing transhepatic dialysis catheter placement[37] and described dislodgement of the catheters in 5 instances. Device failure rate was high, and there was a 29% complication rate, including one death secondary to massive intraperitoneal hemorrhage. Kinking of the catheters between the liver and body wall was frequently observed. Another contemporaneous series of 36 transhepatic dialysis catheters in 12 patients[38] revealed a mean catheter in situ time of 24.3 days, with a catheter thrombosis rate of 2.4 per 100 catheter days, and line sepsis rate of 0.22 per 100 catheter days, with the authors concluding that this approach should only be used as a last resort. A more contemporary series of 127 catheter placements in 22 patients suggests that these catheters require a high degree of maintenance, with frequent exchanges but satisfactory overall safety, citing migration rate of 0.39 per 100 catheter days, sepsis rate of 0.22 per 100 catheter days, and a catheter thrombosis rate of 0.18 per 100 catheter days in these patients.[39]

9.7.3 Other Approaches

Many novel approaches have been described in case reports in the IR literature. These include percutaneous access to the azygos vein and use of venous collaterals as conduits for catheters to achieve a central venous tip position, among other techniques. An advantage of a comprehensive IR skill set is that it should prepare the practitioner to recognize opportunities and hazards in unique approaches relevant to a patient's individual circumstance. Novel approaches warrant a review of the literature for guidance, as available, and candid conversation with referring physicians and the patients, themselves, to ensure that the novelty, risk, alternatives, and potential benefits are well understood by all involved prior to embarking on an attempt to achieve a unique access.

9.8 Pearls of Wisdom

- For best patient outcomes, approach to vascular access should be personalized, treating the patient encounter as a consultation, rather than simply placing a device.
- Institutional stewardship of venous access, led by interventional radiologists, has the potential for improving long-term outcomes for patients, as terminal access options in patients with venous occlusions are few.
- Become familiar with, and support, evidence-based guidelines for catheter removal in CRBSIs, to preserve access when appropriate.
- With end-stage, alternative access approaches, it is important to thoroughly review the potential for complications, including death, with patients and referring physicians prior to embarking on unique approaches. However, IR is best suited to achieve best outcomes due to expertise in imaging and procedural techniques.
- Standardized approach to vascular access will facilitate institutional quality improvement efforts.

9.9 Unanswered Questions

Many questions remain regarding placement and management of vascular access, some of which may be addressed through utilization of developing databases, and through efforts such as the VANGuaRD initiative. Important questions that remain include the optimal catheter tip position and best strategies for reduction of thrombosis and fibrin sheaths in long-term access. Development of definitive algorithms for management of thrombosed and occluded access sites would be welcomed, to improve decision making regarding when to attempt recanalization of occluded segments prior to achieving contralateral or alternative site access. The risk of aggressive recanalization versus the long-term risk of exhausting access options is not known.

References

[1] Ruesch S, Walder B, Tramèr MR. Complications of central venous catheters: internal jugular versus subclavian access–a systematic review. Crit Care Med. 2002; 30(2):454–460

[2] McGee DC, Gould MK. Preventing complications of central venous catheterization. N Engl J Med. 2003; 348(12):1123–1133

[3] Fonkalsrud EW, Murphy J, Smith FG, Jr. Effect of pH in glucose infusions on development of thrombophlebitis. J Surg Res. 1968; 8(11):539–543

[4] Di Costanzo J, Cano N, Martin J, Vadon D. Venous thrombosis during total parenteral nutrition with central venous catheters–role of nutritive solutions. Clin Nutr. 1982; 1(3):201–205

[5] Duszak R, Jr, Bilal N, Picus D, Hughes DR, Xu BJ. Central venous access: evolving roles of radiology and other specialties nationally over two decades. J Am Coll Radiol. 2013; 10(8):603–612

[6] Pisoni R, Plattner B, Saran R, Woodside K. Vascular Access. United States Renal Data System. 2015 USRDS Annual Data Report: Epidemiology of Kidney Disease in the United States. Bethesda, MD: National Institutes of Health, National Institute of Diabetes and Digestive and Kidney Diseases; 2015

[7] O'Grady NP, Alexander M, Dellinger EP, et al. Centers for Disease Control and Prevention. Guidelines for the prevention of intravascular catheter-related infections. MMWR Recomm Rep. 2002; 51 RR-10:1–29

[8] Trerotola SO, Stavropoulos SW, Mondschein JI, et al. Triple-lumen peripherally inserted central catheter in patients in the critical care unit: prospective evaluation. Radiology. 2010; 256(1):312–320

[9] Kusminsky RE. Complications of central venous catheterization. J Am Coll Surg. 2007; 204(4):681–696

[10] Teichgräber UK, Benter T, Gebel M, Manns MP. A sonographically guided technique for central venous access. AJR Am J Roentgenol. 1997; 169(3):731–733

[11] Randolph AG, Cook DJ, Gonzales CA, Pribble CG. Ultrasound guidance for placement of central venous catheters: a meta-analysis of the literature. Crit Care Med. 1996; 24(12):2053–2058

[12] Gordy S, Rowell S. Vascular air embolism. Int J Crit Illn Inj Sci. 2013; 3(1):73–76

[13] Vesely TM, Ness PJ, Hart JE. Bench-top evaluation of air flow through a valved peelable introducer sheath. J Vasc Interv Radiol. 2005; 16(11):1517–1522

[14] Stuart RK, Shikora SA, Akerman P, et al. Incidence of arrhythmia with central venous catheter insertion and exchange. JPEN J Parenter Enteral Nutr. 1990; 14(2):152–155

[15] Fiaccadori E, Gonzi G, Zambrelli P, Tortorella G. Cardiac arrhythmias during central venous catheter procedures in acute renal failure: a prospective study. J Am Soc Nephrol. 1996; 7(7):1079–1084

[16] Silberzweig JE, Sacks D, Khorsandi AS, Bakal CW, Society of Interventional Radiology Technology Assessment Committee. Reporting standards for central venous access. J Vasc Interv Radiol. 2003; 14(9 Pt 2):S443–S452

[17] Song YG, Byun JH, Hwang SY, Kim CW, Shim SG. Use of vertebral body units to locate the cavoatrial junction for optimum central venous catheter tip positioning. Br J Anaesth. 2015; 115(2):252–257

[18] Merport M, Murphy TP, Egglin TK, Dubel GJ. Fibrin sheath stripping versus catheter exchange for the treatment of failed tunneled hemodialysis catheters: randomized clinical trial. J Vasc Interv Radiol. 2000; 11(9):1115–1120

[19] Jean G, Charra B, Chazot C, et al. Risk factor analysis for long-term tunneled dialysis catheter-related bacteremias. Nephron. 2002; 91(3):399–405

[20] Chaiyakunapruk N, Veenstra DL, Lipsky BA, Saint S. Chlorhexidine compared with povidone-iodine solution for vascular catheter-site care: a meta-analysis. Ann Intern Med. 2002; 136(11):792–801

[21] Venkatesan AM, Kundu S, Sacks D, et al. Practice guideline for adult antibiotic prophylaxis during vascular and interventional radiology procedures. J Vasc Interv Radiol. 2010; 21:1611–1630

[22] Johnson E, Babb J, Sridhar D. Routine antibiotic prophylaxis for totally implantable venous access device placement: meta-analysis of 2154 patients. J Vasc Interv Radiol. 2016; 27(3):339–343, quiz 344

[23] Rabindranath KS, Bansal T, Adams J, et al. Systematic review of antimicrobials for the prevention of haemodialysis catheter-related infections. Nephrol Dial Transplant. 2009; 24(12):3763–3774

[24] Mermel LA, Allon M, Bouza E, et al. Clinical practice guidelines for the diagnosis and management of intravascular catheter-related infection: 2009 update by the Infectious Diseases Society of America. Clin Infect Dis. 2009; 49(1):1–45

[25] Anil G, Taneja M. Revascularization of an occluded brachiocephalic vein using Outback-LTD re-entry catheter. J Vasc Surg. 2010; 52(4):1038–1040

[26] Ferral H, Bjarnason H, Wholey M, Lopera J, Maynar M, Castaneda-Zuniga WR. Recanalization of occluded veins to provide access for central catheter placement. J Vasc Interv Radiol. 1996; 7(5):681–685

[27] Farrell T, Lang EV, Barnhart W. Sharp recanalization of central venous occlusions. J Vasc Interv Radiol. 1999; 10(2 Pt 1):149–154

[28] Athreya S, Scott P, Annamalai G, Edwards R, Moss J, Robertson I. Sharp recanalization of central venous occlusions: a useful technique for haemodialysis line insertion. Br J Radiol. 2009; 82(974):105–108

[29] Guimaraes M, Schonholz C, Hannegan C, Anderson MB, Shi J, Selby B, Jr. Radiofrequency wire for the recanalization of central vein occlusions that have failed conventional endovascular techniques. J Vasc Interv Radiol. 2012; 23(8):1016–1021

[30] Sivananthan G, MacArthur DH, Daly KP, Allen DW, Hakham S, Halin NJ. Safety and efficacy of radiofrequency wire recanalization of chronic central venous occlusions. J Vasc Access. 2015; 16(4):309–314

[31] Kenney PR, Dorfman GS, Denny DF, Jr. Percutaneous inferior vena cava cannulation for long-term parenteral nutrition. Surgery. 1985; 97(5):602–605

[32] Butros SR, Walker TG, Salazar GM, et al. Direct translumbar inferior vena cava ports for long-term central venous access in patients with cancer. J Vasc Interv Radiol. 2014; 25(4):556–560

[33] Nadolski GJ, Trerotola SO, Stavropoulos SW, Shlansky-Goldberg RD, Soulen MC, Farrelly C. Translumbar hemodialysis catheters in patients with limited central venous access: does patient size matter? J Vasc Interv Radiol. 2013; 24(7):997–1002

[34] Liu F, Bennett S, Arrigain S, et al. Patency and complications of translumbar dialysis catheters. Semin Dial. 2015; 28(4):E41–E47

[35] Crummy AB, Carlson P, McDermott JC, Andrews D. Percutaneous transhepatic placement of a Hickman catheter. AJR Am J Roentgenol. 1989; 153(6):1317–1318

[36] Kaufman JA, Greenfield AJ, Fitzpatrick GF. Transhepatic cannulation of the inferior vena cava. J Vasc Interv Radiol. 1991; 2(3):331–334

[37] Smith TP, Ryan JM, Reddan DN. Transhepatic catheter access for hemodialysis. Radiology. 2004; 232(1):246–251

[38] Stavropoulos SW, Pan JJ, Clark TW, et al. Percutaneous transhepatic venous access for hemodialysis. J Vasc Interv Radiol. 2003; 14(9 Pt 1):1187–1190

[39] Younes HK, Pettigrew CD, Anaya-Ayala JE, et al. Transhepatic hemodialysis catheters: functional outcome and comparison between early and late failure. J Vasc Interv Radiol. 2011; 22(2):183–191

10 Pelvic and Gonadal Venous Reflux

Douglas A. Murrey, Bill S. Majdalany, and Minhaj S. Khaja

Summary

Pelvic and gonadal venous reflux syndromes are underdiagnosed and undertreated pathologic entities. As demonstrated in this chapter, reflux and obstruction of the gonadal and pelvic veins are significant causes of morbidity in men and women. Minimally invasive, percutaneous image-guided therapies offered by interventional radiologists are efficacious for these syndromes, and are characterized by low periprocedural complications and rapid recovery. This chapter describes the epidemiology of these disorders, symptom complex, and patient presentation, with details of patient evaluation and development of a treatment plan. Included in the chapter are procedural details to assist the new or experienced interventional radiologist in managing this patient population, and the text describes a plan for follow-up after a therapeutic intervention.

Keywords: pelvic congestion syndrome, varicocele, gonadal vein embolization, gonadal vein reflux, ovarian vein embolization, nutcracker syndrome, pampiniform venous plexus

10.1 Introduction

Pelvic and gonadal venous reflux syndromes are poorly understood in the general medical community, leading to misdiagnosis or frequent delays in diagnosis. The central underlying pathologic process that unifies this group of disorders is pelvic venous hypertension caused by primary pelvic venous insufficiency and/or mechanical venous obstruction. Chronic pelvic venous hypertension can lead to dilation and engorgement of various venous collateral pathways within the pelvis. The clinical manifestations of each syndrome are specific to the particular venous structures affected and can significantly impact a patient's quality of life, psychosocial wellbeing, and reproductive health. Consequently, a substantial economic impact is realized when large populations are considered. Herein, pelvic and gonadal venous reflux will be discussed with a focus on pelvic congestion syndrome, varicocele, and nutcracker syndrome.

10.2 Pelvic Congestion Syndrome

Pelvic congestion syndrome (PCS) is defined by chronic pelvic pain (CPP) lasting longer than 3 to 6 months, which is caused by incompetent or obstructed gonadal veins and/or pelvic branches of the iliac venous system.[1] The precise mechanism by which venous congestion causes pain in PCS remains somewhat unclear but is likely multifactorial.[1] Historically, the earliest reports of PCS date to 1831 by Gooch and subsequently in 1857 by Richet as a "tubo-ovarian varicocele."[2,3] In 1928, Cotte further elaborated on the phenomenon of impaired circulation and drainage leading to enlarged venous complexes involving the reproductive tissues.[4] The effect on the female reproductive organs was described in 1949 by Taylor, correlating the dilated pelvic veins with symptoms of CPP, which was ultimately established by Beard et al in 1984.[5,6]

Presently, between 30 and 40% of women will suffer from CPP throughout their life. Additionally, 10 to 15% of asymptomatic women have radiographically demonstrable pelvic varices, which arise from the ovarian, internal iliac, or parauterine veins.[7] While both pelvic pain and venous varices are often present in multiparous women of childbearing age, they may not be related. As such, accurately discriminating PCS from alternative etiologies of CPP can be challenging. A thorough workup with history and physical examination, laboratory results, and imaging studies can narrow the differential diagnosis.

10.3 Case Vignette

10.3.1 Patient Presentation

A 25-year-old woman presents with a primary complaint of pelvic pain, describing it as a dull heaviness that worsens over the course of the day. The pain has been ongoing for several months and worsens before menstruation and during/after intercourse. She is otherwise healthy with a negative review of systems and negative gynecologic workup. With the exception of two pregnancies with normal spontaneous vaginal deliveries, she has no past medical, surgical, or pertinent family history.

10.3.2 Physical Exam

Notable for tenderness at the ovarian points bilaterally and superficial vulvar varicosities.

10.3.3 Imaging

Ultrasonography reveals multiple tortuous vessels around the uterus, which increase in size with Valsalva's maneuver (▶ Fig. 10.1a, b). Pelvic CT reveals an enlarged left gonadal vein, prominent parauterine veins, and vulvar varicosities (▶ Fig. 10.1c). Pelvic MRI reveals retrograde flow in the left gonadal vein (▶ Fig. 10.1d).

10.3.4 Specifics of Consent

The procedure and technical approach, whether from internal jugular or femoral veins, is presented. In addition to reviewing potential complications associated with moderate sedation, venography, embolization, and sclerotherapy, it is important to set appropriate expectations for procedure outcomes and the potential need for additional treatment of internal iliac veins, if not treated concurrently, or superficial varicose veins. Lastly, discuss the available evidence and note that there are no data to support a negative effect on ovarian function, menstruation, or fertility.

10.3.5 Details of Procedure

Through a right internal jugular approach, the left renal vein (LRV) was selected for venography (▶ Fig. 10.2a), after which the left gonadal vein was selected. Left gonadal venography demon-

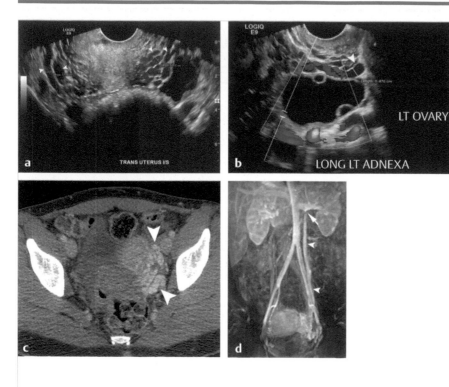

Fig. 10.1 (a) Transvaginal grayscale ultrasound image of the uterus demonstrating large tubular-shaped anechoic structures in the periuterine region measuring approximately 3.8 mm in diameter (*white arrowheads*). (b) Transvaginal ultrasound image of the left adnexa with color Doppler overlay demonstrating large tubular anechoic structures (*arrowhead*) with flow on color Doppler, confirming their vascular nature. The dilated pelvic venous structures measure approximately 4.8 mm on this image, which are abnormal (normal < 4 mm). Note that these dilated venous structures increased in size on Valsalva (*not shown*). (c) Axial postcontrast CT image of the pelvis demonstrating enlarged serpiginous venous structures in the left adnexa that correspond to the abnormally dilated gonadal veins demonstrated on the transvaginal US in Fig. 10.2 (*white arrowheads*). This CT also demonstrated prominent parauterine veins and vulvar varices (*not shown*). (d) Maximum intensity projection (MIP) of an MR venogram (MRV) of the abdomen and pelvis demonstrating a large left ovarian vein (*arrowheads*) with contiguous dilated left parauterine veins, all of which correspond to the US and CT images in ▶ Fig. 10.1, ▶ Fig. 10.2, and ▶ Fig. 10.3.

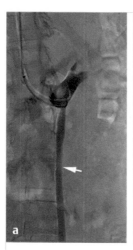

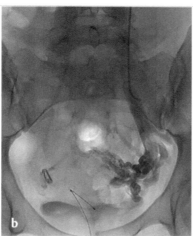

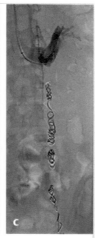

Fig. 10.2 (a) Left renal venogram performed from a right internal jugular approach demonstrating reflux into a dilated left ovarian vein (*arrow*). (b) Selective left gonadal venogram performed through a 5-French angled glide catheter within the mid-left ovarian vein demonstrating retrograde flow into the left ovarian vein, filling of the left parauterine veins, opacification of the myometrial veins, and subsequent opacification of the right parauterine veins. A Foley catheter is noted within the bladder. (c) Left renal venogram obtained after left gonadal vein sclerotherapy documenting the lack of venous reflux into the left ovarian vein after sclerotherapy. The sclerotherapy was performed using foamed sclerosant comprised of equal parts of 3% sodium tetradecyl sulfate and iodinated contrast. The sclerosant was alternated with coils in a "sandwich" technique.

strated retrograde flow into the pelvic varices (▶ Fig. 10.2b). The catheter was advanced into the pelvis, and after venography, sclerotherapy was performed utilizing foamed sclerosant (equal parts 3% sodium tetradecyl sulfate and iodinated contrast, agitated with air through a three-way stopcock) "sandwiched" with mechanical occlusion (▶ Fig. 10.2c).

10.3.6 Follow-up

For most patients, this is an outpatient procedure since it is not associated with significant postprocedural symptoms beyond mild pain and nausea. Approximately 1 week after the procedure, the patient returned for an outpatient clinic visit to evaluate for early complications, review the procedure, and answer any questions. Routinely, a 3-month return visit is scheduled for reevaluation of symptoms and to determine procedural success or need for further intervention.

10.4 Epidemiology and Scope of the Problem

CPP in women is a significant global health issue, which affects an estimated 2 to 24% of all women worldwide (according to a published review from the World Health Organization in 2006).[8,9] In the United States, it is estimated that approximately 30% of all outpatient gynecological visits are specifically for the evaluation of CPP.[10] The economic burden of diagnosing and treating CPP is estimated at $1.2 billion annually, with an additional $15 billion lost due to lack of economic production.[11] Of those suffering from CPP, 30% are thought to be secondary to PCS. According to a 2014 U.S. census, there are 63 million women in the United States between the ages of 25 and 53, which should, presumably, equate to an incidence of approximately 5 to 6 million women suffering from PCS. In addition to the micro- and macroeconomic burden, these patients frequently suffer a significant psychological toll as increased levels of anxiety, stress, and depression have all been liked to PCS.[10]

10.4.1 Patient Presentation and Evaluation

Often, PCS patients visit several physicians and are misdiagnosed before presenting for endovascular therapy. Unfortunately, the differential diagnosis of CPP in women is extensive. Excluding alternative etiologies is paramount, and the differential diagnosis can be narrowed with a thorough history and physical examination, laboratory exams, and imaging.

Most commonly, patients are multiparous, premenopausal, and suffer from several months of pelvic heaviness or a dull diffuse ache. Symptoms may reproducibly worsen with prolonged standing and improve while recumbent. The pain should not be strictly cyclical or only coinciding with menses. Patients may also describe dyspareunia or postcoital pain if vulvar or vaginal veins are involved. Bladder and bowel symptoms can also be present, including urinary frequency, urinary hesitancy, and symptoms similar to irritable bowel syndrome.[1]

On physical exam, ovarian point tenderness may be elicited. In a study by Beard et al, the combination of ovarian point tenderness on physical exam with postcoital pain was 94% sensitive and 77% specific for diagnosing PCS, though these findings have not been reproduced to date.[12]

Vulvar, perineal, and upper thigh varicosities can be visualized, and made more prominent with the patient standing or performing a Valsalva maneuver. Since PCS remains a diagnosis of exclusion, the caregiver should pursue additional imaging if any combination of the above symptoms or physical exam findings is present.

Imaging is performed in order to document the characteristic pelvic venous changes of PCS, which support the diagnosis but do not define it. Imaging is also performed in order to exclude other causes of CPP. Traditionally, ultrasound (US) has been widely regarded as the modality of choice; characteristic findings include dilation of the ovarian veins (>4 mm in diameter), slow (<3 cm/s), or retrograde flow in the ovarian veins that may worsen with Valsalva, presence of tortuous and dilated pelvic venous plexuses, dilated arcuate veins (>5 mm) crossing the uterine myometrium and communicating with the pelvic venous plexuses, and polycystic changes of the ovary.[13] An additional advantage of US is the ability to perform the examination in the semi-supine or upright position, as some patients' symptoms and venous dilation will remit in a fully supine position. Time-resolved pelvic magnetic resonance imaging (TrMRI) has recently been shown to accurately demonstrate pelvic venous reflux while simultaneously providing excellent anatomic detail of the pelvis (▶ Fig. 10.3). However, evaluation of the vasculature by TrMRI is slightly limited in that it requires the patient to lie in a supine position, and it is less cost-effective when compared to US. Computed tomography venography

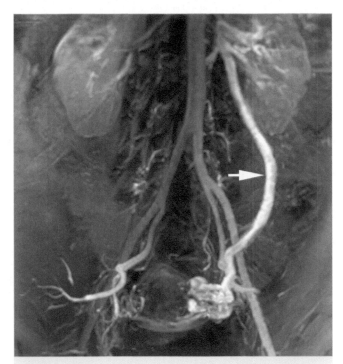

Fig. 10.3 Maximum intensity projection (MIP) of a time-resolved MR venogram (TrMRV) of the abdomen and pelvis demonstrating contrast refluxing from the left renal vein into an enlarged left ovarian vein (*arrow*) with contiguous dilated left parauterine veins.

(CTV) can be of some benefit as it can provide excellent anatomic vascular detail. However, CT is unable to produce the requisite dynamic information necessary to diagnose venous reflux, which limits its utility in PCS. On the other hand, CT can be beneficial in the general workup of CPP secondary to its ability to provide anatomic detail and quick acquisition times (▶ Fig. 10.4a,b). Direct venography (DV) is classically the test of choice for diagnosing venous reflux; however, given the invasive nature of venography and the excellent accuracy of US, DV has been largely replaced by US in the diagnostic setting.

The American Venous Forum has published clinical practice guidelines, which address varicose veins and chronic venous disease.[14] At present, noninvasive imaging with US, CT, and MRI receives the highest grade of recommendation with retrograde ovarian and iliac venography reserved for patients in whom an intervention is planned. Ultimately, patients with a suspicious clinical history and concordant imaging findings of pelvic/gonadal venous insufficiency should be considered for treatment, assuming alternative diagnoses of CPP have been excluded. Additionally, if a patient has a compelling history and physical without correlative imaging findings, a definitive diagnosis can be pursued with semi-upright venography or with Valsalva at the time of venography.

10.4.2 Preparation for Procedure

After the clinic visit, which should include reviewing patient clinical status, allergies, labs, and imaging, no other specific preprocedural testing is needed. Preprocedural medications may include a single dose of an antibiotic to cover skin flora, but no other medications are necessary. Nursing should acquire intravenous access that can be used for the administration of

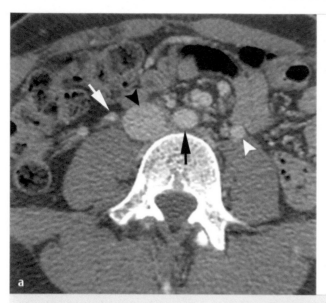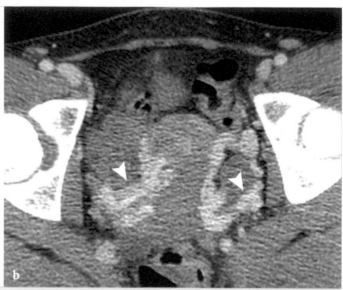

Fig. 10.4 **(a)** Axial postcontrast CT image of the lower abdomen demonstrating an asymmetrically enlarged left gonadal vein (*white arrowhead*). The right gonadal vein has been labeled with a *white arrow* for size comparison. Also note the size of the left gonadal vein in comparison to the adjacent aorta (*black arrow*) and IVC (*black arrowhead*) at the same level. **(b)** Axial postcontrast CT image of the pelvis demonstrating enlarged bilateral parauterine veins (*arrowheads*) in the same patient as was shown in (a). Note that despite the normal caliber of the right gonadal vein in this patient, bilateral parauterine veins are enlarged. This is most likely secondary due to retrograde flow (reflux) from the left renal vein into the left ovarian vein, into the left parauterine veins, across the myometrial veins, and into the right parauterine veins.

moderate sedation as needed, fluids for hydration, and antiemetics. General anesthesia is not required unless there are comorbid conditions that warrant it. Placement of a urinary catheter is also not required.

The patient is positioned supine in an interventional suite, and sterile preparation and draping is performed for the access site, commonly the right internal jugular and/or right common femoral vein. A tilt table may be helpful to accentuate the findings on venography, but is not required. No special equipment is needed beyond the standard repertoire found in most interventional radiology suites. As with any endovascular procedure, the operator should be mindful of contrast volume and radiation dose. Fluoroscopic image saves should be utilized in lieu of standard digital subtraction runs during the endovascular procedure, if possible. These radiation safety measures are particularly important for this patient population, many of whom are still of childbearing age.

10.4.3 Technical Tips and Tricks and Procedural Details

Preferred access site is the right internal jugular vein, since this allows evaluation and possible treatment of the bilateral gonadal and the bilateral internal iliac veins. However, these veins may all also be selected from a common femoral approach. The approach to selection and treatment of the gonadal veins and internal iliac veins is slightly different, and each is discussed separately.

Gonadal Vein Embolization

A 5- to 7-French vascular sheath is placed at the access site, through which a 4- to 5-French angled tip catheter is used to gain access to the veins. The left gonadal vein is usually larger

and more easily accessed than the right gonadal vein. Care should be taken to minimize potential spasm or injury to the veins during selection. The left gonadal vein arises from the LRV, which is selected for venography to demonstrate incompetence of the gonadal venous valves. Subsequently, the left gonadal vein is selected with a guidewire, and the catheter is advanced into the pelvis, close to the varicosities, for additional venography (▶ Fig. 10.5a). In contrast to the left, the right gonadal vein terminates directly as a confluence with the inferior vena cava (IVC), and can be accessed with an angled catheter from the jugular approach or a reverse-curve catheter, such as a Simmons 1, from a femoral approach. As with the left, the catheter is navigated into the pelvis, close to the varicosities, for additional venography. If there is difficulty advancing a 4- or 5-French catheter, a coaxial microcatheter (2.4–2.8 French) can easily reach deep into the pelvis.

Once positioned in the pelvis and following venography, adjacent to the varicosities, embolization can be performed with a combination of coils, plugs, and sclerosants. Sclerosants can be either liquid or foamed, and, when used, allow for deeper penetration of the treatment area. The use of occlusion balloons is dependent on operator preference. Embolization is performed from the upstream (most caudal) pelvic veins in ascending fashion to the termination of the gonadal vein. Sclerosant is alternated with mechanical occlusion every few centimeters, which creates an embolic "sandwich" allowing for complete embolization while additionally helping to prevent collateralization of the reflux circuit (▶ Fig. 10.5b).

Internal Iliac Vein Embolization

If symptoms are refractory after treatment of the gonadal veins, the potential for internal iliac venous incompetence should be assessed. Some operators choose to evaluate internal iliac vein

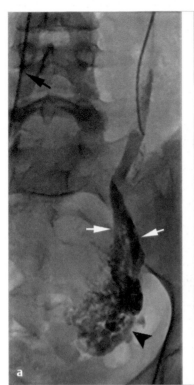
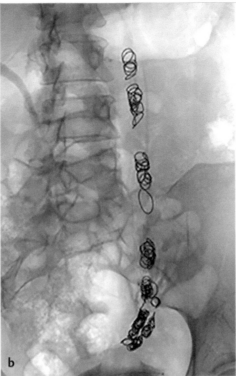
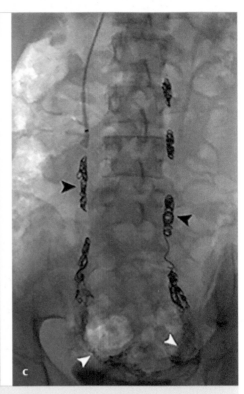

Fig. 10.5 **(a)** Selective left gonadal venogram performed through a 5-French angled glide catheter within the mid left ovarian vein which was performed via a right femoral venous access (*black arrow* shows the catheter in the IVC). The venogram demonstrates a dilated distal left gonadal vein with an accessory gonadal venous branch (*white arrows*) feeding dilated parauterine venous complex (*black arrowhead*). Both main gonadal venous branches will need treated to increase the likelihood of treatment success. **(b)** Posttreatment radiograph of the abdomen and pelvis obtained in the PA projection obtained after left gonadal vein sclerotherapy documenting the treatment of both the main left gonadal vein and the accessory gonadal venous tract using a combination of coils and foamed sclerosant (comprised of equal parts of 3% sodium tetradecyl sulfate and iodinated contrast) in alternate fashion. This method of gonadal vein embolization is commonly referred to as the "sandwich" technique. **(c)** Posttreatment radiograph of the abdomen and pelvis obtained in the PA projection obtained after bilateral gonadal vein sclerotherapy. Note that embolization was performed using a combination of coils (*black arrowheads*) and foamed sclerosant (*white arrowheads*) comprised of equal parts of 3% sodium tetradecyl sulfate and iodinated contrast. The coils and sclerosant are placed in and alternating fashion, commonly referred to as the "sandwich" technique. Also note the presence of a 2.4-French microcatheter within the right gonadal vein.

incompetence during a separate procedure, while others treat both the gonadal and internal iliac veins on the same day without consequence. After selecting each internal iliac vein, venography is performed (▸ Fig. 10.6a). Balloon occlusion venography is performed to better visualize the varicosities (▸ Fig. 10.6b); in the absence of balloon occlusion, the brisk inflow into the circulation may not allow visualization of the multiple draining veins. With balloon occlusion, the tributary veins are visualized with test injections prior to subsequent balloon-occluded sclerotherapy. After a dwell time of approximately 10 minutes and with fluoroscopic monitoring, the occlusion balloon may be deflated. This is repeated on both sides, or may be done concurrently with bilateral access. Mechanical occlusion of the internal iliac veins has been previously reported, and is performed in some practices, depending on operator preference.

10.4.4 Potential Complications or Pitfalls

Major complications are uncommon and can include nontarget embolization of coils or plugs to the pulmonary circulation. This can be prevented by using detachable plugs or coils at the rostral portion of the ovarian vein and by oversizing the mechanical

embolics by 30 to 50% to account for venous distensibility due to patient volume status and supine intraprocedural positioning. Migration of the coil or plug can be treated with snaring and removal if necessary. Other complications may include vessel perforation, pelvic venous thrombophlebitis, pelvic pain, and recurrence of varices. The overall reported rates for all complications are less than 4%.[9,13,15,16]

10.4.5 Postprocedural Management and Follow-up

Patients are observed for approximately 2 to 4 hours postprocedure in order to recover from sedation. Pain management, antiemetics, and intravenous hydration are all important components of postprocedural care. Patients are discharged with prescriptions for pain medications and antiemetics, though ibuprofen and naproxen are encouraged as a first-line therapy. Transient pelvic pain, particularly if sclerosants are used, is not unusual and may represent a degree of phlebitis. Generally, this will subside in a few days and can be managed conservatively. A minority of patients may require overnight admission for debilitating pain.[17,18,19]

Normal activity may be resumed after 72 hours. No special labs or unique monitoring is required in the postprocedural

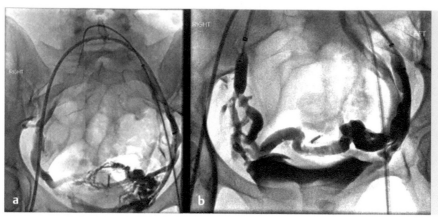

Fig. 10.6 (a) Angiography of left internal iliac vein without balloon occlusion demonstrates reflux into pelvic venous plexus, uterine veins, and spontaneous reflux across midline into right internal iliac venous outflow. (b) Bilateral balloon-occluded internal iliac venography demonstrates large transpelvic collateral veins.

setting. Postoperative pain scores should be obtained and compared with preoperative scores, though pain improvement times can vary widely. The literature suggests that immediate improvements should not be expected, as the earliest reports of pain improvement occur at 1 week after the procedure but may lag for up to 3 months postprocedure. An early follow-up, in the range of 2 weeks, is performed in order to assess for complications, review the procedure and expectations, and monitor recovery. A second clinic visit is scheduled at approximately 12 weeks to reassess pelvic pain and to determine if additional treatment is warranted. Afterward, patients may return as needed on an annual basis or earlier if symptoms recur. These visits include standardized pain assessments, and specifically address overall pain, pain on standing, pain on lying down, dyspareunia, menstrual pain, and urinary alterations. Repeat imaging is not routinely performed and should be pursued only if symptoms warrant further evaluation.

10.4.6 Outcomes

Ovarian vein embolization for PCS was first described in a case report in 1993.[20] Subsequently, multiple observational case series and meta-analyses have been published describing the technique and outcomes. These studies were summarized in a recent meta-analysis by Mahmoud et al, which demonstrated an overall immediate technical success rate of 99%, improvement in symptoms categorized by the patients as "significant improvement" in 88.1% at 1 to 3 months postprocedure, and 86.6% long-term symptomatic relief. Follow-up times ranged from 7 months to 5 years.[21] Finally, the rate of ovarian vein recanalization requiring repeat embolization is estimated at approximately 2 to 4% based on the largest available series.[19,21]

10.5 Pearls of Wisdom

- Patient evaluation and exclusion of alternative etiologies of CPP is paramount to increase technical and clinical success of embolization procedures.
- Treatment of the entire length of the ovarian vein helps prevent collateralization of retroperitoneal veins to the refluxing pelvic veins.
- Using sclerosants, in addition to mechanical occlusion devices, can more deeply ablate interconnected pelvis venous plexuses.

- PCS has a complex etiology that requires multimodality treatment. Endovascular embolization and sclerotherapy are successful in eliminating the physical cause, but psychosocial supportive therapy and medical treatment may also be necessary to achieve the best results for patients.

10.6 Unanswered Questions

PCS continues to be a misunderstood and underdiagnosed cause of pelvic pain. Timely diagnosis and prompt endovascular treatment can effectively mitigate the somatic, psychological, and economic consequences of the disease. While large, prospective randomized trials are lacking, emerging case series and meta-analyses suggest high rates of clinical success and low rates of complications when patients undergo endovascular embolization. Prospective trials comparing medical management and invasive therapies would be helpful to delineate which management strategy would best serve this diverse patient population and provide convincing outcomes data. Moreover, refinement of the diagnostic imaging criteria, investigations of optimal embolic choice and technique, and outcomes data comparing different techniques (unilateral vs. bilateral ovarian vein embolization, and ovarian vein vs. combined ovarian and internal iliac vein embolization) could further guide practitioners and optimize patient care.

10.7 Varicocele

The first description of varicocele is attributed to Celsus, a Greek physician in the first century, who described veins that were "swollen and twisted over the testicle."[22] Currently, varicoceles are defined as an abnormal distension of the pampiniform venous plexus and are the male equivalent of PCS. Like PCS, it is thought to be a result of gonadal vein incompetence, which may be from primary venous insufficiency or secondary to venous compression/obstruction. Varicoceles are a common cause of scrotal pain, predispose to infertility, and may arrest testicular growth in adolescents and adult males that may lead to decreased testosterone levels.[23]

The connection between varicocele and male infertility dates back to the late 19th century, but documentation of improved semen parameters and subsequent successful pregnancies after treatment were not reported until 1955.[24,25] The ultimate goal of treatment relies on the disruption or occlusion of the dilated

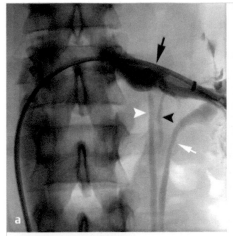
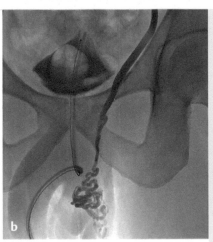
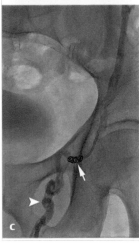
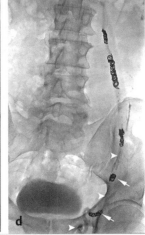

Fig. 10.7 **(a)** Left renal venogram performed through a 5-French catheter from a right femoral approach with a 5-French sheath extending through the IVC and terminating in the left renal vein (*black arrow*). The venogram demonstrates reflux into the left gonadal/testicular vein (*white arrowhead*). There is also reflux into a second, incidental, left gonadal vein, which originates more distally from the left renal vein and connects with the proximal aspect of the main left renal vein (*black arrowhead*). The left ureter is also noted incidentally (*white arrow*). **(b)** Fluoroscopic image of the pelvis taken during left gonadal vein sclerotherapy using a sclerosant solution comprise of equal parts of 3% Sotradecol and contrast (Isovue 300), showing a dilated left gonadal vein (single channel) as well as opacification of the left pampiniform plexus. Note the subtle filling defects and relative lucencies within the varicocele representing the sclerosing agent. A Foley catheter is noted in the bladder. **(c)** Fluoroscopic image of the left pelvis demonstrating a coil pack in the distal left gonadal vein (*white arrow*). Just distal to the coil, the sclerosant solution can be seen dwelling within the distal aspect of the left gonadal vein (*white*) **(d)** Completion fluoroscopic image of the left abdomen and pelvis demonstrating a series of coil packs along the entire course of the left gonadal vein consisting of a combination of 8–12 mm pushable coils (*white arrows*). Sandwiched in between in coil packs, sclerosing solution can be faintly seen (*white arrowheads*).

veins that drain the testis. Currently, in North America urologic microsurgery is the most commonly employed treatment technique, but a growing body of evidence suggests that percutaneous embolization is a safe alternative offering the potential of improved patient safety, lower morbidity (hydroceles and impotence), and lower costs.[24,26,27]

10.8 Case Vignette

10.8.1 Patient Presentation

An otherwise healthy 29-year-old man initially presented to his urologist for infertility. The patient complained of left testicular pain that was exacerbated by prolonged periods of sitting. His review of symptoms and past medical history were otherwise negative.

10.8.2 Physical Exam

The patient was noted to have a grade III left-sided varicocele, which was visible without Valsalva.

10.8.3 NonInvasive Testing

Semen analysis revealed slow or sluggish progressive sperm motility despite an adequate sperm concentration.

10.8.4 Imaging

Scrotal US identified anechoic tubular structures with vascular flow adjacent to the left testis. The vessels measured greater than 3 mm in size and enlarged with Valsalva's maneuver. The right side was unremarkable.

10.8.5 Specifics of Consent

The procedure and technical approach, whether from internal jugular or femoral veins, is presented. In addition to reviewing potential complications generally associated with moderate sedation, venography, embolization, and sclerotherapy, setting appropriate expectations for procedure outcomes and the potential for continued difficulty conceiving (clinical failure) is important.

10.8.6 Details of Procedure

The procedure was performed via the right femoral vein using a long, hydrophilic 6-French sheath (although internal jugular access could have been used as well). A left renal venogram was performed on a tilt table positioned in reverse Trendelenburg 20 degrees, with a catheter beyond the orifice of the left gonadal vein and the patient performing a Valsalva maneuver (▶ Fig. 10.7a). After confirmation of retrograde flow into the gonadal vein, the catheter was advanced to the midleft gonadal vein and repeat venography was performed, confirming the varicocele (▶ Fig. 10.7b). Next, a combination of coils and sclerosant (3% sodium tetradecyl sulfate solution mixed with contrast) were used for embolization and sclerosis. Some operators put an emphasis on placing coils most distally to avoid deposition of sclerosant into the pampiniform plexus. However, some believe that improved efficacy may be achieved with deposition of sclerosant into the varicocele (▶ Fig. 10.7c,d). A prominent right gonadal vein could not be visualized.

10.8.7 Follow-up

The immediate postprocedure course was uneventful. On 3-month follow-up, the patient no longer had a varicocele and the couple was able to conceive. A scrotal US at that time was unremarkable.

10.9 Epidemiology and Scope of Problem

Varicoceles are present in 15 to 20% of young, healthy, asymptomatic men, but the prevalence increases with age, reaching as high as 42% in the elderly population. However, the incidence of a varicocele in men who present for evaluation of infertility is disproportionately high (35–40%).[28] While the majority of males with a varicocele are asymptomatic, there is a growing body of evidence linking varicoceles with progressive decline in testicular function; this culminates in impaired semen parameters, infertility, and decreased serum testosterone levels.[29]

According to the World Health Organization, infertility is defined by the inability of a sexually active couple to conceive after 1 year of unprotected intercourse[30]; it is estimated that 15% of all couples are infertile under this definition. Further, male factors are solely responsible for the couples infertility in about 20% of cases and a contributing factor in an additional 30 to 40% of cases.[31] Most cases of infertility are idiopathic, but varicoceles are the most commonly identified cause of male factor infertility, accounting for 15% of all cases. When only azoospermic patients are considered, varicoceles are the second most common underlying diagnosis, behind maldescended testes (10.9 and 17.2%, respectively).[32,33]

While most varicoceles are asymptomatic, 2 to 10% are associated with pain; this equates to an estimated 35 million men worldwide.[34,35] In fact, varicoceles have been reported to be the cause of pain in 2 to 14% of all men suffering from chronic scrotal pain.[36] Much like its female counterpart, PCS, chronic scrotal pain can significantly impact the daily activities of those suffering from this entity and can lead to significant psychosocial issues.

10.9.1 Patient Presentation and Evaluation

Men with a varicocele present with a variety of clinical scenarios, and treatment of each has unique therapeutic goals and diagnostic workup. Thus, proper patient management is tailored to the presenting clinical situation. The three primary indications for intervention are infertility, testicular atrophy in the adolescent or pediatric patient, and pain. Clinical evaluation begins with a history, physical examination, and scrotal ultrasonography.

Most often, varicoceles are asymptomatic and patients present for infertility. According to the American Urological Association (AUA) and the American Society for Reproductive Medicine (ASRM), routine evaluation of infertile men with a varicocele should include a medical and reproductive history, a physical exam, and a minimum of two semen analyses.[37,38] On physical exam, upon palpation the clinician may appreciate a "bag of worms" within the scrotum, irrespective of the presence or absence of pain. Physical exam is best performed with the patient in the standing position, and a Valsalva maneuver should be performed during the exam in order to accentuate dilation of the pampiniform plexus and properly grade the varicocele.[23] Varicoceles are then classified as Grade I (palpable only with Valsalva), Grade II (palpable without Valsalva), and Grade III (visible from a distance).

Treatment of a varicocele in the setting of infertility is advocated when the following criteria are met in the adult male: the couple has known infertility; the female partner has been evaluated and has no identifiable abnormality or has a potentially treatable cause of infertility; the varicocele is palpable on physical examination; and the male partner has abnormal semen parameters or abnormal results on sperm function tests. Treatment should also be offered to any adult men who are not currently attempting to conceive but desire future fertility, have a palpable varicocele, and abnormal semen analyses. Of note, the AUA and the ASRM do not currently recommend treatment in adult men if semen analysis is normal or the varicocele is not palpable (i.e., "subclinical"), pointing to the fact that "only palpable varicoceles have been documented to be associated with infertility."[37] Given the controversial link between varicoceles and reduced ipsilateral testicular size and function, the AUA and ASRM suggest that treatment should be "considered" in adolescent males with unilateral or bilateral varicoceles and with objective evidence of reduced ipsilateral testicular size.[37] These associations suggest annual follow-up with US to document testicular size and/or annual semen analysis in order to detect the earliest sign of varicocele-related testicular dysfunction.

Scrotal US with pulsed and color Doppler images is an invaluable tool in the evaluation of a suspected varicocele (**see** ▶ Fig. 10.8a–c). On grayscale US, the dilated pampiniform venous plexus is apparent as serpiginous, tubular-shaped anechoic structures. Threshold vein diameters of 2.5 mm at rest and 3.0 mm during Valsalva have been shown to be over 80% predictive of clinically-apparent varicoceles (Grades I-III).[39] Varicoceles are noted on US, but those that are occult on physical exam are categorized as Grade 0 or "subclinical." It is worth noting that the AUA and the ASRM have both recommended reserving US for those cases of inconclusive physical examination in the setting of infertility; however, some authors have advocated for the use of US in the evaluation of male infertility and pediatric varicoceles. These authors argue that US can be used to follow pre- and posttreatment measurements as a measure of clinical success and to evaluate for postoperative complications such as hydrocele or testicular atrophy secondary to inadvertent testicular artery ligation.[23,32,37,38,40]

Patients presenting with pain describe a "dull" and/or "throbbing" scrotal pain that extends to the ipsilateral inguinal region.

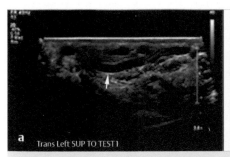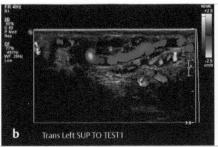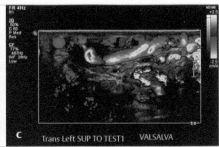

Fig. 10.8 **(a)** Grayscale ultrasonographic image of the left scrotum demonstrating a tubular anechoic structure within the left scrotal sac measuring > 3 mm in diameter (*arrow*). **(b)** Color Doppler ultrasound image of the left scrotum confirming nonpulsatile venous flow within the dilated anechoic tubular structure noted in **(a)** consistent with a dilated vein in the pampiniform plexus. This image was taken prior to Valsalva's maneuvers. **(c)** Color Doppler ultrasonographic image of the left scrotum during a Valsalva maneuver demonstrating accentuated flow and further dilation of the left pampiniform plexus, characteristic of gonadal venous reflux and diagnostic for a left-sided varicocele.

Much like its PCS counterpart, the pain associated with a varicocele tends to worsen with straining, exercise, and long periods of standing.[35] US evaluation in these cases can exclude alternative diagnoses and confirm the diagnosis of varicocele as the sole abnormality. A new, right-sided unilateral varicocele is concerning for an intra-abdominal mass and cross-sectional imaging and evaluation is recommended. No specific criteria exist for the treatment of varicocele in the setting of pain, provided that the history, physical exam, and imaging findings are concordant.

10.9.2 Preparation for Procedure

As with ovarian vein embolization for PCS, testicular vein embolization can be performed in an outpatient setting utilizing a combination of local anesthesia and IV moderate sedation. General anesthesia is not required and is utilized only if needed to help manage comorbid conditions. No particular preprocedural testing or medications are required, and no special or unique equipment outside the standard IR repertoire is required for this procedure. A tilt table may be helpful to accentuate the findings on venography, but is not required. Patients should be positioned supine in the procedure room and the operator's preferred vascular access wire and sheath combinations should be available. Every effort should be made to reduce the radiation exposure to the pelvis and gonads, and radiation shielding may be used. To decrease radiation dose, fluoroscopic image saves should be utilized in lieu of standard digital subtraction runs during the endovascular procedure, if possible.

10.9.3 Technical Tips and Tricks and Procedural Details

A 5- to 7-French vascular sheath is placed, through which a 4- to 5-French angled tip catheter is used to gain access to the veins. The left internal spermatic vein is usually larger and more easily accessed than the right gonadal vein. Care should be taken to minimize potential spasm or injury to the veins when selecting them. The left internal spermatic vein arises from the LRV, which is selected for venography to evaluate the

competence of the gonadal vein valves (▸ Fig. 10.9a). If access is required of the right internal spermatic vein, a Simmons 1 or other reverse-curved catheter can be used from a femoral approach, whereas an angled catheter can be used if a jugular approach has been utilized. The authors prefer a transjugular access for most patients since the patient can ambulate sooner after the procedure. Additionally, many patients prefer neck access to a groin puncture, which requires flat bed rest for a longer period. However, in patients whose gonadal vein orifice has an acute angle from the renal vein, it is easier to select the left gonadal vein via right groin access. In some patients with difficult angles, it may be easiest to select the gonadal vein while the patient is performing the Valsalva maneuver. Once the internal spermatic vein is selected and venography confirms reflux, the catheter is navigated to the level of the superior pubic ramus and embolization is performed with a combination of sclerosants and mechanical occlusion, which are alternated as the catheter is withdrawn to the orifice of the gonadal vein (▸ Fig. 10.9b–d).

Technical success rates are dependent on each patient's anatomy, vascular access (right-sided, left-sided, or bilateral varicoceles), and sclerosant/embolic agent used. It is important to know that the right internal spermatic vein drains directly into the anterolateral aspect of the IVC in 80% of patients, but can be found emptying into the inferior aspect of the right renal vein as well and is, in general, much more difficult to access when compared to the left gonadal vein.[41] While in more recent reports technical success rates for left-sided unilateral gonadal vein embolization approach 90 to 100%, multiple studies have reported technical failure rates as high as 50% for right-sided gonadal vein embolization attempts.[26,27]

One should also carefully consider the embolization agent to be employed. Mechanical embolic material (coils/vascular plugs), sclerosants (sodium tetradecyl sulfate/polidocanol), glues, and a combination of all have been described in the literature for gonadal vein embolization. However, there are significant differences in the reported clinical success rates with coils alone, consistently leading to the highest rates of clinical failure and recanalization. A report published in 2015 by Favard et al reported on 203 gonadal vein embolizations performed for varicoceles, comparing outcomes using coils alone versus glue alone versus a combination of coils and sclerosants. These

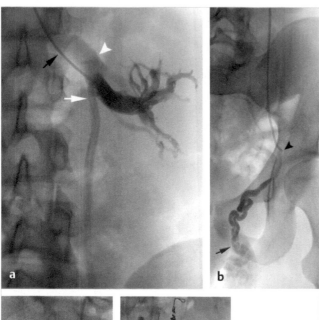

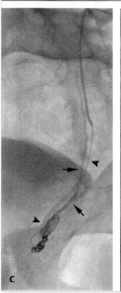

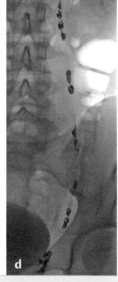

authors found a significantly higher clinical success rate and lower recanalization rates when glue was used in isolation.[42] Incidentally, these authors also found a significantly lower dose of radiation in the glue-only group.[42] While this is one of the only reports to date advocating the use of glue alone, there are multiple reports that demonstrate superior outcomes when using a combination of coils and sclerosant as compared to coils alone.[43,44] As such, the current authors suggest either a combination of coils and sclerosant agent or glue alone, but do not advocate using coils alone. Regardless of the embolic agent, the entire length of the gonadal vein, to approximately 1 to 2 cm from its renal vein orifice should be treated.

10.9.4 Potential Complications or Pitfalls

Major complications from gonadal vein embolization are uncommon, which is an advantage over surgical ligation. Theoretical risks include vascular perforation and subsequent hemorrhage, but clinically significant hemorrhage secondary to vascular perforations has not been reported to date in the literature. Coil migration and/or distal embolization of embolic material is the main risk when performing gonadal vein embolization. This can lead to renal vein thrombosis, or more central thrombosis of the IVC or pulmonary arteries.[45] Coil oversizing by 30 to 50% of the diameter of the gonadal vein is recommended to avoid this potential complication. Pampiniform plexus thrombophlebitis occurs in approximately 0.5% of cases and is thought to be secondary to nontarget sclerosis of the pampiniform plexus but can be easily treated with anti-inflammatory agents and antibiotics.[46]

Minor complications are noted in around 11% of all procedures. Some patients may experience ongoing periprocedural pain for up to 10 days, which can be managed with anti-inflammatory medications; however, there have been no reports of developing chronic scrotal pain after embolization. Allergic reactions to contrast media and access site hematomas have also been reported, but are not unique to this particular procedure. Finally, gonadal radiation exposure is of specific concern with this procedure. In 2000, Chalmers et al demonstrated in a retrospective study that the average lifetime cancer risk in patients who had undergone gonadal vein embolization was approximately 0.1%.[47]

10.9.5 Postprocedural Management and Follow-up

Three months after treatment, patients should be evaluated for persistence or recurrence of the varicocele with both US and physical exam. Repeat venography should be reserved to evaluate persistent patency of the testicular vein or for identification of additional collateral veins missed during the initial procedure. Semen analyses and hormone levels should also be reassessed at 3-month intervals for at least 1 year following the procedure if the procedure was performed for infertility. If the procedure was undertaken for pain management, standardized pain assessments should be performed in the postprocedural clinic visit(s).

Fig. 10.9 **(a)** Fluoroscopic image of the left mid-abdomen demonstrating a 6-French catheter (*black arrow*) within the IVC and terminating in the left renal vein (*white arrowhead*) via a right internal jugular venous approach (*black arrow*). The venogram, performed form the distal main left renal vein, demonstrates reflux into the left gonadal/testicular vein (*white arrow*). **(b)** Selective left gonadal venogram demonstrating a dilated pampiniform plexus, consistent with a varicocele (*black arrow*). Note the classic "bag of worms" appearance of the varicocele. The venogram also shows an additional venous channel communicating with the mid left gonadal vein near the C2 catheter tip (*black arrowhead*). **(c)** Fluoroscopic image if the pelvis in the right anterior oblique (RAO) projection again demonstrating the main left gonadal vein (*black arrows*) after coil embolization of the distal aspect of this vein. The additional venous channel noted in figure 9b is better appreciated on this image after it has been selected with a microwire (*black arrowheads*). It is important to identify all additional venous channels to be sure they are excluded, as these can be a cause of gonadal vein recanalization and subsequent embolization failure. **(d)** Completion radiograph of the left abdomen and pelvis after embolization of the entire length of the main left gonadal vein and the additional venous channel noted more distally within the pelvis in **(b)** and **(c)**.

10.9.6 Outcomes

Most recent publications report technical success rates for gonadal vein embolization of 90 to 100%. Based on US or clinical assessment, recurrence rates at 6 weeks postembolization range from 7 to 16%. However, it should be noted that some authors have shown a disconnect between ultrasonographic and clinical success rates, noting that long-term clinical successes may still be achieved despite ongoing or recurrent ultrasonographic findings.[35]

When technically successful, the clinical outcomes of gonadal vein embolization vary depending on the goal of treatment and are similar to those obtained with surgical procedures. Patients presenting with painful varicoceles experience significant improvement in symptoms 83 to 93% of the time, whereas 70 to 97% report complete resolution of their pain.[43,48] Clinical recurrence of pain after embolization is uncommon, and is reported 0 to 3% of the time in most modern studies when either glue or a combination of sclerosant and coils is used as the embolic agents.[23]

Clinical success rates of gonadal vein embolization with respect to fertility are less clear and remain somewhat controversial due to conflicting reports. While multiple studies have demonstrated significant improvements in semen parameters following embolization, pregnancy outcomes following embolization are mixed. While there are larger case series demonstrating significant improvements in pregnancy rates in treated versus untreated men with varicoceles, other reports fail to demonstrate a difference.[48,49,50]

Finally, treatment of adolescent patients with varicoceles and low testicular volumes has been shown to have "catch-up growth" of the ipsilateral testicle in 80% of treated patients.[51]

10.10 Pearls of Wisdom

- Establish a good working relationship with your local urologist, and discuss preprocedural evaluation and follow-up plans.
- Develop a technical "kit" for these types of cases and approach them in a similar fashion with exceptions to your protocol as needed. Consider using the same sheath, catheter, sclerosing agents, and coils to maximize efficiency and minimize procedural time and radiation dose.
- Using sclerosants in addition to mechanical occlusion devices can treat more deeply interconnected channels.
- Treatment of the entire length of the left gonadal vein helps prevent collateralization of retroperitoneal veins and the formation of secondary channels.

10.11 Unanswered Questions

Varicoceles result in significant morbidity for affected patients. Patients may be treated with surgical or endovascular means. While large prospective randomized trials are lacking, emerging case series and meta-analyses suggest high rates of clinical success and low rates of complications when patients undergo endovascular sclerosis/embolization. Additionally, studies comparing sclerosant and embolic agents as well as outcomes data between unilateral versus bilateral gonadal vein treatment may be helpful in determining the optimal treatment of these patients.

10.12 Nutcracker Syndrome

The "fork-like" anatomical relationship that the superior mesenteric artery (SMA) shares with the abdominal aorta was described in 1937 as being analogous to that of a "nutcracker."[52] The anatomic compression of the LRV within the acute angle made between the aorta and the SMA was first identified in patients in 1950 by El-Sadr and Mina, who named this phenomenon "left renal vein entrapment syndrome."[53] In 1971, Chait was the first to apply to the term *nutcracker* to describe entrapment of the LRV by the aorta and the SMA in patients.[54] However, it was not until the following year that de Schepper, a Belgian physician, coined the term *nutcracker syndrome* (NCS) to describe the clinical scenario of symptomatic entrapment of the LRV.[55]

The term *nutcracker syndrome* is now used to describe any anatomic variant or other pathologic circumstance that leads to compression of the LRV that is significant enough to cause LRV hypertension, which manifests clinically as hematuria, flank pain, or occasionally PCS in women or varicoceles in men. The term *nutcracker phenomenon* should be reserved for asymptomatic LRV entrapment.

Entrapment of the LRV between the SMA and aorta is the most frequently encountered cause of NCS. However, multiple anatomic variations and nonanatomic causes of NCS have been described, necessitating more detailed nomenclature. The classic scenario of LRV compression between the SMA and abdominal aorta has been referred to as "anterior NCS."[56,57] Additional variants include compression of the LRV between the aorta and vertebral body (typically in the setting of a retroaortic LRV), which is termed "posterior NCS," and "lateral NCS" describing compression of the LRV between the SMA and proximal aspect of the right renal vein.[56,58] A combination of anterior and posterior NCS has also been described in the setting of a circumaortic LRV in which the anterior venous limb is compressed between the SMA and aorta, while the posterior venous limb is compressed between the aorta and underlying vertebral body.[59] Additional causes of NCS include excessive fibrous tissue at the origin of the SMA, pancreatic and retroperitoneal tumors, and para-aortic lymphadenopathy.[56,60,61]

10.12.1 Case Vignette

Patient Presentation

A 32-year-old woman presents with hematuria and left flank pain. She has a body mass index of 19 and is otherwise healthy with a negative review of systems.

Physical Exam

Slender, well-developed woman with normal abdominal and pelvic exam.

Imaging

Abdominal CT imaging was performed which revealed normal hollow and solid viscera. No suspicious masses are identified. There is a paucity of retroperitoneal fat with a narrow aortomesenteric diameter (AMD) and acute aortomesenteric angle (AMA) (▶ Fig. 10.10a).

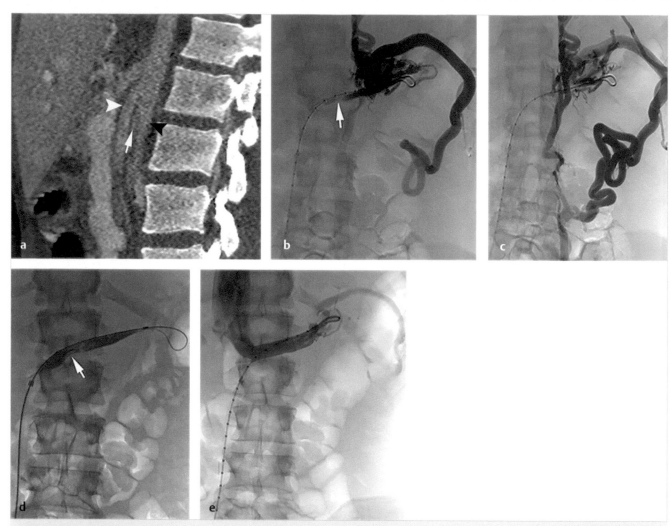

Fig. 10.10 (a) Sagittal postcontrast CT image of the upper abdomen demonstrating significant compression of the left renal vein (*white arrow*) between the underlying aorta (*black arrowhead*) and the overlying superior mesenteric artery (SMA) (*white arrowhead*). Note that the aortomesenteric distance (AMD) was less than 3 mm and the aortomesenteric angle (AMA) was under 16 degrees (b) Left renal venogram performed through a 5 French Omni Flush catheter demonstrating significant venous reflux into the left gonadal vein and an abrupt stenosis (*arrow*) along the medial aspect of the left renal vein at the expected level of the overlying superior mesenteric artery. These finding correspond and confirm the findings of the CT shown in **a**. Of note, pressure measurements taken across the lesion demonstrated a gradient greater than 3 mmHg and intravascular ultrasound (IVUS) images also confirmed significant stenosis of the left renal vein between the underlying aorta and overlying SMA. (c) Delayed images of the left renal venogram shown in **b** demonstrating dilated collateral lumbar veins in addition to the dilated left gonadal vein. Once again, the abrupt stenosis along the medial aspect of the left renal vein at the expected level of the overlying superior mesenteric artery is evident. (d) Fluoroscopic image of the mid abdomen during balloon venoplasty of the stenotic left renal vein described in (**a; b; c**). Note the significant impression that the overlying SMA is creating on the angioplasty balloon (*white arrow*). (e) Left renal venogram performed after venoplasty and stenting of the medial left renal vein demonstrating resolution of the previously noted left gonadal venous reflux and nonfilling of the significant collateral veins in the lumbar plexus. Note the free antegrade flow of contrast out of the left renal vein and into the IVC.

Specifics of Consent

The procedure and technical approach, whether from internal jugular or femoral veins, is presented with general procedural risks including sedation and access site hematoma. Venography, manometry, intravascular ultrasound (IVUS), stenting, and venoplasty are all discussed as possible interventions during the procedure. The potential complications associated with these interventions can include venous injury, venous thrombosis, and stent maldeployment/migration.

Details of Procedure

A right common femoral approach was used, and an 8-French vascular sheath was placed. The left common femoral vein was accessed and a multi-side hole catheter was advanced deep into the renal vein for venography (▶ Fig. 10.10b,c). Initial venography reveals a robust collateral venous network draining the renal vein away from the IVC. Little, if any, anterograde flow is noted. Manometry from the LRV to the IVC was performed revealing a gradient > 3 mm Hg. IVUS was performed across the

LRV to the IVC confirming near-complete compression of the LRV.

A 12 mm diameter by 4 cm high pressure balloon was used for venoplasty across the LRV stenotic segment, in order to pre-dilate the vein for subsequent stent placement (▶ Fig. 10.10d). IVUS was again used to accurately measure venous diameter and needed treatment length. A 14 mm × 60 mm self-expanding stent was deployed within the vein. Completion venography reveals brisk anterograde flow from the LRV to the IVC, with concomitant collapse of the collateral venous network (▶ Fig. 10.10e). Manometry confirms resolution of gradient.

Follow-up

After overnight observation, the patient was discharged uneventfully the next day. Aspirin 81 mg and clopidogrel 75 mg daily therapy was initiated. At 2-week follow-up, the patient confirmed that her hematuria had resolved. After 2 months, the patient was maintained on aspirin alone. Follow-up CT imaging was performed at 1 year, which demonstrated persistent patency.

10.12.2 Epidemiology and Scope of the Problem

The incidence of symptomatic NCS is unknown.[62] This is in part due to the lack of consensus regarding what specific symptoms, or constellation of symptoms, are severe enough to suggest an underlying syndrome as opposed to normal anatomic variation.[56] Asymptomatic dilation of the LRV (so-called "nutcracker physiology") has been reported to occur in up to 50 to 70% of the population.[63] Similarly, hematuria, the most common presenting symptom of NCS, is a common medical problem occurring in up to 18% of asymptomatic individuals.[64] Further, Shin et al reported that approximately 30% of individuals with isolated hematuria in the pediatric population were found to have nutcracker physiology on renal US.[65]

10.12.3 Patient Presentation and Evaluation

NCS most commonly presents with intermittent macroscopic hematuria.[66,67] Other symptoms are much less common and may include nonspecific left flank pain, upper abdominal pain, and/or orthostatic proteinuria. Infrequently, NCS can lead to varicoceles in men or PCS in women, each presenting with their own unique clinical symptoms. The typical patient is a woman in her second or third decade of life with above average height and an asthenic build.[61] Diagnostic criteria for NCS include both invasive and noninvasive imaging techniques. On duplex US, the ratio of peak systolic velocity (PSV) of the aortomesenteric segment of the LRV to the hilar portion of greater than 4 has been shown to have a sensitivity and specificity of 80 and 94%, respectively.[68,69] In addition, the ratio of the anteroposterior (AP) diameter of the LRV at the hilum to the aortomesenteric segment > 5 has been shown to have a sensitivity and specificity of 69 and 89%, respectively, on US but has also been extrapolated to CT and MRI. In combination, an AP diameter ratio and PSV ratio of > 5 portends a 90% sensitivity and a specificity approaching 100%.[69] Additional findings on CT and MRI include

a significantly reduced AMD (< 3 mm), and an AMA under 16 degrees.[70] However, because variations in anatomy vary widely in normal subjects, venography with renocaval pressure gradients (> 3 mm Hg) is widely considered the gold standard for diagnosis.[61,71] Ultimately, imaging findings alone are insufficient for making the diagnosis and are used more in a confirmatory capacity.

10.12.4 Preparation for Procedure

After careful evaluation of the patient's history, physical exam, and imaging, an outpatient venogram may be scheduled with the intent of measuring pressure gradients across the suspected stenosis at the level of the SMA, and intravenous interrogation with IVUS. IVUS is particularly helpful for defining and measuring the left renal venous luminal narrowing, properly sizing stent diameter and length, and optimizing stent placement. Self-expanding stents are generally preferred in the setting of all compressive venous diseases because of their superior radial strength. No additional special equipment is required for stenting in the setting of NCS.

Preprocedure preparation follows the standard preparation for venography with the intention for venous stenting. These preparations include nothing by mouth (NPO) status the night prior to the procedure, and basic labs (creatinine, PT, INR, PTT, platelets, and a baseline hemoglobin level). Moderate sedation is sufficient for most patients unless additional comorbidities necessitate anesthesia support.

Both internal jugular and common femoral venous approaches have been described and are acceptable. Selection of the LRV can be achieved with any number of catheter and wire combinations, and after determining that treatment is warranted, a self-expanding stent with high radial force is recommended.

10.12.5 Technical Tips and Tricks and Procedural Details

The endovascular procedure can be performed with moderate sedation. Some patients may have comorbid conditions that require general anesthesia, but these are noted in the minority of patients. Percutaneous access of the right common femoral vein is obtained and selective catheterization of the LRV is performed. Access can also be obtained from the left common femoral vein or the right internal jugular vein for easier access into the LRV. Confirmation of the diagnosis can be made with venography (using the Valsalva maneuver) by visualization of contrast washout and well-developed collaterals, renocaval pressure gradient measurements, and with IVUS to obtain accurate measurements of the renal vein diameter. As mentioned above, IVUS can be used for proper stent sizing and positioning.

Once the diagnosis has been confirmed, a wire is directed into the left gonadal vein to allow sufficient purchase for sheath delivery. After sheath positioning across the stenosis, IVUS can be used to define precisely where the LRV stent is to be optimally deployed. The stent is centered across the stenosis and is deployed after the sheath is partially withdrawn. Self-expanding stents are suggested, partially due to their excellent radial force. A second reason is their elasticity, which accommodates the adjacent arteries and avoids overcompression of the SMA and aorta by the venous stent. Partial protrusion of the stent into the IVC is generally advocated, as this may prevent displacement fully into the renal vein. Distal landing of the stent just lateral to the first large branch of the LRV has been suggested in order to reduce the risk of migration. However, the long-term implications of stent placement across the first large branch on renal function and symptom recurrence are not well known.

Poststenting angioplasty is typically needed for full stent expansion. Antiplatelet therapy is recommended, although the duration of therapy should be individualized.

10.12.6 Potential Complications or Pitfalls

Major complications after NCS repair are uncommon but generally include those typical to venous angioplasty and stenting. These specifically include bleeding from the access site (most common), thrombosis at the angioplasty site (LRV), vein rupture, and stent migration or misplacement. All of these are extraordinarily rare.

10.12.7 Postprocedural Management and Follow-up

Patients are discharged the same day or after an overnight observation. Few symptoms are associated with stenting, although transient back or abdominal pain has been encountered following stent placement, which may possibly be due to pressure on the aorta and SMA by the stent. Medical management is centered on antiplatelet therapy. Dual antiplatelet agents (aspirin 81 mg and clopidogrel 75 mg) may be used daily for 2 months, at which time clopidogrel is discontinued. Aspirin therapy is continued indefinitely. The need for systemic anticoagulation is decided on a case-by-case basis. Clinical follow-up at 2 weeks postprocedure and at 6 months is routine, with annual follow-up thereafter. If symptoms return, initial evaluation is performed with CT imaging and followed by repeat venography, manometry, and stent revision if necessary.

10.12.8 Outcomes

There are no large prospective randomized trials assessing the efficacy of endovascular stenting as a treatment option for NCS. However, there are several cohort studies that report favorable and compelling long-term outcomes. One of the largest cohort studies to report long-term follow-up results after endovascular stenting of the LRV demonstrated that 97% of patients experienced resolution of their symptoms while having only one reported complication (1.6%) in the 64-month follow-up period. The single complication was reportedly a nonfatal stent migration that was successfully retrieved without incident.[72]

10.12.9 Pearls of Wisdom

- Manometry is useful to help confirm the diagnosis. A gradient of > 3 mm Hg across a stenotic area in the LRV caused by the compressive SMA is highly suggestive of NCS.

- IVUS is the most accurate measure of vessel size, which will minimize the risk of stent migration.
- IVUS is useful to identify the precise location of the compression and the landing zone for the stent. This is helpful to reduce stent malpositioning, which can reduce the potential for stent migration and increase patency rates.

10.12.10 Unanswered Questions

NCS is a rare entity, and diagnosis requires attention to the history and physical examination, noninvasive imaging, and confirmation with conventional venography and manometry. While many treatment options have been proposed and described in the literature, endovascular therapies, namely endovascular stenting, have become the preferred method of treatment. However, because of the low incidence of NCS, no head-to-head randomized trials exist to definitively show superiority of one treatment option over another. As such, it is paramount that every effort be taken to optimize outcomes and reduce complications, especially stent migration and thrombosis. The liberal use of IVUS, in addition to good interventional technique, may help the operator achieve this goal.

References

[1] Richardson G. Pelvic congestion syndrome: diagnosis and treatment. In: Bergan JJ, Bunke-Paquette N, Bunke N, eds. The Vein Book. New York, NY: Oxford University Press; 2013
[2] Gooch R. An account of some circumstances, under which a hæmorrhage may occur, sufficient to produce alarming symptoms, though the uterus feels contracted in the ordinary degree. Med Chir Trans. 1823; 12(Pt 1):152–166
[3] Richet A, Traité pratique d'anatomie médico-chirurgicale. Paris: F. Chamerot, Libraire-Éditeur; 1855
[4] Cotte G. Les troubles functionelles de l'appareil genital de la femme. Paris: Masson et Cie; 1928
[5] Beard RW, Highman JH, Pearce S, Reginald PW. Diagnosis of pelvic varicosities in women with chronic pelvic pain. Lancet. 1984; 2(8409):946–949
[6] Taylor HC, Jr. Vascular congestion and hyperemia; their effect on function and structure in the female reproductive organs; etiology and therapy. Am J Obstet Gynecol. 1949; 57(4):654–668
[7] Stones RW. Pelvic vascular congestion-half a century later. Clin Obstet Gynecol. 2003; 46(4):831–836
[8] Latthe P, Latthe M, Say L, Gülmezoglu M, Khan KS. WHO systematic review of prevalence of chronic pelvic pain: a neglected reproductive health morbidity. BMC Public Health. 2006; 6:177
[9] Koo S, Fan CM. Pelvic congestion syndrome and pelvic varicosities. Tech Vasc Interv Radiol. 2014; 17(2):90–95
[10] O'Brien MT, Gillespie DL. Diagnosis and treatment of the pelvic congestion syndrome. J Vasc Surg Venous Lymphat Disord. 2015; 3(1):96–106
[11] Perry CP. Current concepts of pelvic congestion and chronic pelvic pain. JSLS. 2001; 5(2):105–110
[12] Beard RW, Reginald PW, Wadsworth J. Clinical features of women with chronic lower abdominal pain and pelvic congestion. Br J Obstet Gynaecol. 1988; 95(2):153–161
[13] Borghi C, Dell'Atti L. Pelvic congestion syndrome: the current state of the literature. Arch Gynecol Obstet. 2016; 293(2):291–301
[14] Gloviczki P, Comerota AJ, Dalsing MC, et al. Society for Vascular Surgery, American Venous Forum. The care of patients with varicose veins and associated chronic venous diseases: clinical practice guidelines of the Society for Vascular Surgery and the American Venous Forum. J Vasc Surg. 2011; 53(5) Suppl:2S–48S
[15] Angle JF, Siddiqi NH, Wallace MJ, et al. Society of Interventional Radiology Standards of Practice Committee. Quality improvement guidelines for percutaneous transcatheter embolization: Society of Interventional Radiology Standards of Practice Committee. J Vasc Interv Radiol. 2010; 21(10):1479–1486
[16] Rundqvist E, Sandholm LE, Larsson G. Treatment of pelvic varicosities causing lower abdominal pain with extraperitoneal resection of the left ovarian vein. Ann Chir Gynaecol. 1984; 73(6):339–341

[17] Kim HS, Malhotra AD, Rowe PC, Lee JM, Venbrux AC. Embolotherapy for pelvic congestion syndrome: long-term results. J Vasc Interv Radiol. 2006; 17(2 Pt 1):289–297

[18] Venbrux AC, Chang AH, Kim HS, et al. Pelvic congestion syndrome (pelvic venous incompetence): impact of ovarian and internal iliac vein embolotherapy on menstrual cycle and chronic pelvic pain. J Vasc Interv Radiol. 2002; 13 (2 Pt 1):171–178

[19] Andrews R. Pelvic congestion syndrome. In: Geschwind J, Dake M, eds. Abrams' Angiography: Interventional Radiology. Philadelphia, PA: Wolters Kluwer Health; 2013

[20] Edwards RD, Robertson IR, MacLean AB, Hemingway AP. Case report: pelvic pain syndrome–successful treatment of a case by ovarian vein embolization. Clin Radiol. 1993; 47(6):429–431

[21] Mahmoud O, Vikatmaa P, Aho P, et al. Efficacy of endovascular treatment for pelvic congestion syndrome. J Vasc Surg Venous Lymphat Disord. 2016; 4(3): 355–370

[22] Kantartzi PD, Goulis ChD, Goulis GD, Papadimas I. Male infertility and varicocele: myths and reality. Hippokratia. 2007; 11(3):99–104

[23] Kwak N, Siegel D. Imaging and interventional therapy for varicoceles. Curr Urol Rep. 2014; 15(4):399

[24] Akman A. Varicocele. In: Geschwind J, Dake M, eds. Abrams' Angiography: Interventional Radiology. Philadelphia, PA: Wolters Kluwer Health; 2013

[25] Tulloch WS. Varicocele in subfertility; results of treatment. BMJ. 1955; 2 (4935):356–358

[26] Cassidy D, Jarvi K, Grober E, Lo K. Varicocele surgery or embolization: which is better? Can Urol Assoc J. 2012; 6(4):266–268

[27] Halpern J, Mittal S, Pereira K, Bhatia S, Ramasamy R. Percutaneous embolization of varicocele: technique, indications, relative contraindications, and complications. Asian J Androl. 2016; 18(2):234–238

[28] Masson P, Brannigan RE. The varicocele. Urol Clin North Am. 2014; 41(1): 129–144

[29] Pastuszak AW, Wang R. Varicocele and testicular function. Asian J Androl. 2015; 17(4):659–667

[30] Rowe PJ, Comhaire FH, Hargreave TB, Mellows HJ; World Health Organization. WHO Manual for the Standardized Investigation and Diagnosis of the Infertile Male. Cambridge, MA: Cambridge University Press; 2000

[31] Thonneau P, Marchand S, Tallec A, et al. Incidence and main causes of infertility in a resident population (1,850,000) of three French regions (1988–1989). Hum Reprod. 1991; 6(6):811–816

[32] Jungwirth A, Giwercman A, Tournaye H, et al. European Association of Urology Working Group on Male Infertility. European Association of Urology guidelines on male infertility: the 2012 update. Eur Urol. 2012; 62(2):324–332

[33] Nieschlag E, Behre HM, Nieschlag S. Andrology: Male Reproductive Health and Dysfunction. Berlin: Springer; 2010

[34] Peterson AC, Lance RS, Ruiz HE. Outcomes of varicocele ligation done for pain. J Urol. 1998; 159(5):1565–1567

[35] Puche-Sanz I, Flores-Martín JF, Vázquez-Alonso F, Pardo-Moreno PL, Cózar-Olmo JM. Primary treatment of painful varicocoele through percutaneous retrograde embolization with fibred coils. Andrology. 2014; 2(5):716–720

[36] Karademir K, Senkul T, Baykal K, Ateş F, Işeri C, Erden D. Evaluation of the role of varicocelectomy including external spermatic vein ligation in patients with scrotal pain. Int J Urol. 2005; 12(5):484–488

[37] Practice Committee of American Society for Reproductive Medicine. Report on varicocele and infertility. Fertil Steril. 2008; 90(5) Suppl:S247–S249

[38] Jarow JP, Sharlip ID, Belker AM, et al. Male Infertility Best Practice Policy Committee of the American Urological Association Inc. Best practice policies for male infertility. J Urol. 2002; 167(5):2138–2144

[39] Pilatz A, Altinkilic B, Köhler E, Marconi M, Weidner W. Color Doppler ultrasound imaging in varicoceles: is the venous diameter sufficient for predicting clinical and subclinical varicocele? World J Urol. 2011; 29(5):645–650

[40] El-Haggar S, Nassef S, Gadalla A, Latif A, Mostafa T. Ultrasonographic parameters of the spermatic veins at the inguinal and scrotal levels in varicocele diagnosis and post-operative repair. Andrologia. 2012; 44(3):210–213

[41] Lechter A, Lopez G, Martinez C, Camacho J. Anatomy of the gonadal veins: a reappraisal. Surgery. 1991; 109(6):735–739

[42] Favard N, Moulin M, Fauque P, et al. Comparison of three different embolic materials for varicocele embolization: retrospective study of tolerance, radiation and recurrence rate. Quant Imaging Med Surg. 2015; 5(6):806–814

[43] Gandini R, Konda D, Reale CA, et al. Male varicocele: transcatheter foam sclerotherapy with sodium tetradecyl sulfate–outcome in 244 patients. Radiology. 2008; 246(2):612–618

[44] Jargiello T, Drelich-Zbroja A, Falkowski A, Sojka M, Pyra K, Szczerbo-Trojanowska M. Endovascular transcatheter embolization of recurrent post-

[45] Chomyn JJ, Craven WM, Groves BM, Durham JD. Percutaneous removal of a Gianturco coil from the pulmonary artery with use of flexible intravascular forceps. J Vasc Interv Radiol. 1991; 2(1):105–106

[46] Wunsch R, Efinger K. The interventional therapy of varicoceles amongst children, adolescents and young men. Eur J Radiol. 2005; 53(1):46–56

[47] Chalmers N, Hufton AP, Jackson RW, Conway B. Radiation risk estimation in varicocele embolization. Br J Radiol. 2000; 73(867):293–297

[48] Bittles MA, Hoffer EK. Gonadal vein embolization: treatment of varicocele and pelvic congestion syndrome. Semin Intervent Radiol. 2008; 25(3):261–270

[49] Abdel-Meguid TA, Al-Sayyad A, Tayib A, Farsi HM. Does varicocele repair improve male infertility? An evidence-based perspective from a randomized, controlled trial. Eur Urol. 2011; 59(3):455–461

[50] Evers JH, Collins J, Clarke J. Surgery or embolisation for varicoceles in subfertile men. Cochrane Database Syst Rev. 2009(1):CD000479

[51] Salzhauer EW, Sokol A, Glassberg KI. Paternity after adolescent varicocele repair. Pediatrics. 2004; 114(6):1631–1633

[52] Grant JCB. Method of Anatomy: Descriptive and Deductive. Baltimore, MD: The Williams and Wilkins Company; 1944

[53] El-Sadr AR, Mina E. Anatomical and surgical aspects in the operative management of varicocele. Urol Cutaneous Rev. 1950; 54(5):257–262

[54] Chait A, Matasar KW, Fabian CE, Mellins HZ. Vascular impressions on the ureters. Am J Roentgenol Radium Ther Nucl Med. 1971; 111(4):729–749

[55] de Schepper A. "Nutcracker" phenomenon of the renal vein and venous pathology of the left kidney. J Belge Radiol. 1972; 55(5):507–511

[56] Kurklinsky AK, Rooke TW. Nutcracker phenomenon and nutcracker syndrome. Mayo Clin Proc. 2010; 85(6):552–559

[57] Quevedo HC, Arain SA, Abi Rafeh N. Systematic review of endovascular therapy for nutcracker syndrome and case presentation. Cardiovasc Revasc Med. 2014; 15(5):305–307

[58] Polguj M, Topol M, Majos A. An unusual case of left venous renal entrapment syndrome: a new type of nutcracker phenomenon? Surg Radiol Anat. 2013; 35(3):263–267

[59] Venkatachalam S, Bumpus K, Kapadia SR, Gray B, Lyden S, Shishehbor MH. The nutcracker syndrome. Ann Vasc Surg. 2011; 25(8):1154–1164

[60] Shin JI, Park JM, Lee SM, et al. Factors affecting spontaneous resolution of hematuria in childhood nutcracker syndrome. Pediatr Nephrol. 2005; 20(5): 609–613

[61] Avgerinos ED, McEnaney R, Chaer RA. Surgical and endovascular interventions for nutcracker syndrome. Semin Vasc Surg. 2013; 26(4):170–177

[62] Ahmed K, Sampath R, Khan MS. Current trends in the diagnosis and management of renal nutcracker syndrome: a review. Eur J Vasc Endovasc Surg. 2006; 31(4):410–416

[63] Buschi AJ, Harrison RB, Norman A, et al. Distended left renal vein: CT/sonographic normal variant. AJR Am J Roentgenol. 1980; 135(2):339–342

[64] Grossfeld GD, Litwin MS, Wolf JS, et al. Evaluation of asymptomatic microscopic hematuria in adults: the American Urological Association best practice policy–part I: definition, detection, prevalence, and etiology. Urology. 2001; 57(4):599–603

[65] Shin JI, Park JM, Lee JS, Kim MJ. Effect of renal Doppler ultrasound on the detection of nutcracker syndrome in children with hematuria. Eur J Pediatr. 2007; 166(5):399–404

[66] Kim SH, Cho SW, Kim HD, Chung JW, Park JH, Han MC. Nutcracker syndrome: diagnosis with Doppler US. Radiology. 1996; 198(1):93–97

[67] Nishimura Y, Fushiki M, Yoshida M, et al. Left renal vein hypertension in patients with left renal bleeding of unknown origin. Radiology. 1986; 160(3): 663–667

[68] Park SJ, Shin JI. Renal Doppler ultrasonography in the diagnosis of nutcracker syndrome. Eur J Pediatr. 2013; 172(1):135–136

[69] Wendel RG, Crawford ED, Hehman KN. The "nutcracker" phenomenon: an unusual cause for renal varicosities with hematuria. J Urol. 1980; 123(5): 761–763

[70] Lamba R, Tanner DT, Sekhon S, McGahan JP, Corwin MT, Lall CG. Multidetector CT of vascular compression syndromes in the abdomen and pelvis. Radiographics. 2014; 34(1):93–115

[71] Menard MT. Nutcracker syndrome: when should it be treated and how? Perspect Vasc Surg Endovasc Ther. 2009; 21(2):117–124

[72] Chen S, Zhang H, Shi H, Tian L, Jin W, Li M. Endovascular stenting for treatment of Nutcracker syndrome: report of 61 cases with long-term followup. J Urol. 2011; 186(2):570–575

11 Portal and Mesenteric Venous Disorders

Maria del Pilar Bayona-Milano and Hector Ferral

Summary

The array and complexity of portal vein interventions represent an area of challenge for the interventional radiologist. These procedures require an in-depth understanding of the relationship between hepatic, cardiac, and renal physiology, and may be intellectually and clinically satisfying when performed well. This chapter reviews the broad spectrum of portal venous interventions performed for a variety of clinical syndromes, providing technical guidance as well as clinical management tools for the beginning and advanced practitioner.

Keywords: portal vein, portomesenteric, splenic vein, TIPS, DIPS, portal hypertension, portal vein embolization, Budd–Chiari, varices, BRTO

11.1 Introduction

Endovascular interventions in the portal venous system have become standard in current medical practice. These procedures range from elective procedures for the management of chronic problems to emergency procedures performed for patients who are in critical condition, such as patients with acute variceal hemorrhage. Interventions in the portal venous system may be technically challenging, laborious, and time consuming. The purpose of this chapter is to discuss the broad range of portal venous interventions as well as their planning.

11.2 Case Vignette

11.2.1 Patient Presentation

A 53-year-old man with a history of cirrhosis secondary to non-alcoholic steatohepatitis and refractory ascites requiring frequent large-volume paracentesis presented emergently with upper gastrointestinal bleeding. The patient had a preexisting occluded transjugular intrahepatic portosystemic shunt (TIPS), with cavernous transformation of the portal vein. Attempts to open his shunt at the outside hospital had been unsuccessful. On presentation, esophagogastroduodenoscopy was performed to treat an active area of bleeding from the esophageal varices, and gastric antral vascular ectasia was treated with epinephrine injection and clip placement. Attempts to sclerose the esophageal varices failed, and the interventional radiology team was consulted to evaluate the TIPS and attempt recanalization or new TIPS creation.

11.2.2 Physical Exam

The patient was critically ill, with jaundice and abdominal distension due to ascites. Laboratory values were as follows: prothrombin time/international normalized ratio (INR), 2.0; creatinine, 2.2 mg/dL; bilirubin, 2.1 mg/dL; alanine aminotransferase, 160 U/L; aspartate aminotransferase, 102 U/L; albumin, 2.5 g/dL; sodium level, 135 mmol/L; and platelets, 65 k/uL. The calculated corrected Model for End-Stage Liver Disease (MELD) score for the patient was 25 (estimated 3-month mortality: > 50%).

11.2.3 Imaging

Contrast-enhanced CT of the abdomen was performed and demonstrated chronic portal vein thrombosis (PVT). The TIPS was occluded. There was nonocclusive thrombus in the superior aspect of the superior mesenteric vein (SMV). The splenic vein and left portal vein were patent. Multiple small collaterals were identified around the anticipated anatomic location of the right portal vein.

11.2.4 Specifics of Consent

The following risks were discussed with the patient prior to proceeding:
- Procedure failure due to PVT or because of other technical difficulties.
- Bleeding, either from capsular disruption or from fistula creation.
- Liver failure due to portal venous shunting. In such cases, liver transplant must be considered as a therapeutic alternative.
- Deterioration of renal function. A mild elevation in creatinine level increases the risk, and this risk is increased in patients with acute anemia secondary to bleeding. This risk was discussed with the patient.
- Infection of the TIPS stent graft. In cases of spontaneous bacterial peritonitis or other known infection, a bare metal stent can be used in place of a covered stent.

The patient's MELD score was 25, a high-risk patient. The clinical predictive value of MELD decreases in the emergent setting, but risk of mortality should be discussed with the patient.

PVT increases the difficulty of TIPS placement, so preprocedural planning was extremely important.

11.2.5 Details of Procedure

The procedure performed was a TIPS with portal vein recanalization. The procedure was performed under general anesthesia. Recanalization of the preexisting TIPS was not attempted as it was thought it would be technically difficult and potentially not useful. The procedure was performed with simultaneous transjugular and transarterial approaches. The most important role for the transarterial approach was to perform a superior mesenteric artery (SMA) injection to identify the largest collaterals suitable for transhepatic puncture. Once the most suitable collaterals were identified, a transhepatic puncture was performed, aiming to the largest suitable collateral. After a successful entry into a large collateral, guidewire and catheter manipulation to negotiate the collateral was performed until a large branch of the SMV was entered. An extended shunt was created from the superior mesenteric branch to the right hepatic vein. The most distal aspect of the shunt was created with a noncovered stent and the transhepatic tract was treated with a VIATORR stent graft (W.L. Gore & Associates, Flagstaff, AZ).

11.2.6 Follow-up

Liver function tests are critical to identify immediate changes after TIPS creation. Hemodynamic changes after TIPS are known to affect liver function and the interventionalist should be attentive to those changes. Assessment for postprocedural bleeding is also critical at this stage.

Early and frequent assessment of mental status is recommended to identify signs of hepatic encephalopathy. A TIPS reduction may be necessary if encephalopathy is refractory to medical management. This event occurs in 3 to 7% of cases.

A vascular ultrasound of the liver should be obtained approximately 4 to 5 days postprocedure to assess shunt patency, and repeated every 6 months for early identification of stenosis or thrombosis.

11.3 Portal Hypertension

The liver receives its blood supply predominantly via the portal venous circulation, which accounts for 75 to 80% of the blood flow; the remaining 25% is supplied by the hepatic artery. The portal circulation is a low-pressure system with minimal resistance in which blood traverses the portal triad and the sinusoids before draining into the hepatic veins. The portal vein flow (PVF) follows Ohm's law, where the portal vein pressure (PVP) is the product of the PVF and the intrahepatic venous resistance.[1]

Portal hypertension (PH) occurs as the result of increased resistance to PVF in conditions such as cirrhosis, intra- and extrahepatic tumors, and outflow obstructions such as Budd–Chiari syndrome. Due to these conditions, the PVF directed toward the liver (hepatopetal) is reduced, or may be forced retrograde (hepatofugal). This situation results in a constellation of clinical signs and symptoms caused by increased blood volume in the splanchnic circulation, which induces the development of collateral veins and body fluid redistribution.[2] The major consequences are the development of extensive varices in the gastrointestinal tract that can cause severe or even fatal episodes of bleeding, and refractory ascites or hydrothorax with multiple hemodynamic implications.

Endovascular treatments are typically used as a rescue therapy in patients with PH and variceal gastrointestinal bleeding or refractory ascites who have not responded to more conservative medical treatments.[3] In such cases, endovascular therapies are used to decompress the portal venous system and reduce the PVP, thereby redistributing and redirecting the splanchnic flow.[3]

PH is classified as prehepatic, intrahepatic, or posthepatic based on anatomic levels (▶ Table 11.1; ▶ Fig. 11.1). The etiology of PH and its anatomic correlation are used to determine which endovascular therapeutic approach is optimal. The therapeutic options include: portal vein recanalization with angioplasty and stenting in cases of prehepatic PH (▶ Fig. 11.2; ▶ Fig. 11.3); hepatic vein or inferior vena cava (IVC) interventions in posthepatic PH; and TIPS creation in cases of intrahepatic and posthepatic PH.

Table 11.1 Causes and sites of portal hypertension

Causes of portal hypertension
Anatomic levels and etiologies
Prehepatic: extrinsic compression, stenosis, or thrombosis of the PV
Intrahepatic
Presinusoidal: chronic viral hepatitis, schistosomiasis, primary biliary cirrhosis, idiopathic sarcoidosis, myeloproliferative disease, storing diseases
Sinusoidal: Acute viral hepatitis, alcoholic hepatitis and acute fatty liver
Postsinusoidal: Veno-occlusive disease, sclerosis of the central veins
Suprahepatic: Budd–Chiari syndrome, right heart failure
Hyperdynamic: Increased (arterialized) portal venous flow in arterioportal fistulas

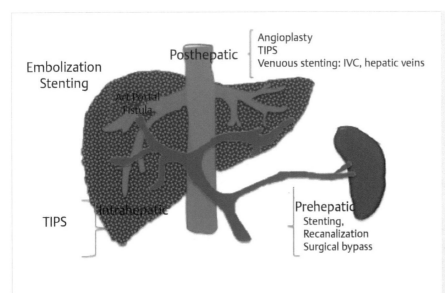

Fig. 11.1 Scheme of causes of portal hypertension and potential treatment.

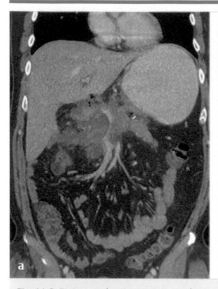
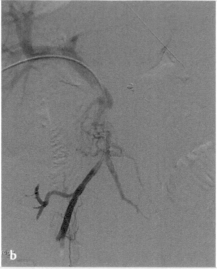
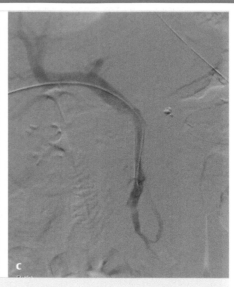

Fig. 11.2 Patient with primary neuroendocrine tumor status post central pancreatectomy complicated by portal vein stenosis and hypertension with bleeding varices. **(a)** Coronal reconstruction of CT abdomen with contrast demonstrating extensive postsurgical changes causing compression of the portal vein. **(b)** Percutaneous portal venogram with occlusion of the SMV confluence and multiple venous collaterals that bypass the stenosis. **(c)** SMV stenting with resolution of the varices and clinical improvement of the bleeding.

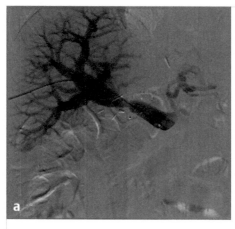
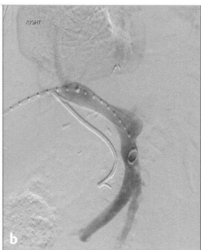

Fig. 11.3 Patient status post liver transplant with severe ascites. **(a)** Post liver transplant direct portogram that demonstrates high degree stenosis at the portal vein anastomotic level with subsequent varices and prehepatic portal hypertension. **(b)** Post stenting of the anastomosis with resolution of the varices and clinical improvement of the ascites.

11.3.1 Patient Presentation and Evaluation

The hepatic venous pressure gradient (HVPG) measures PVP obtained during hepatic vein catheterization. The HVPG measures the gradient between the higher portal venous pressure and the lower hepatic vein pressure; it is this gradient that drives portal blood through the sinusoids and into the hepatic veins.

To calculate the HVPG, the free hepatic vein pressure should be measured approximately 4 cm upstream to the confluence into the IVC, and the wedge pressure should be measured with balloon inflation in the same anatomic region within the hepatic vein. Balloon occlusion should be confirmed by visualizing sinusoidal opacification during contrast injection. In addition to sinusoidal contrast, contrast should be noted filling the portal veins in retrograde fashion. If hepatic vein to hepatic vein collaterals are noted during balloon occlusion injection, the subsequent pressure gradient measurements will be indeterminate since the balloon occlusion measurement will actually be of the collateralized hepatic vein rather than of the portal venous system.

The HVPG corresponds to the difference between the wedge hepatic venous pressure, which is equivalent to the portal venous pressure, and the free hepatic venous pressure, which is similar to the IVC pressure.

HVPG = wedge hepatic pressure – free hepatic pressure

In humans, normal HVPG values range from 1 to 5 mm Hg; an HVPG value > 12 mm Hg represents clinically significant PH.[3,4] Additionally, HVPG can be used as a measure of success of PH treatment, which is typically defined as a decrease in HVPG of > 20% compared to preintervention values, or a posttreatment HVPG value < 12 mm Hg.[3]

11.4 Transjugular Intrahepatic Portosystemic Shunt

11.4.1 Indications for Transjugular Intrahepatic Portosystemic Shunt

The TIPS procedure creates an endovascular, transhepatic shunt that decreases the HVPG. If successfully created, the bypass across the liver decompresses the high pressure mesenteric, splenic, and portal venous system, diverting flow via the stent directly into the systemic circulation via the hepatic veins and right atrium (low-resistance outflow pathway).[3] The procedure is most frequently used to relieve variceal bleeding and ascites refractory to medical treatment. First-line therapy for bleeding varices typically includes nonselective beta-blockers and endoscopic band ligation. Currently, TIPS are usually placed when endoscopic and medical therapies are not successful.[4]

In treating variceal bleeding, TIPS decreases HVPG by directly diverting flow into the systemic circulation. In refractory ascites, TIPS works by increasing natriuresis by reducing proximal tubular sodium resorption in the renin–angiotensin–aldosterone axis. TIPS is more effective in controlling recurrent or refractory ascites when compared to large-volume paracentesis; however, encephalopathy rates are higher in patients undergoing TIPS. Additionally, a significant benefit on survival has not been demonstrated.[5]

In addition to the common indications of variceal bleeding and refractory ascites, TIPS can be used in patients with PH who are to undergo major abdominal surgeries (e.g., hernia repair, colectomy, cholecystectomy). By decompressing the portal system and varices, TIPS is used to prevent intraoperative bleeding. In patients with Budd–Chiari syndrome, TIPS can be used in addition to or after the failure of other interventions, such as hepatic venous thrombectomy, angioplasty, and/or stenting of the hepatic vein outflow.[6]

Transjugular intrahepatic portal vein shunting can also provide safe portal venous access in patients with ascites or peritoneal lesions when a percutaneous transhepatic approach cannot be used. Such indications may include cases in which SMV interventions are required (e.g., SMV thrombosis, stenosis), in cases of posttransplant interventions, or in the operative scenario of pancreatic cell transplantation/infusion into the portal vein.

Some clinicians use TIPS as a bridge to liver transplant in patients with end-stage liver disease; this indication is typically reserved for patients with clinically significant sequelae of their PH (e.g., varices at risk for bleeding). After orthotopic liver transplantation, TIPS can also be used to treat complications of PH, such as Budd–Chiari syndrome, PVT, and recurrent PH.[7] TIPS has also been used in the treatment of hepatic hydrothorax and hepatorenal syndrome; however, its use in these conditions remains controversial.[5,8] The indications and contraindications for TIPS procedures are described in ▶ Table 11.2.

11.4.2 Preparation for Procedure

Careful patient evaluation is essential before proceeding with TIPS. Patient and family members must have a clear understanding of the risks and potential benefits of the procedure. In

Table 11.2 Indications and contraindications for tips procedure

Indications for TIPS procedure
- Unsuccessful endoscopically treated variceal hemorrhage
- Recurrent variceal bleed in high-risk patients
- Portal hypertensive gastropathy
- Refractory ascites
- Hepatic hydrothorax
- Budd–Chiari syndrome
- Hepatorenal syndrome
- Decompression of portosystemic collaterals prior to abdominal or esophageal surgeries

Contraindications for TIPS procedure

Absolute
- Severe liver failure
- Severe right heart failure
- Severe encephalopathy
- Polycystic liver disease

Relative
- Pulmonary hypertension
- Elevated right or left heart pressures
- Clinically significant hepatic encephalopathy
- Uncontrolled systemic infection or sepsis
- Biliary obstruction
- Primary or metastatic hepatic malignancy
- Uncorrectable coagulopathy

critical situations such as massive, acute variceal bleeding, TIPS is performed as a life-saving procedure, and a full patient evaluation may not be feasible.[9] It has been demonstrated that emergent TIPS procedures are associated with a higher mortality rate than those performed electively.[10,11]

Prior to performing the procedure, it is important to obtain a complete history from the patient and evaluate the symptoms. Particular attention should be paid to preexisting hemodynamic and respiratory conditions. Although right heart catheterization and pressure measurements will be obtained during the TIPS procedure, a preintervention echocardiogram is recommended. On echocardiography, the presence of heart failure, abnormal right ventricular function, pulmonary artery hypertension (pulmonary wedge pressure > 45 mm Hg), and tricuspid regurgitation constitute absolute contraindications to TIPS. In addition, the presence of a significant right-to-left shunt can increase perioperative morbidity[10]; an echocardiographic bubble study with vascular ultrasound is recommended to assess whether the risk of paradoxical embolus will be significant (e.g., in cases of acute portal or hepatic vein thrombosis). Other risk factors to assess for during the initial clinical evaluation include increased age, preexisting encephalopathy, elevated liver enzymes, and the presence of ascites.

In current clinical practice, the MELD score is used for pre-TIPS risk stratification. This score is the most accepted predictor for post-TIPS short- and intermediate-term mortality and post-TIPS outcomes.[3,12] The variables used in calculating the MELD score are serum total bilirubin, INR, and serum creatinine level. With this score, TIPS procedures are classified as low risk (MELD score ≤ 18), intermediate risk (MELD score 19–25), or high risk (MELD score > 25), with corresponding 3-month mortality rates of 15, 33, and 80%, respectively.[3,13]

The most recent laboratory values, including complete serum electrolytes, complete blood count, liver and kidney function panel, coagulation tests including INR, and blood type matching, in case blood products are required, should be obtained. In the context of suspected infection, the recommendation is to obtain prior blood and body fluid cultures. If current infection exists, the risk of performing the procedure versus waiting should be determined. Even in the setting of no ongoing infection, prophylaxis with wide-spectrum antibiotics before the TIPS procedure is recommended routinely.[14]

Paracentesis may be performed in the days prior to the procedure to reduce ascites volume, and should be repeated immediately before the procedure to reduce the risk of bleeding, hypotension, and dehydration.[5] Infusion of intravenous concentrated albumin may assist with intravascular volume retention when large volumes of ascitic or pleural fluid are drained; this infusion may also help prevent contrast-induced nephropathy or worsening prerenal failure. Exceptional situations include cases of large-volume pleural effusion or ascites in the perioperative period that limit adequate ventilation or preclude prompt postoperative extubation. In these settings, more aggressive preoperative fluid removal may be indicated.

The decision to use general anesthesia versus moderate sedation should be based on the mental, hemodynamic, and respiratory status of the patient, the risk of aspiration, the estimated time required for the intervention, and the preference of the operating physician.

Pre-TIPS Imaging Evaluation

A recent liver vascular ultrasound and cross-sectional imaging of the abdomen with or without contrast are useful tools for assessing the portal and hepatic venous anatomy as well as the presence of venous collaterals and spontaneous portosystemic shunts. Imaging can also be used to exclude or confirm the presence of focal liver lesions that may interfere with intra- or transhepatic access. The operating interventional radiologist should also evaluate the patency of the hepatic artery and celiac trunk on these imaging studies. A significant arterial stenosis is considered a relative contraindication for TIPS since the hepatic arterial flow compensates for the liver blood flow that is shunted from the portal system.

Mapping the Portal Vein Target

The proposed intrahepatic pathway may be planned to use anatomic details obtained from a 3D multiplanar reconstruction (MPR) to evaluate the spatial relationship between the hepatic and portal veins (▶ Fig. 11.4). The trajectory of the access is traced from the hepatic vein to the chosen intrahepatic portal venous branch. The preferred exit site in the hepatic vein should be approximately 1 to 2 cm from the IVC confluence to avoid difficult angles when the sheath is advanced across the liver parenchyma.

The orientation of the entry needle can also be determined depending on which hepatic vein is chosen. For instance, from the right hepatic vein, the needle must be directed ventrally in order to obtain access into the right portal vein. From the middle hepatic vein, the needle can be oriented dorsally if the puncture is made far from the portal bifurcation but should be oriented anteriorly if the puncture is very close to the bifurcation. From the left hepatic vein, the needle should be oriented ventrally and medially (▶ Fig. 11.5).

All useful landmarks, including ribs, gallstones, and surgical clips, can be used as references. Those landmarks that are within the abdominal cavity are preferred over those outside the abdomen (e.g., bones), since the former will move with the liver during respiration. Obtaining preprocedure CT or MRI is useful if fusion software is to be used during the TIPS procedure. With this technology, across-sectional image can be used to reconstruct the vascular anatomy and bony landmarks, and the image can be fused with an image obtained by cone-beam acquisition of the upper abdomen during the TIPS procedure. The advantage of using such fusion technology is that this overlapped 3D image also rotates with fluoroscopy used in real time (▶ Fig. 11.6).

Technical Tips and Tricks and Procedural Details

Once access is obtained in the jugular vein, a 10-French-long vascular sheath is advanced into the right atrium, and the central venous pressures (including the right atrial, right ventricle, and pulmonary venous pressures) are measured. If elevation of the pressures is demonstrated (e.g., > 15 mm Hg), a wedge pulmonary artery pressure should be obtained to determine the degree of pulmonary hypertension.

The standard and most frequent approach to creating a TIPS involves right hepatic to right portal vein access; this is considered the safest way to avoid puncture of the hepatic artery, extrahepatic main portal vein, or biliary ducts. A left hepatic to left portal vein access has been correlated with a lower risk for encephalopathy development, but the reasons for this are not clearly understood.[15] Even with this advantage, a right hepatic vein to right portal vein approach is preferred due to favorable anatomic relationships.

In cases of challenging access to the hepatic vein, one may attempt transcaval access, parenchymal access via hepatic venous stumps, or direct intrahepatic portocaval shunt (DIPS) creation using fluoroscopy or intravascular ultrasound (discussed later in this chapter).[16] Strategies for accessing the hepatic veins are shown in ▶ Table 11.3.

Once in the hepatic vein, a wedge portogram, sometimes with improved visualization using carbon dioxide instead of iodinated contrast, viewed in at least two different obliquities should be obtained at an acquisition rate of at least four frames/second and set as a reference. By obtaining at least two obliquities, the anatomic relationship between the hepatic veins and portal veins can better be determined.

Conventional alternatives to acquiring a portogram for portal venous mapping include SMA angiogram with delayed venous portal phase and percutaneous access in a patent umbilical vein used in order to advance the catheter into the left portal vein (▶ Fig. 11.7). If access into the portal vein is challenging despite the use of multiple techniques, a percutaneous access into a varix (▶ Fig. 11.8) or transhepatic approach into the portal vein, with combined transjugular access in the hepatic vein, should facilitate access by providing a direct target for portal venous puncture.

After the TIPS needle is passed across the liver, gentle pullback aspiration is performed until significant blood return is obtained. This should be followed by portal venogram to confirm the position of the needle. If access is deemed suitable for

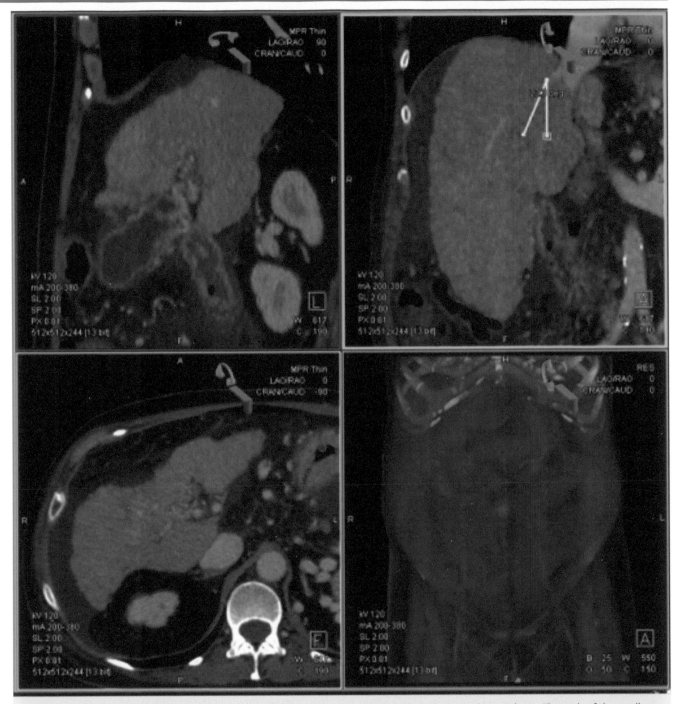

Fig. 11.4 Line parallel to the spine in the coronal and sagittal planes (on MPR) and a hypothetical tract to the portal vein. The angle of the needle can be estimated.

eventual TIPS placement, a hydrophilic wire in combination with a catheter should be negotiated distally followed by exchange for a stiff wire; catheter access is then obtained over the stiff wire. Once catheter access into the portal vein has been obtained, it is essential to perform a portogram to confirm that there is no contrast extravasation at the portal vein entry site, and measure direct portal venous pressures to determine the gradient. If the access is deemed appropriate, and the gradient and anatomy support the decision to proceed, the tract should be predilated with a 6- to 8-mm-diameter angioplasty balloon,

with progressive advancement of the sheath immediately after or during balloon deflation until the portal vein is accessed with the sheath. If a severe angulation in the entry site to the portal vein is present, multiple maneuvers may be performed to advance the vascular sheath into the portal vein (▶ Table 11.4). Extrahepatic access in the portal vein should be carefully evaluated and aborted if the operator determines that there is the high risk of peritoneal bleeding. By using a covered stent, extravasation around the portal vein entry site can be successfully treated by placing the graft segment across the vascular injury.

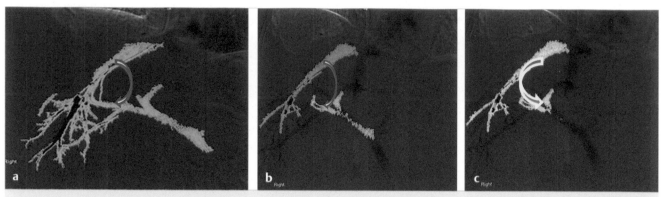

Fig. 11.5 CO_2 wedge portogram with portal vein and hepatic vein colorization and hypothetical pathway of the needle. **(a)** An AP projection with an *arrow* that indicates how lateral or medial the needle has to be directed depending on the selected target. **(b, c)** An RAO projection in which the needle pathway can be simulated pointing the needle anterior **(a)** or posterior **(b)** depending on how far the exit site in the hepatic vein from the IVC confluence will be.

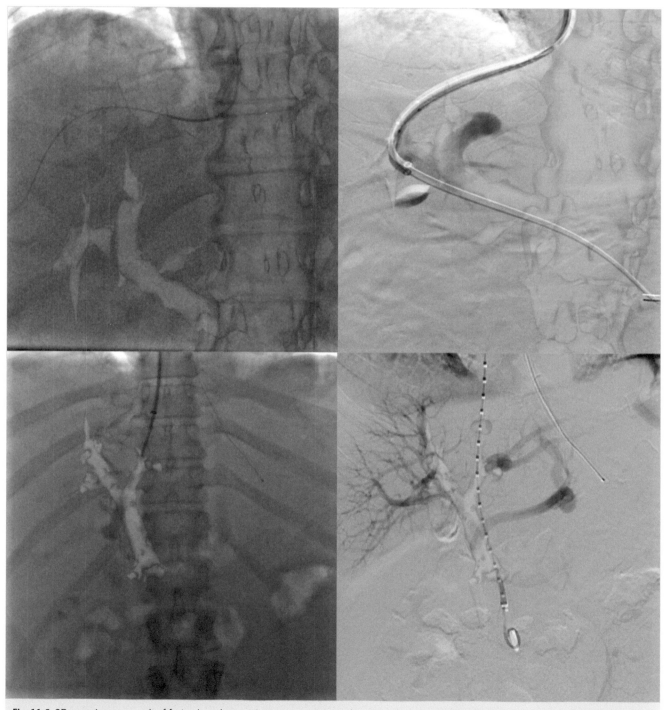

Fig. 11.6 3D mapping as a result of fusion based on axial CT image overlapped with a cone-beam evaluation. A 3D map of the portal vein is available in real time during fluoroscopy and can be used as a target.

Table 11.3 Techniques for access to challenging hepatic venous anatomy

- Sustained deep inspiration can be performed while the catheter is advanced with the wire to the confluence to engage the hepatic vein
- If the angle of the vein appears very acute, a 4-French glide C2 or Cobra catheter can be used to gain access
- If there is a small hepatic vein already accessed, an injection of carbon dioxide may show the confluence of the three hepatic veins
- Intravascular ultrasound guidance can be used to guide the catheter into the hepatic vein
- The vein can be mapped on cross-sectional imaging if fusion software is available

Table 11.4 strategies for advancing a sheath across unfavorable angulation to portal vein

- Start tract dilation into the liver parenchyma with a small-diameter, low-profile balloon (4–6 mm)
- Use sustained deep inspiration (controlled by the anesthesia team or by the patient) while the balloon is deflated and the sheath is advanced
- If the needle is still in position, advance the sheath as far as possible over the needle and its introducer
- Carefully advance the sheath over its inner dilator and the wire
- If the sheath appears floppy and looping during the process, it can be changed for a vascular sheath that gives more support (e.g., Cordis Brite Tip sheath)
- Use a superstiff wire to have more support (e.g., Amplatz superstiff wire)

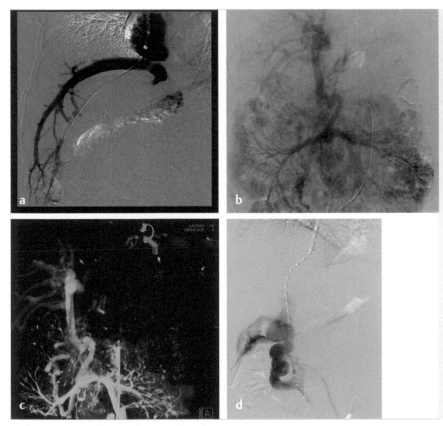

Fig. 11.7 (a) Wedge CO_2 portogram in a patient with portal vein thrombosis that failed to demonstrate the venous anatomy given collateral pathways in the hepatic vein, unable to obtain a wedge image. **(b)** Superior mesenteric angiogram with acquisition in delayed venous phase that showed the portal vein anatomy including the portomesenteric vein confluence. **(c)** 3D reconstruction after cone-beam acquisition in the delayed SMA portogram. **(d)** Portal vein access after using the SMA portogram as a target.

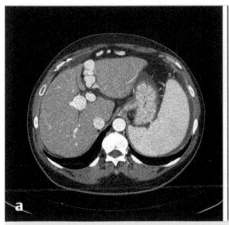
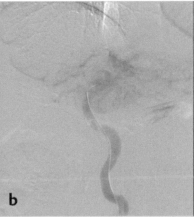
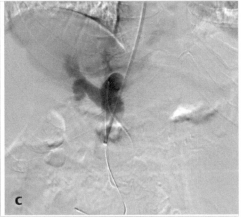

Fig. 11.8 (a) Patient with recanalized umbilical vein. CT of the abdomen with contrast demonstrating the prominent left portal vein recanalizing through umbilical vein. **(b)** Percutaneous access into the umbilical vein. **(c)** A catheter was advanced into the left portal vein, obtaining a direct portogram, used to map the target pre- TIPS procedure.

Table 11.5 Recommendations for inserting stent

- If the stent is a VIATORR (PTFE-covered), avoid inserting the covered portion of the stent within the right and left portal vein confluences, as this can cause thrombosis
- The leading and trailing ends of the shunt should parallel the long axis of the vessels without angulation and flow turbulence, which can cause TIPS dysfunction
- During stent dilation, the use of a 20-mm-length balloon is recommended; longer balloons can straighten the stent and cause undesired angulation of the ends within the vessel
- Undesired angulation of the stent at the portal vein end can be corrected with an overlapping bare metal or PTFE-covered (VIATORR) stent

Direct PVP is obtained to establish a baseline portosystemic gradient (PSG) and to determine the appropriate diameter of the stent as well as the diameter of the angioplasty balloon. A PSG < 12 mm Hg may be misleading and raises the question of the presence of a potential unidentified spontaneous portosystemic shunt. In this scenario, it is very important to identify the spontaneous shunt on prior studies (CT or MRI) or in delayed venous phase SMA angiography. If the spontaneous shunt is not visualized during the maneuvers or during direct contrast portography, the decision to proceed with TIPS is based on whether signs and symptoms related to PH will be improved with TIPS placement.

Before stent placement, a portal venogram with a calibrated pigtail catheter is performed in order to plan the length of the stent and to determine where to deploy the covered and uncovered portions of the stent. If calibrated pigtail catheters are not available, the measurement may possibly be obtained directly by measurements from the angiographic software.

The VIATORR stent graft is often used during TIPS procedures due to its long history with such procedures, ease of use, and unique design combining covered and noncovered stent designs. The VIATORR is deployed with the uncovered portion advanced into the portal vein or right or left branches, and the downstream end deployed across the hepatic vein to the level of the hepatic vein–IVC confluence (▶ Table 11.5).

Bare metal stents are still used in multiple institutions and, due to not being covered, are effective in cases of emergent TIPS when infection is suspected. Since 2004, when polytetrafluoroethylene (PTFE)-covered stent grafts were first approved by the U.S. Food and Drug Administration (FDA), multiple studies have shown decreased shunt dysfunction rates, increased long-term patency, decreased transmural permeation, and improved clinical outcomes with PTFE-covered stents compared to bare metal stents.[17,18,19]

11.5 Hemodynamic Changes after TIPS Procedures

In the short term, the increased volume shunted to the heart through a TIPS can cause pressure elevation beyond the normal reserve of the right and left ventricle, elevating the pulmonary arterial pressure. Kovács et al[20] reported persistent transient post-TIPS enlargement of the left and right atria on cardiac MRI with normalization of cardiac dimensions 3 to 6 months after TIPS placement. Filì et al suggested that the volume expansion

and hemodynamics following TIPS, including elevation of the cardiopulmonary pressures in patients with refractory ascites, returned to baseline at 24 hours postintervention[21]; however, the number of patients in this study was limited. Colombato et al reported that after the increased volume load post-TIPS, a compensatory vasodilatory effect from splanchnic vessels decreases the peripheral and pulmonary circulation resistance. This mechanism helps explain the progressive hemodynamic adaptation noted after TIPS placement.[22]

11.5.1 Combined TIPS and Variceal Embolization

There are differing opinions regarding the necessity for variceal embolization following TIPS. Some operators chose to evaluate patients angiographically following TIPS placement to evaluate whether varices have resolved with the performance of shunting and forego embolization if there is no opacification of the varices (▶ Fig. 11.9). Several studies have suggested that TIPS in combination with variceal embolization decreases the risk of recurrent variceal bleeding. Chen et al compared 106 patients with TIPS, including patients with and without variceal embolization, and concluded that the combination of TIPS and embolization decreased the risk of recurrent bleeding during the first few months post-TIPS.[23]

Additionally, a recent meta-analysis suggested the benefit of performing variceal embolization during the TIPS procedure versus performing the TIPS procedure alone in the treatment of patients with variceal bleeding.[18] Adding variceal embolization at the time of the TIPS was found to reduce the incidence of variceal rebleeding (▶ Fig. 11.10). Additionally, distal embolization of the varices using liquid embolic agents in combination with coils may help with long-term durability of embolization, preventing the possibility of recanalization. In contrast, a separate study concluded that the combination of TIPS with embolization was not beneficial in patients with a PSG < 12 mm Hg.[24] Some authors recommend performing variceal embolization before the TIPS procedure to prevent systemic migration of the embolic material.[19] The long-term outcomes of this technique are still unclear, as the variability in available embolization techniques and materials makes it difficult to compare study results.

11.5.2 TIPS and Chronic PVT

Cavernous transformation of the portal vein (cavernoma) acts as a compensatory mechanism after PVT. In this condition, multiple venous collaterals develop to supply and bypass the occluded portal vein. During this process, the native portal vein regresses, eventually degenerating into a fibrotic cord.[25] If the collateral pathways are not sufficiently large, PH may develop. Several classifications have been proposed for chronic PVT (▶ Table 11.6), but predictors for successful recanalization of the vein have not been clearly defined.[26]

Multiple techniques have been described for the treatment of PH caused by chronic PVT, including a conventional TIPS procedure, transhepatic or transsplenic portal recanalization, and DIPS placement.[27] TIPS can be very difficult if the portal vein has been transformed to a fibrotic cord.[28]

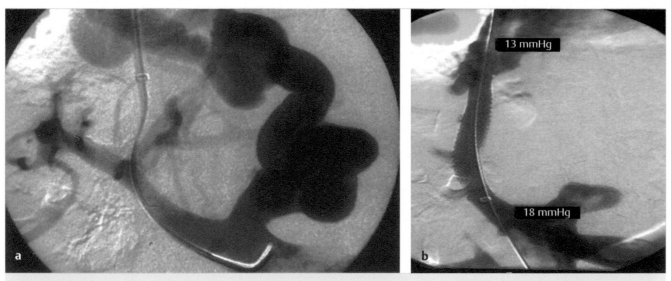

Fig. 11.9 Patient with ulcerative colitis and portal hypertension. The TIPS procedure was requested to decrease portal pressure for a planned, elective colectomy. **(a)** Pre-TIPS portography demonstrating prominent varix in the left coronary vein. **(b)** Direct portography after TIPS demonstrated complete resolution and decompression of the varix, not requiring embolization. The patient underwent an uneventful colectomy.

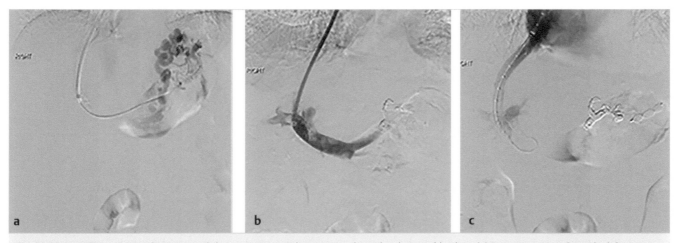

Fig. 11.10 Post TIPS varices with gastrorenal shunt in patient with severe esophageal and gastric bleeding. **(a)** Extensive varices from the left coronary and splenic vein territory opacified though TIPS venogram. **(b)** Embolization of the varices using Amplatzer plug and coils in the emergent scenario, without further visualization of the portosystemic shunt. **(c)** Patent TIPS.

Table 11.6 Classifications of chronic PVT

- Type I: Partial PVT without cavernoma
- Type II: Partial PVT with cavernoma
- Type III: Complete PVT without cavernoma
- Type IV: Complete PVT with cavernoma

When a TIPS procedure is performed in the setting of cavernous transformation, the operator must first determine the feasibility of gaining access into a high-flow venous collateral, and must then determine where to insert the stent. The stent must be inserted in a collateral that will sufficiently decompress the varices and mesenteric circulation, while ensuing enough flow to keep the shunt patent. Prior to the procedure, cross-sectional imaging should be performed to determine the potential target vein.

The initial part of the TIPS procedure for chronic PVT is identical to that of conventional TIPS procedures. A wedge hepatic portogram is used to establish a reference from at least two different angles. An SMA or splenic artery angiographic study can be used to evaluate whether an appropriate collateral vessel is present, and to determine where to place the stent (▶ Fig. 11.11). The angiogram can be combined with cone-beam acquisition in a delayed venous phase to trace the proposed needle course and to identify the potential target vein. After evaluation of the imaging, a suitable collateral for access for TIPS placement can be selected (▶ Table 11.7).

A transhepatic approach–assisted TIPS can be performed via percutaneous puncture of an intrahepatic portal vein, if there are no contraindications (e.g., severe ascites or varices around the access) to the procedure. In the case of severe ascites, a paracentesis should be performed immediately prior to percutaneous

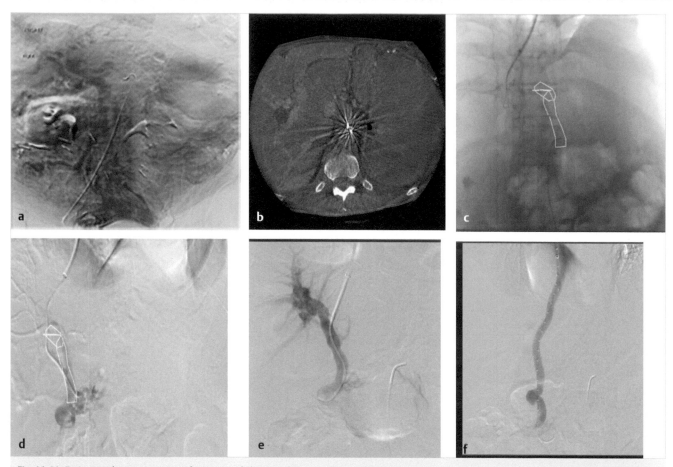

Fig. 11.11 Patient with cavernous transformation of the portal vein requiring TIPS for intractable ascites. **(a)** Superior mesenteric angiogram with delayed portal venous phase showing extensive collateral veins at the hepatic hilum consistent with cavernous transformation of the PV. **(b)** Cone-beam evaluation in the delayed phase demonstrated multiple collateral vessels in an intrahepatic location amenable to be safely accessed for recanalization and TIPS creation. **(c)** A 3D map was created based on the cone-beam findings. **(d, e)** The selected branch was accessed and again the 3D map was used for stent insertion optimizing the portomesenteric vein confluence. **(f)** The stent was deployed from the collateral vein draining the portomesenteric vein confluence into the hepatic vein confluence.

Table 11.7 Characteristics of a collateral vein that can be used for TIPS stenting

- Intrahepatic portal venous collaterals are preferred as they confer a lower risk of bleeding when compared to extrahepatic. Safer access if the collateral is in intrahepatic location to avoid the risk of severe bleeding

- Collateral vessels demonstrating drainage of the superior mesenteric and splenic vein territories are ideal. When this is not possible, collaterals in communication with SMV are preferred

- Moderate **or large** size of the collateral vessel is preferred, although smaller branches can be successfully cannulated. Very small branches are not amenable to recanalization

- Collaterals draining directly into the remaining main portal vein are preferred

hepatic access. Once access into a portal branch is gained with a 21-gauge Chiba needle, a microwire can be directed centrally. At the authors' institution, a 6-French Neff introducer (Cook Medical, Bloomington, IN) is inserted, and using a 4-French Glidecath (Terumo Interventional Systems, Somerset, NJ), access is obtained in the main portal vein. At this point, a direct portogram should be acquired to establish a target venous branch for the TIPS placement. In some cases, operators have inserted a low-profile

angioplasty balloon into the thrombosed portal vein and inflated the balloon with contrast to highlight the target for the TIPS needle approach.[29]

Transsplenic access involves a direct parenchymal approach through the spleen using a contrast injection to opacify the splenic vein and to advance a catheter retrograde into the portomesenteric vein confluence. Once access into the portal vein is achieved, a 10-mm gooseneck snare is placed within the peripheral intrahepatic portal branch to be targeted by the TIPS needle. Once the needle is place through the snare, an exchange length wire can be advanced from the jugular vein to the splenic access (through and through access), followed by tract dilation in the liver parenchyma and VIATORR stent deployment in normal fashion. Some operators perform embolization of the splenic access tract using coils or Amplatzer plugs, although some authors choose to use manual compression only.[30]

The "gunsight technique" uses two gooseneck snares, one in the portal branch that is placed via the percutaneous approach, and one in the hepatic vein that is placed via transjugular access. The snares are crossed with a 21-gauge Chiba needle, and a microwire is inserted. The wire is manipulated through the jugular access to advance a catheter into the portal vein.[26]

Once access is obtained in a portal venous collateral, manipulation of a 4-French catheter and hydrophilic wire can be performed until the splenomesenteric confluence is reached. In certain circumstances, a 0.018-inch microcatheter may be required to negotiate the vein.

A stent graft is generally recommended for deployment in the collateral vessel[31]; however, a bare metal stent can also be used, specifically when the main collateral vessel receives inflow from other collaterals.

11.6 Potential Complications or Pitfalls

Capsular perforation is one of the main complications that can cause hemodynamic instability during or after TIPS procedures. This perforation can occur secondary to a laceration during a forced wedge hepatic venogram, or as an accidental extracapsular puncture with the TIPS needle.

Portal venous bleeding, especially when an extrahepatic puncture leading to intraperitoneal bleeding is the source, must be treated immediately by the deployment of a covered stent graft (▶ Fig. 11.12). If perforation occurs from wedge venography, contrast is injected through the catheter to localize extravasation in the vein. If the bleeding site is visualized, transcatheter embolization using coils can be performed (with a diameter upsize of at least 50% of the vessel diameter), or balloon-assisted Gelfoam injection to avoid the possibility of systemic migration.[32]

Most frequently, extracapsular punctures are clinically silent or are sufficiently treated with decompression of the portal system following stent deployment. However, in the setting of persistent hemodynamic compromise from an extracapsular puncture without clear contrast extravasation on venography, an arterial source of bleeding must be excluded by hepatic angiogram and, if required, transcatheter embolization performed (▶ Fig. 11.13).

The clinical presentation of hepatic arterial puncture in a patient undergoing TIPS can range from irrelevant (no hemodynamic changes) to severe hemorrhage, hemobilia, arterioportal fistula (APF), and liver infarction with subsequent liver failure. If a catheter is positioned across the hepatic artery during percutaneous transhepatic access, gentle pullback injection with Gelfoam slurry is recommended to embolize the tract. If the main hepatic artery requires embolization, the surgical or transplant team should be consulted.

Stent migration retrograde into the main portal vein and the SMV confluence can be problematic for the potential anastomosis when the patient is a liver transplant candidate. In this situation, a second overlapping stent must be deployed to secure the migrated stent and prevent further retrograde movement.

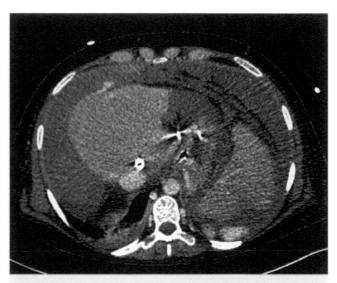

Fig. 11.13 Subcapsular hematoma post TIPS creation. Subcapsular hematoma, small pseudoaneurysm, and active contrast extravasation in the anterior aspect of the liver capsule, requiring embolization of a branch from the hepatic artery.

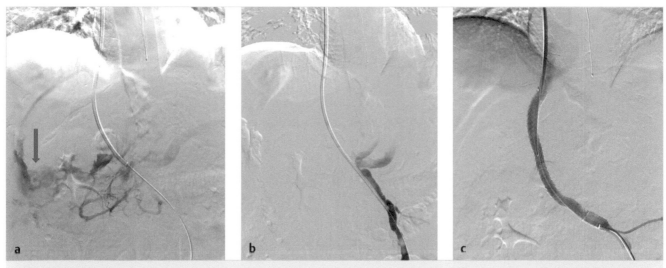

Fig. 11.12 (a) Contrast extravasation (*blue arrow*) post vascular introducer insertion after extrahepatic puncture of the portal vein branch. **(b)** The 10-French sheath was advanced into the portal venous system immediately after the extravasation episode. **(c)** Stent insertion for TIPS creation with complete resolution of the extravasation.

If the potential migration will be toward the right atrium, wire access should be maintained and the stent should be removed with a snare to prevent migration into the right ventricle or pulmonary arteries.[33]

The most important adverse consequence after TIPS is hepatic encephalopathy, which can be seen in approximately 30% of cases. Hepatic encephalopathy has a direct effect on overall mortality following nonemergent TIPS procedures.[34,35] Clinically, encephalopathy is evaluated with psychometric tests, electroencephalogram, evoked potentials, and critical flicker frequency. The presentation of this condition ranges from minimal, in which mild cognitive impairment is present, to overt, which is associated with long-term sequelae of coma and death.[34,36] Recent studies have suggested that advanced age, the occurrence of encephalopathy before the TIPS procedure, and decreased liver function (assessed with Child–Pugh score) are the most important risk factors predicting the post-TIPS encephalopathy.[35] The most widely accepted pathophysiologic explanation for the occurrence of this condition is increased shunting of ammonia products from the splanchnic circulation. Ammonia and other splanchnic venous components behave as neurotoxins, and are normally cleared through hepatic metabolism. Additionally, some medications have been postulated to cause hepatic encephalopathy, including flumazenil and bromocriptine, through binding of gamma aminobutyric acid receptors.[35,37]

Hepatic encephalopathy can be prevented by not overshunting the portal circulation. This means that the desired HVPG gradient after TIPS must be carefully measured and correlated with the MELD score and clinical condition to avoid overdilation of the stent. The presence of a concomitant spontaneous portosystemic shunt can aggravate encephalopathy by increasing the amount of ammonia products going into the systemic circulation and brain. The optimum post-TIPS HVPG depends on the indication for TIPS; the gradient expected to decrease recurrent bleeding should be reduced to < 12 mm Hg,[38,39] and to decrease recurrent ascites, the gradient should be reduced to < 8 mm Hg. If the gradient drops to < 5 mm Hg, the risks of overshunting increase and therefore the risk of hepatic encephalopathy is elevated. However, Gaba et al reported self-expansion of TIPS stents over time and questioned the advantages of intraprocedural underdilation.[37] Initial therapy for encephalopathy is based on restricting dietary proteins, and increasing the clearance and decreasing the production of ammonia with nonabsorbable disaccharides such as lactulose. Lactulose acidifies the gut and inhibits the ammoniagenic enzyme (urease), decreasing ammonia production.

In addition, antibiotics such as rifaximin inhibit urease-producing bacteria and decrease ammonia production.[35] When medical therapy fails and significant encephalopathy persists, reduction of the TIPS should be considered (described below).

11.6.1 TIPS Reduction versus Occlusion

Interventional radiologists use a variety of techniques to reduce the TIPS diameter for patients with inadequate response to medical treatment for encephalopathy. Endovascular procedures are used to reduce the stent diameter or completely occlude the shunt to improve hepatopetal portal flow into the liver, indirectly decreasing the availability of the ammonia

derivatives in the blood stream and blood–brain barrier. Because of the theory that TIPS outflow occlusion can cause a severe decrease in cardiac output, leading to sudden life-threatening shock,[37] careful evaluation using a balloon-occlusion test in the shunt is recommended before permanent occlusion is performed. With this technique, a baseline measure of the central venous pressure is obtained before an occluding balloon is temporarily inflated at the stent level. Immediately after temporary occlusion with the balloon, central venous pressure is remeasured to evaluate the effect of the shunt occlusion on the patient's hemodynamic status.

As a temporary measure, occlusion of the stent with a balloon for 48 hours has been described; however, this procedure is associated with a high risk of recurrent variceal bleeding and PVT. More acceptable techniques are described below.

One technique for reduction of TIPS flow is that of placement of a self-expanding stent graft placed in parallel with a balloon-expandable stent (▶ Fig. 11.14). To accomplish this, two long sheaths are placed via the internal jugular vein, one to deploy the stent graft and the second to insert the balloon-expandable stent. Once the stent graft is deployed, within the existing TIPS stent, the balloon-expandable stent is deployed between the new just-deployed stent graft and the prior TIPS stent. The balloon-expandable stent causes an hourglass configuration of the new stent graft, thereby limiting flow. If the flow is too restricted by the stent, it can be crushed by inflating a balloon inside the new TIPS graft.

Another technique for TIPS reduction involves placement of a suture-constrained self-expandable stent graft within the shunt. A suture is tied midstent to create an hourglass-shaped stent. The suture should be placed to match with the portion of the TIPS shunt across the liver parenchyma. Other techniques include placement of two parallel stents within the TIPS followed by coil embolization of one of the stents, or deployment of a balloon-expandable bare metal stent or a balloon-expandable stent graft within the TIPS for minor narrowing of the lumen.

To permanently occlude a TIPS, coils and Amplatzer plugs can be safely used once the patient's hemodynamic stability is confirmed with temporary balloon occlusion.

11.6.2 TIPS Dysfunction and Parallel TIPS

A long-term recurrence of PH sequelae may represent either TIPS dysfunction or the need for placement of a second parallel TIPS (more common when ascites or hepatic hydrothorax is a symptom) (▶ Fig. 11.15). In the first instance, Doppler ultrasound should be performed to evaluate for velocities of the main portal vein and shunt.[5] Multiple Doppler findings may indicate TIPS dysfunction. These include: velocities anywhere in the TIPS stent of < 90 cm/s or > 190 cm/s; a gradient across the TIPS of > 50 cm/s; or a change in velocity measurements of > 50 cm/s from one Doppler examination to another (e.g., between annual follow-up ultrasound examinations). In the case of abnormal ultrasound findings, patients should undergo a TIPS catheter evaluation and revision with further angioplasty or stenting if the MELD score is appropriate (ideal MELD score ≤ 18). When the original stent is a bare metal stent, an overlapping stent graft may be placed instead. If a patient

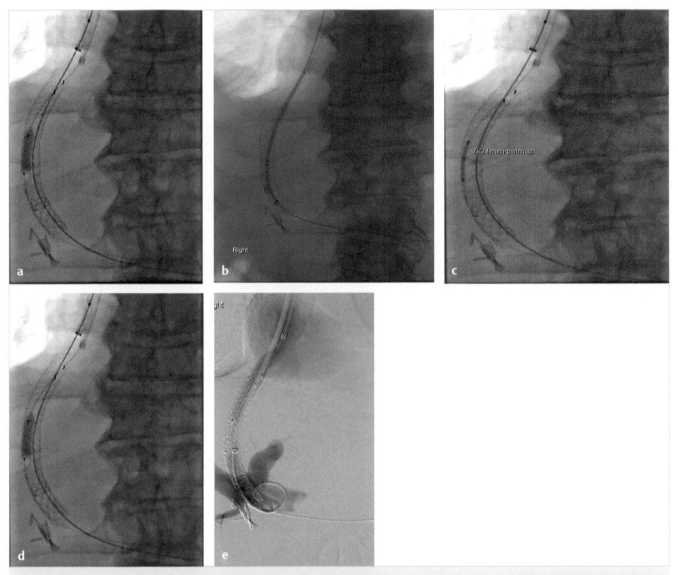

Fig. 11.14 TIPS reduction on a patient with overt encephalopathy post TIPS. **(a)** Portogram demonstrating flow across the TIPS with mild opacification of the right and left intrahepatic portal venous branches. **(b)** Two different accesses were obtained via transjugular approach into the TIPS, one using a 10-French vascular introducer and the second one with a 35-cm, 7-French sheath. **(c, d)** A 7-mm balloon-mounted stent was placed alongside the 10-French vascular sheath, through a 7-French sheath. Simultaneously through the 10-French sheath, a 10-mm VIATORR stent graft was inserted and deployed. Once the VIATORR stent graft was deployed, the balloon-mounted stent was progressively deployed adjacent, with intermittent evaluation of the desired portoatrial gradient. **(e)** Post TIPS reduction portogram demonstrated a waist at the level of the bare metal stent with persistent flow across the TIPS.

presents post-TIPS with sequelae of PH and an elevated HVPG, but the TIPS appears patent and is maximally dilated, the patient may require a second, parallel TIPS. The procedure for a parallel TIPS is identical to placement of the original TIPS; however, often a different anatomic approach using the left or middle hepatic vein may be necessary.

11.7 DIPS (Direct Intrahepatic Portocaval Shunt)

DIPS is an alternative to TIPS for cases in which the anatomy precludes a transjugular approach and for cases of Budd–Chiari syndrome, in which the hepatic veins are occluded. With this technique, a side-to-side portal vein to IVC access is obtained through the caudate lobe. Some authors suggest that this may be a safer pathway than TIPS.[40,41]

Multiple options are available for imaging guidance when performing DIPS. By using a 9-MHz intravascular ultrasound, the needle can be guided to puncture the portal vein directly from the IVC. In this technique, femoral access is obtained while a transjugular long sheath is positioned in the IVC through which a Colapinto or Rosch Uchida needle is placed[40]; portal access is thereby obtained through the caudate lobe. Conversely, percutaneous access can be obtained from the portal vein to the IVC with a 21-gauge Chiba needle under sectorial ultrasonographic guidance. An exchange-length wire can then be advanced and snared from the IVC access. If the transjugular

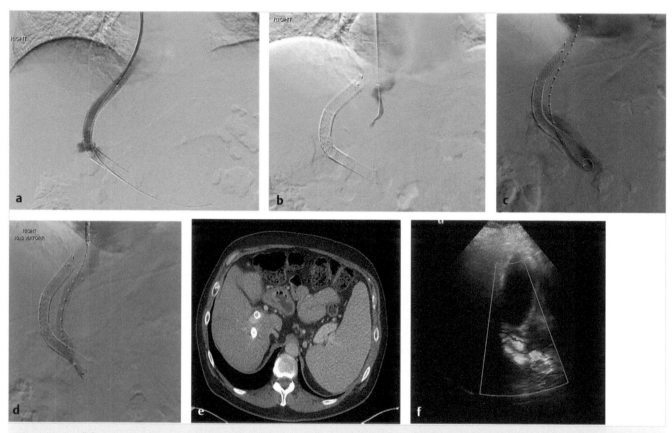

Fig. 11.15 Parallel TIPS creation in a patient with refractory ascites without improvement after initial TIPS. **(a)** Portogram through preexisting stent. **(b)** Middle hepatic vein access with venogram. **(c)** Parallel TIPS access into the left portal vein using the initial TIPS and portogram as a reference for the new puncture. **(d)** Contrast opacification of two parallel stents after injection at the main portal vein level. **(e)** CT scan with contrast demonstrating parallel TIPS stents. **(f)** Hepatic duplex ultrasound demonstrating flow through two stents.

sheath can be advanced into the hepatic vein, a parallel Chiba needle can be used to target the portal vein to the hepatic vein (▶ Fig. 11.16).

In a series of 19 patients undergoing DIPS, the long-term patency of PTFE-covered stent grafts was superior to that of bare metal or homemade stent grafts.[42] In general, the decision regarding which stent to use should be made on a case-by-case basis. If DIPS dysfunction is identified, careful angioplasty can be performed.

11.8 Balloon-Occluded Transvenous Obliteration

Transvenous obliteration is an alternative therapy for the treatment of gastric varices that can be performed either through systemic or portal venous access. The technique that uses portal vein access is termed balloon-occluded antegrade transvenous obliteration (BATO), and that using systemic venous access is referred to as balloon-occluded retrograde transvenous obliteration (BRTO). Antegrade obliteration can be performed through percutaneous transhepatic access, through a TIPS, or surgically by using ileocolic vein access. In many circumstances, BATO is performed via a preexisting TIPS. If the percutaneous route is an option, the technique is basically the same as that used for percutaneous transhepatic cholangiogram, accessing portal

venous branches (more frequently on the right) and manipulating a wire into the main portal vein.[43] The technique for occlusion is the same as that described below in the performance of BRTO (▶ Fig. 11.17).

BRTO involves transvenous sclerosis of gastric (cardio-fundal) and mesenteric varices through systemic veins via a patent gastrorenal shunt.[44] The goal of this intervention is to control bleeding and reduce rebleeding rates in gastric varices caused by PH. While the purpose of TIPS is to decompress the portal circulation, BRTO has the opposite effect. Native gastrorenal shunts occur in the setting of PH, and represent a spontaneous naturally occurring decompression of the portal venous system. Occluding these spontaneously occurring portosystemic shunts effectively raises the portal venous pressure. The sclerosis of the gastrorenal shunt and varices that occurs during BRTO confers low rates of recanalization.

Originally, BRTO was considered an alternative to TIPS in cases with unfavorable anatomy, tumoral invasion of the portal vein, MELD score > 18, high risk of hepatic encephalopathy, or failure of endoscopic treatment. However, more recent studies have assessed the use of TIPS (to relieve PH) combined with BRTO (to treat the underlying gastric varices) and found that the combination improves portal flow and leads to superior outcomes.[45,46] The downside of performing BRTO alone is the possibility of exacerbating PH, which can aggravate sequelae such as esophageal varices, ascites, and hepatic hydrothorax.[47]

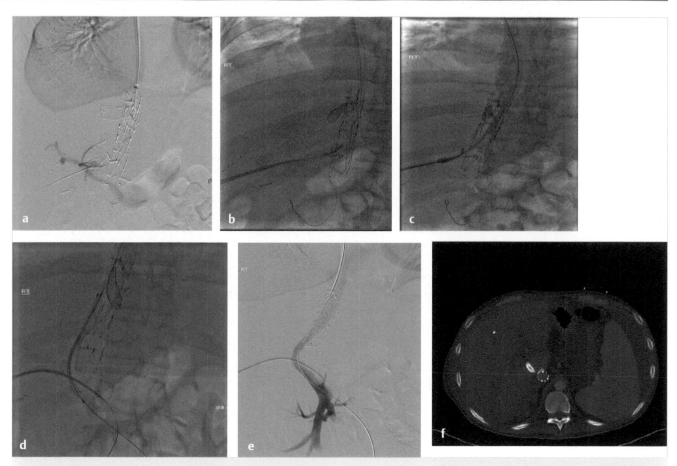

Fig. 11.16 DIPS in patient status post liver transplant with prior IVC and hepatic vein stenting. **(a)** Direct percutaneous portogram. **(b)** Parallel percutaneous access across the portal vein into the IVC stent. **(c)** Simultaneous manipulation of gooseneck snare across transjugular access positioning an exchange length wire from the percutaneous transhepatic access through jugular access. **(d)** After angioplasty of the IVC stent the wire and vascular introducer were manipulated from the transjugular access into the main portal vein. **(e)** Stent insertion. **(f)** CT post DIPS demonstrating stent across the segment I of the liver.

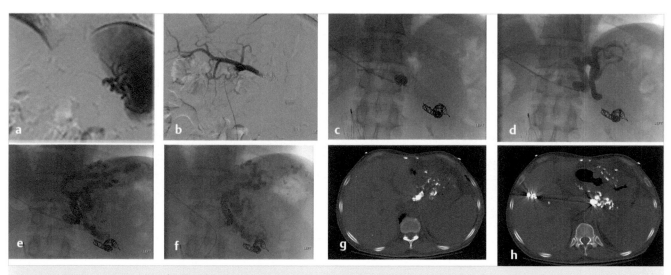

Fig. 11.17 BATO in a patient with history of gastric varices persistent bleeding via gastric varices, splenic vein thrombosis without evidence of gastrorenal shunt, and not candidate for TIPS. **(a, b)** Initial proximal splenic artery embolization to decrease the venous flow into the varices. **(c–e)** Direct transhepatic coronary (left gastric vein) venous access with balloon-assisted occlusion of the varices using sodium tetradecyl sulfate, ethiodized oil, and coils through microcatheter. **(f)** Post balloon deflation image showing occlusion of the varices. **(g, h)** Noncontrast CT of the liver that confirms the presence of the embolization material in the gastric wall at the desired embolized vascular territory.

A second risk of BRTO is the potential migration of sclerosant into the portal vein with subsequent PVT. However, a benefit of BRTO in the setting of TIPS is the improvement of flow into the TIPS shunt, which otherwise could be competitive with porto-systemic shunts, potentially increasing the risk of TIPS failure.[46]

Depending on the clinical scenario (emergent or elective), candidates for BRTO may require hemodynamic stabilization with fluid resuscitation and local compressive therapies such as intragastric Sengstaken–Blakemore or Minnesota balloons, prior to proceeding.

Planning for BRTO should be based on imaging to evaluate for signs of PH, patency of the portal and splenic veins, and signs of gastrorenal or other spontaneous portosystemic shunts. Concomitant PVT with or without cavernous transformation is a contraindication to the occlusion of the gastrorenal shunt if the shunt is the only venous drainage available for the mesenteric circulation. If no collateral vessels have developed around the thrombosed portal vein, BRTO can precipitate mesenteric vein thrombosis and subsequent bowel ischemia. On the other hand, hemodynamics around partial occlusion of the portal vein may be improved after BRTO, given the flow redirection toward the portal system. Imaging results should also be assessed for signs of left epiphrenic veins, azygos tributaries, left pericardial veins, and possible shunts into the iliac veins so that undesired migration of the sclerosant into the systemic circulation can be prevented during injection.

BRTO must be performed with the patient sedated and carefully monitored, with special attention paid to any respiratory compromise (due to the potential for nontarget embolization of the systemic veins). Access into the shunt can be obtained from the femoral or jugular veins using long sheaths to stabilize the system. A Cobra configuration catheter is used, with an over-the-wire exchange for the occluding balloon. Some authors suggest that a 9-French TIPS sheath should be advanced into the left renal vein from a femoral approach.[48] A reverse curve catheter such as a Simmons II can also be very useful for gaining access in the left renal vein and gastro-adrenal-renal shunt. The sheath ideally should be positioned in the left renal vein in close proximity to the gastrorenal shunt origin. Throughout the procedure, the Sengstaken–Blakemore balloon, if present, should be intermittently deflated to avoid misregistration of the veins secondary to extrinsic compression. Once the gastro-renal or splenorenal shunt is identified, multiple venograms including cone-beam acquisition should be performed to verify the anatomy and to evaluate the flow and potential portal draining collaterals. A combined BATO–BRTO, if feasible, may be the safest alternative if significant collateral vessels are visualized; those collaterals may require coil embolization or balloon-assisted sclerosis to prevent systemic or portal vein migration. If portal vein access is available, a sheath and a catheter should be manipulated across the main portal vein and direct portal, splenic, and variceal venograms should be obtained to map the anatomy and flow direction, and to plan the embolization of prominent portal venous afferent feeders (usually the left coronary, posterior gastric, and short gastric veins).[43] When the caliber of the varix is small, coil embolization should be used; if the varix is prominent, balloon-assisted sclerosis can be used. Multiple techniques have been described to optimize embolization of the portal venous feeders (referred to as "debranching" by some authors). Some reports describe a "splenic vein–sparing" technique in which the short gastric veins are embolized so that occlusion of the splenic vein can be avoided.

Once the potential outflow of sclerosant through portal feeders is controlled, an occluding balloon is inflated within the portosystemic (gastrorenal) shunt. This should be followed by a venogram to exclude reflux or escape of material into other collaterals and to confirm stagnation of flow in the gastric varices. If the position of the balloon is optimal, a microcatheter can be inserted through the balloon catheter, and the sclerosant can be injected starting as downstream as possible. Multiple sclerosants have been used for this procedure, including ethanolamine oleate and 3% sodium tetradecyl sulfate. Ethanolamine oleate can cause hemoglobinuria; this is one of the main reasons that foam sclerosants are preferred. The foam sclerosant is reconstituted by mixing one fraction of lipiodol, two fractions of 1% (or diluted 3%) sodium tetradecyl sulfate, and three fractions of carbon dioxide or air. This optimizes the volume of the injection and increases the surface area of the sclerosant to which the vein wall is exposed. During sclerosant injection, the operator must be aware of opacification of untreated portal vein feeders (e.g., left coronary vein, posterior gastric vein), so that the injection can be stopped and sclerosant can be aspirated if necessary to prevent the risk of material being spilled into the portal vein circulation.

After sclerosis, the standard time for balloon inflation can range from 12 to 24 hours; however, with the advent of sodium tetradecyl sulfate, this time has decreased to 6 hours. The time required for inflation depends on the size of the vessels, with longer inflation times and occasionally multiple injections required for larger veins.

TIPS combined with BATO and BRTO has also been used to treat stomal and parastomal varices caused by PH. The same techniques are used for this indication, with detailed evaluation of portosystemic feeders and balloon occlusion–assisted sclerosis with foam.[49]

11.9 Splenic Arterial Embolization to Treat Gastric Varices Secondary to Splenic Vein Thrombosis

Segmental, sinistral, or "left-sided PH" is an entity associated with splenic vein thrombosis or arteriovenous fistulas in the splenic vessels. Such entities result in collateralization through the short gastric veins and prehepatic PH, bypassing the venous flow from the spleen into the portal vein through enlarged splenoportal collaterals. As a consequence, retrograde flow from the short gastric veins into the coronary vein as well as from the left gastroepiploic vein into right gastroepiploic and SMVs is identified. The primary etiology is usually secondary to pancreatic disease (e.g., pancreatitis or pancreatic tumor), with extrinsic compression of the pancreatic veins. Such entities can also be secondary to hematologic disorders, trauma, or immunological problems. The diagnosis is based on clinical and imaging findings when a patient develops isolated gastric or gastroesophageal varices without evidence of liver disease.[50]

The major complication of splenic vein–associated varices is bleeding, which has been estimated to be up to 50% of such

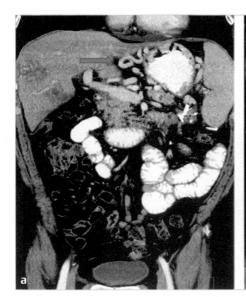
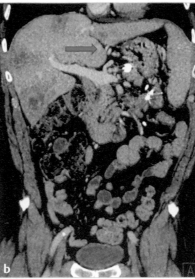

Fig. 11.18 Patient with splenic vein thrombosis and gastric varices. **(a)** Multiple varices around the gastric fundus (*blue arrow*). **(b)** CT scan with contrast 1 week following proximal splenic artery embolization demonstrates significant improvement and decompression of the short gastric varices (*blue arrow*).

patients.[51] Multiple reports have combined surgical and endovascular treatments, namely splenic artery embolization prior to splenectomy.[50,52,53] The most accepted endovascular treatment consists of embolization of the mid- and proximal splenic artery to reduce splenic venous return in an attempt to decompress the varices (▶ Fig. 11.18). This procedure has been reported as life-saving in patients where endoscopic control of variceal bleeding has failed. One of the most devastating complications related with splenic artery embolization is splenic abscess in the territory of splenic infarction. This complication is rare, and can largely be prevented by avoiding distal embolization.

Alternative endovascular treatments have been proposed, such as splenic vein stenting. There is limited experience using this technique in splenic vein thrombosis, but it has been more frequently described for splenic vein stenosis in pediatric patients secondary to neonatal umbilical vein catheterization.

11.10 Thrombolysis and Mechanical Thrombectomy for Acute Portal Vein Thrombosis

PVT is an uncommon entity that includes thrombosis of the main portal vein with or without extension into the intrahepatic portal branches. The thrombosis can extend into the mesenteric and splenic veins. It can occur in the setting of cirrhotic and noncirrhotic livers, as well as in malignancy and inflammatory disorders. Some of the common causes are myeloproliferative disease, intra-abdominal infection, sepsis, surgery, trauma, hypercoagulable states, oral contraceptives, and liver tumors.[53] Although spontaneous resolution can occur, serious or even lethal complications are noted in the acute setting due to bowel ischemia and infarction. In the long term, it can result in cavernous transformation with resultant PH and devastating outcomes.

Depending on the clinical condition and CT findings, the treatment of acute portomesenteric vein thrombosis can vary from systemic anticoagulation to prevent thrombus propagation, to emergent bowel resection.[54] Endovascular treatment

options have two main goals: remove the thrombus, and reestablish portal flow. One way these goals can be accomplished is through indirect thrombolytic injection into the SMA. Thrombolysis via the SMA is performed with a catheter placed in the SMA for lytic infusion. In theory, injecting thrombolytic medications into the SMA results in lysis on the venous side; thrombolytic infusion can be used as adjunctive therapy in combination with systemic anticoagulation.[55] With this treatment, infusion can be prolonged, increasing to some degree the risk of bleeding.[56]

It is suggested that lysis is most efficient through direct portal venous thrombolytic infusion and mechanical thrombectomy. Several endovascular approaches for recanalization of the portal vein have been proposed, most notably percutaneously via transhepatic or transsplenic approaches, transjugular following a TIPS approach. The TIPS approach has two main objectives: one is to provide a pathway to intervene on the portal vein, and the second is to establish outflow in the system after partial thrombectomy when residual intrahepatic PVT is identified.

Prior to the procedure, lab evaluation includes complete blood count, comprehensive metabolic panel, type and screen, baseline fibrinogen level, and partial thromboplastin time. Blood products and an intensive care unit bed should be immediately available. As detailed earlier in the chapter, evaluation of the CT or MRI cross-sectional imaging is important to plan the procedure and to establish the approach. Again, the fusion of a preexisting study with a cone-beam evaluation during the intervention can be used as an alternative to map the portal vein and to guide the access.

Other valuable tools in visualizing the portal system are wedge CO_2 portography and indirect portography via SMA or splenic artery injection. When a TIPS approach is used, it may be obtained in the conventional way (▶ Fig. 11.19). Once access into the portal vein is obtained, the wire should be negotiated into the SMV if possible.

After accessing the vein, a 7-French-long sheath is introduced over a wire, followed by acquisition of a venogram. Initial 10-mg bolus of tissue plasminogen activator (tPA) is injected through the catheter allowed to dwell for about 10 minutes

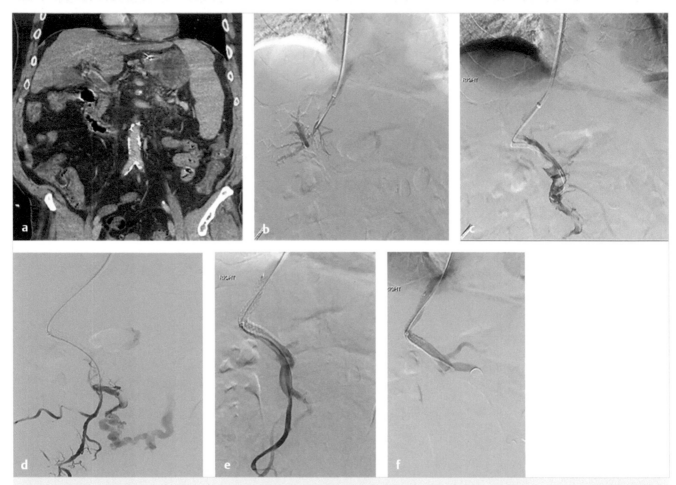

Fig. 11.19 Patient with acute portal vein thrombosis requiring thrombectomy. **(a)** Coronal view CT of the abdomen that demonstrates extensive filling defect in the main portal vein. **(b, c)** Transjugular puncture into a portal vein branch with access into the SMV confluence. **(d)** Venogram of the SMV demonstrated thrombosed confluence with venous collateral. **(e, f)** Mechanical thrombectomy and TIPS insertion with final portogram demonstrating patency of the SMV, main portal vein, and TIPS with resolution of the collateral vessels.

(initial half-life of tPA is 5 minutes, with a terminal half-life of 72 minutes). An aspiration can be performed though the sheath using a 6-French guiding catheter. Other alternatives for aspiration are the Indigo device (Penumbra, Alameda, CA) and Angiojet (Boston Scientific, Waterton, MA); however, experience with these devices in the portal vein is limited. Balloon angioplasty and clot fragmentation are also very useful adjuncts to reestablish the flow.

An alternative approach is to insert an infusion catheter or ultrasound-accelerated thrombolysis catheter, either via TIPS approach or via transsplenic or percutaneous transhepatic approach (▶ Fig. 11.20), and start with an infusion of tPA at a dose of 0.5 to 1 mg/h. Infusion generally occurs for 24 hours, and is monitored by serial serum fibrinogen levels. Fibrinogen levels of < 150 mg/dL are associated with an increased risk of major bleeding, and may be used as a threshold for discontinuation of infusion therapy.[57] Simultaneously, heparin is administered through the sidearm of the sheath at a dose of 300 to 500 units/hour. After the infusion, the patient returns for a venogram and to define if recanalization is complete, as well as to verify portomesenteric flow. If residual clot is present, the infusion can be initiated again for 6 to 24 hours.

Balloon angioplasty will be necessary if stenosis of the vein is identified. Some authors report the use of a variety of thrombectomy devices to remove the residual clot. A similar alternative to this device is the Cleaner device (Argon Medical, Plano, TX), which has limited experience reported in the portal vein.[58]

Once the procedure is complete, it is common practice to remove the sheath with embolization of the liver or transsplenic access tract to avoid further bleeding; this is particularly important in the context of anticoagulation. Such embolization can be accomplished using coils, Amplatzer plugs, or Gelfoam pledgets. The use of catheter-directed thrombolysis has been also effective in the management of extrahepatic portal venous thrombosis in the perioperative period following liver transplant. However, in this circumstance the risk of bleeding has to be carefully assessed, and if the procedure is performed immediate availability of the surgical team is recommended.

TIPS with or without thrombolysis is a safe alternative, and helps create a low pressure outflow for the portal vein as well as promoting endogenous lysis due to reestablishment of blood flow.[59]

Although systemic infusion of tPA has been reported as a promising alternative in the treatment of acute PVT,[60] some

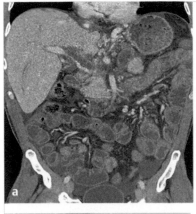
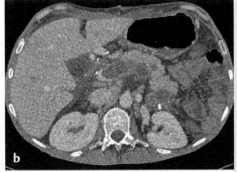
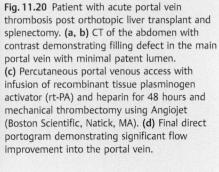
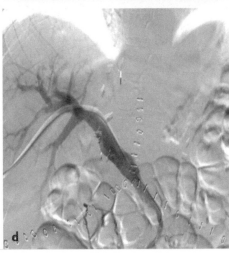
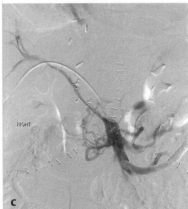

Fig. 11.20 Patient with acute portal vein thrombosis post orthotopic liver transplant and splenectomy. **(a, b)** CT of the abdomen with contrast demonstrating filling defect in the main portal vein with minimal patent lumen. **(c)** Percutaneous portal venous access with infusion of recombinant tissue plasminogen activator (rt-PA) and heparin for 48 hours and mechanical thrombectomy using Angiojet (Boston Scientific, Natick, MA). **(d)** Final direct portogram demonstrating significant flow improvement into the portal vein.

studies suggest long-term anticoagulation (6 months) with Doppler surveillance every 3 months as the standard of care.

11.11 Portomesenteric Venous Recanalization and Stenting

During the treatment for periampullary tumors and cholangiocarcinoma, multiple combined therapies for local control and to prevent local recurrence are used, including chemotherapy, radiation therapy, and surgical resection. Portomesenteric stenosis can occur as a short- or long-term complication of these treatments with subsequent PH. Liver transplantation can also cause stenoses at the portal venous anastomotic level. A percutaneous transhepatic approach for recanalization of the portal vein and endovascular treatment following pancreaticoduodenectomy and radiation has been reported.[61]

The procedure is performed under moderate sedation or general anesthesia, depending on the clinical condition. Percutaneous access is obtained into right portal vein branches under ultrasound or fluoroscopic guidance, and after confirming position appropriate access site, a 6-French microintroducer is placed. A 4-French hydrophilic catheter in combination with a hydrophilic wire is advanced beyond the stenosis. Indirect portography via an SMA/splenic artery injection (with or without cone-beam evaluation) can help as a reference if advancement of the wire across the stenosis is challenging. Once the catheter is placed across the stenosis, a direct portogram is obtained in order to depict the anatomy and characterize the stenosis as well as to calculate the size of the stent. It is important to

consider prophylactic anticoagulation while treating a severe stenosis before angioplasty or stenting in order to prevent intraprocedural thrombosis (▶ Fig. 11.21).

The diameter of the stent is oversized about 2 mm larger than the diameter of the normal vein. Self-expandable stents are used, followed by angioplasty and measurement of the pressure gradient. Once the result is satisfactory, the transparenchymal tract is embolized using Gelfoam pledgets, coils, or Amplatzer plugs to prevent access site bleeding.

In case of restenosis, the stent can be reintervened upon. The most common cause of restenosis is recurrence of the original tumor.[61]

11.12 Portal Venous Pancreatic Cells Infusion

Percutaneous injection of isolated beta islet cells of the pancreas into the portal vein represents a minimally invasive procedure that has been used in the treatment of type I diabetes mellitus. Islet cell transplants have the advantage of decreased morbidity relative to whole organ pancreas transplant. Although the results appear variable in different reports, Gaba et al reported a 1-year insulin-free rate of 60 to 70%.[62] Pancreatic cell transplantation has been performed alone or in combination with kidney transplant in patients with renal failure, having the advantage of using the same immunosuppression regimen for both transplants. The absolute and relative contraindications to pancreatic cell transplant are described in ▶ Table 11.8.

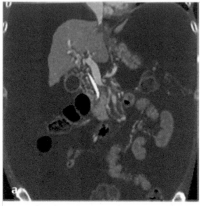
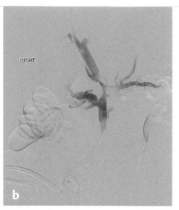
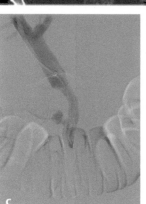
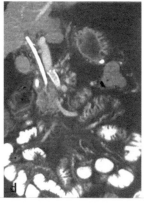
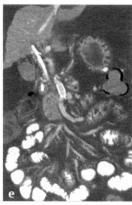

Fig. 11.21 Patient with pancreatic cancer status post radiation therapy with prehepatic portal hypertension. **(a)** Coronal view of CT of the abdomen with contrast that demonstrated severe stenosis at the SMV confluence with extensive ascites. **(b)** Direct portogram via transjugular approach demonstrated severe stenosis at the SMV–splenic vein and portal vein confluence with some degree of collateralization. **(c)** Post bare metal stent placement favoring the portomesenteric confluence. **(d, e)** Coronal CT images of the abdomen demonstrating the stent location and contrast flow through the patent stent. The patient demonstrated significant clinical improvement post treatment.

Table 11.8 Absolute and relative contraindications to pancreatic islet cell transplantation

Absolute contraindications
1. Age < 18 y or > 70 y
2. Diabetes mellitus with duration < 5 y
3. Residual C-peptide level > 0.5 ng/dL
4. Untreated proliferative diabetic retinopathy
5. Portal hypertension
6. Coexisting cardiovascular disease
7. Active infection (hepatitis C, hepatitis B, HIV, and tuberculosis)
8. Alcohol or substance abuse
9. Positive pregnancy test

Relative contraindications
1. Obesity (body mass index > 28 kg/m²)
2. Relative insulin resistance (insulin requirement > 0.8 IU/Kg body weight)
3. Abnormal liver function test
4. Chronic or acute pancreatic

Percutaneous or transvenous access into the portal vein is useful, although the most frequently used is the percutaneous approach.[62] Moderate sedation is generally considered sufficient. Once access into the portal vein is obtained, an initial pressure measurement in the main portal vein is obtained. The pancreatic cell infusion is by gravity, given risk of damage of the cells by pushing them with a syringe. The recommended minimum inner diameter of the infusion catheter is 700 μm in order to avoid damage to the cells from shear stress.[62] The 6-French microintroducer can be used; however, a 4-French catheter system is optimal for infusion. The tip of the catheter is positioned in the mid-main portal vein to allow a homogeneous distribution of the cells, thereby preventing thrombosis in small branches due to cell aggregation. In addition, minimal manipulation of the catheter is recommended in order to avoid endothelial injury that can contribute to thrombosis. Some authors recommend a systemic heparin drip throughout the procedure, although this must be weighed against the risk of bleeding requiring tract embolization at the end of the procedure. The portal venous pressure should be measured initially in order to establish a baseline, and measured again after each injection. If after any infusion the pressure doubles or measures more than 20 mm Hg, the infusion must be suspended, as this represents cell stagnation and the risk of PH. Contrast injection must be reserved for the initial and final portogram because of the risk of aggregation of the cells due to contrast viscosity.

Following completion of the infusion, a final portogram is obtained in order to evaluate patency of the veins. The percutaneous tract requires embolization, which can be achieved with Gelfoam, coils or an Amplatzer plug. The most common described complications of islet cell transfusion include bleeding (hemoperitoneum, hemothorax, hemobilia) and PVT. Vasovagal reaction is also reported as a potential complication. Postprocedure follow-up imaging can be performed with vascular ultrasound or CT scan of the liver.

11.13 Portal Vein Embolization

Liver resection, including segmentectomy, right hepatectomy, and extended hepatectomy, may be the therapeutic option for patients with liver metastases. Resectability criteria include free resection margins and sufficient liver remnant to avoid liver

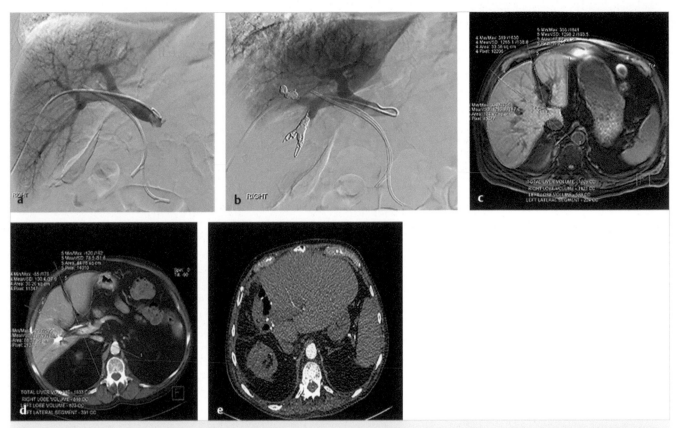

Fig. 11.22 Right portal vein embolization. **(a)** Percutaneous access with portogram. **(b)** Portogram demonstrating patency and increased flow through the left portal vein after embolization of the right portal vein using coils and 900–1,200-μm particles. **(c)** CT of the liver with preembolization volume measurements. **(d)** CT of the liver with postembolization volume measurements of the left hepatic lobe. **(e)** CT post right hepatectomy demonstrating significant enlargement of the left hepatic lobe.

dysfunction.[63] In noncirrhotic patients, the threshold for hepatic resectability is a functional liver remnant (FLR) of 25% of total liver volume, while in patients with liver disease the threshold is higher (at 30–40%).[63,64] In anticipation of surgery and to prevent postsurgical liver failure, as well as taking advantage of the regenerative capacity of the liver, endovascular selective portal vein embolization (PVE) has been performed in order to improve the volume of the FLR. PVE involves embolization of the ipsilateral portal vein branch prior to hepatectomy to cause hypertrophy of the contralateral, nonresected lobe.

Percutaneous vascular access for PVE can be ipsilateral or contralateral; however, the ipsilateral approach has the advantage of noninstrumentation of the healthy FLR, avoiding the risk of thrombosis or vascular injury (▶ Fig. 11.22). An alternative surgical approach requires minilaparotomy and transileocolic venous catheterization. Multiple techniques have been described using different embolization material including gelatin sponges, n-butyl cyanoacrylate (NBCA), polyvinyl alcohol particles (PVA), trisacryl spheres, coils, Amplatzer vascular plugs, absolute alcohol, and polidocanol.[64]

The use of PVE is guided by the expected size of the resection and the resulting liver remnant, with embolization performed with a resection of more than 70 to 75% of liver anticipated (or 60–65% in patients with cirrhosis).[65] Preprocedure evaluation includes cross-sectional imaging of the liver to measure the volumes of total liver, the anatomic segments to be resected, and the FLR. In addition, the tumor volume can be evaluated. A useful formula for calculation of the FLR is:

$$\%FLR = (FLRV/TLV - TV)\times100$$

where FLR = future liver remnant; FLRV = future liver remnant volume; TLV = total liver volume; TV = tumor volume.[65]

Experience has shown that the percentage of FLR is a better predictor of outcomes than are absolute volume measurements, since it takes into account issues such as size of the patient.

The procedure can be performed under moderate sedation. Prophylactic antibiotics may be used according to operator preference. Percutaneous access to the portal vein is obtained under ultrasound and fluoroscopic guidance using a microintroducer set. A 6-French, 25-cm vascular sheath is inserted, and a portogram is obtained to evaluate the portal venous anatomy. If an ipsilateral approach is used, a reverse curve catheter can be useful to access all the portal venous branches and segment IV, if needed. Using a contralateral approach, injection of the embolic material can be performed through standard catheters, or using an occlusion balloon placed in the portal vein of the segment to be resected, with embolic and coils delivered through this catheter.

There is still controversy about the ideal embolic material. Gelatin sponge alone is absorbable, and portal recanalization has been described after 2 to 3 weeks. The most frequent materials used are a combination of NBCA and lipiodol, and PVA with coils/plugs. Fischman et al reported technical success in 97.1% using sodium tetradecyl sulfate foam, using an ipsilateral approach and the occluding balloon technique.[64] The NBCA gives excellent results with a greater FLR volume increase when compared with other embolic materials; however, early polymerization and risk of nontarget embolization require experience of the interventionalist. In addition, NBCA can cause a severe inflammatory reaction. When coils or Amplatzer plugs are used, it is important to avoid deployment close to the bifurcation, which may cause difficulty during operative clamping.

Maximal rate of hypertrophy is expected to occur in the first 3 weeks following embolization, with plateau phase reached after this point, with continued growth of the remnant observed with longer observation period.[66] Predictors for poor outcomes have been described, such as insufficient embolization or portal vein recanalization, as well as interval time between embolization and surgery.[66] In patients with failed hypertrophy of the contralateral liver, neoadjuvant therapies like transcatheter arterial chemoembolization (TACE) or ablation can be used. A double-stage hepatectomy has been described for colorectal metastases involving both lobes, with TACE or ablation prior to PVE in order to improve the outcome.[67] Complications of the procedure include subcapsular hematoma, PVT, cholangitis, or other infection.

11.14 Embolization of Intrahepatic Arterioportal Fistulas

APF is an abnormal communication between the hepatic artery and the portal vein, which can result in PH due to the high-pressure arterialized flow in the venous bed. APFs can be congenital (associated with Osler–Weber–Rendu syndrome, Ehlers–Danlos syndrome, or biliary atresia) or acquired. Acquired APF may be iatrogenic (e.g., post liver biopsy), secondary to blunt or penetrating trauma, due to rupture of the hepatic artery, or can develop in the clinical context of tumoral invasion or infectious process.

APFs may be intra- or extrahepatic.[68] Symptoms can vary from clinically insignificant to severe PH requiring prompt diagnosis and treatment. Once the APF is suspected, diagnosis can be made using a liver vascular ultrasound, MRA or CTA of the liver can be diagnostic, and angiography, which also allows treatment in a minimally invasive manner, can be confirmatory. On the MRA/CTA, early opacification of the portal vein or its branches can be seen in the arterial phase. Hepatofugal portal flow can be present.[69] Other associated findings, such as splenomegaly, ascites, hydrothorax, or varices, can also be present and may indicate PH.

Percutaneous embolization has been increasingly performed before resorting to surgery (▶ Fig. 11.23).[69] The endovascular treatment for APF consists of embolization of the hepatic artery branches supplying the fistula using coils, plugs, or Gelfoam. In

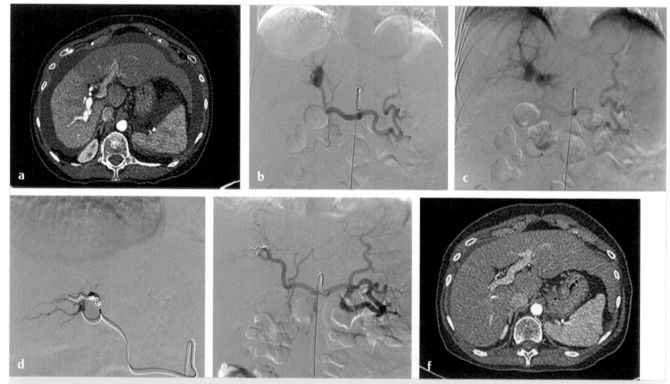

Fig. 11.23 Patient with portal hypertension secondary to hepatic artery to portal vein fistula. **(a)** CT abdomen with contrast demonstrates early arterial enhancement of the right portal vein suspicious for arterial to portal vein fistula. Ascites is also identified. **(b)** Early and **(c)** late images from celiac angiogram shows a fistula supplied by a branch of the right hepatic artery with opacification of the portal vein. **(d)** Embolization of the branch of the right hepatic artery using a microcatheter and multiple microcoils. **(e)** Celiac angiogram postembolization demonstrated resolution of the fistula. **(f)** CT of the abdomen 1-month postembolization demonstrated resolution of the fistula, with almost complete improvement of the ascites.

failed embolization cases, angiography allows definition of the anatomy and hemodynamic behavior of the fistula as part of presurgical planning.

11.15 Budd–Chiari Syndrome

Budd–Chiari syndrome is defined as an obstruction of the hepatic venous outflow at any level, resulting in postsinusoidal PH. The obstruction can occur at multiple levels including the small veins in the liver parenchyma, hepatic veins, or IVC. As shown in ▶ Table 11.9, Budd–Chiari has been classified into three types depending on the level of venous obstruction. The prognosis without therapy is poor, with an estimated 3-year survival of 10%. Most common causes of mortality in patients with Budd–Chiari include gastrointestinal bleed, liver failure, and encephalopathy.[70,71]

Primary Budd–Chiari is caused by venous thrombosis, intravenous stenosis, or webs. The secondary type refers to extrinsic compression of the veins, in the setting of tumors, cysts, or hyperplastic nodules.[71] Obstruction of venous outflow leads to

Table 11.9 Budd–Chiari classification according to the level of the obstruction

- Type I: Limited to the IVC
- Type II: Lesions are limited to the hepatic veins
- Type III: Mixed type involving the IVC and hepatic veins

venous congestion with parenchymal edema and hypoxic damage of the hepatocytes. Clinical presentation may range from asymptomatic to acute liver failure. Intrahepatic venous collateralization is an imaging hallmark of Budd–Chiari syndrome. The medical treatment is based on treating the underlying cause, with anticoagulation being hallmark therapy.

Diagnosis and treatment for Budd–Chiari can be achieved by endovascular means, starting with obtaining a hepatic venogram through transjugular or transfemoral approach. In cases in which these options are not available, percutaneous hepatic vein access can be considered. The angiographic diagnosis can be made by the presence of stenosis or occlusion of the hepatic veins with extensive collateralization in the parenchyma ("spider web appearance") of the vessels (▶ Fig. 11.24). In addition, a high degree stenosis of the IVC can be noted, which can be aggravated by extrinsic compression by a hypertrophied caudate lobe.

Endovascular treatments include angioplasty of the veins, stenting, catheter-directed thrombolysis, and TIPS insertion (▶ Fig. 11.25). TIPS and angioplasty have improved the long-term survival rates without liver transplantation, in some reports exceeding 75%.[69] DIPS can be considered as a safe alternative when hepatic vein recanalization is not possible. A direct percutaneous access into the portal vein, followed by transcaudate puncture of the IVC, can be an option when the hepatic veins are completely occluded.

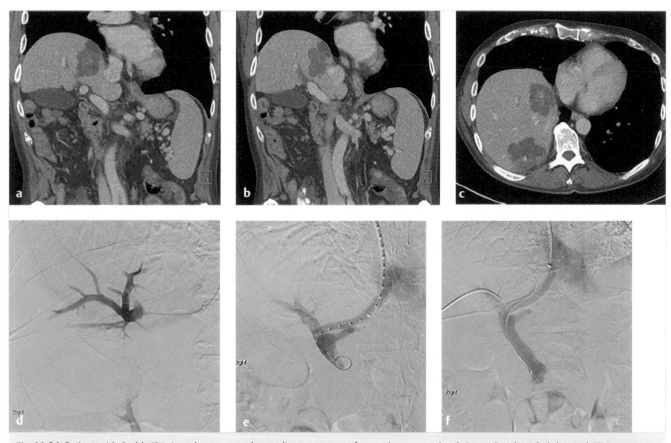

Fig. 11.24 Patient with Budd–Chiari syndrome secondary to liver metastases from colon cancer. (a–c) Coronal and axial abdominal CT images demonstrating liver lesion infiltrating the confluence of the hepatic veins. (d–f) DIPS procedure with direct percutaneous portal venous access into the IVC, bypassing the hepatic veins confluence.

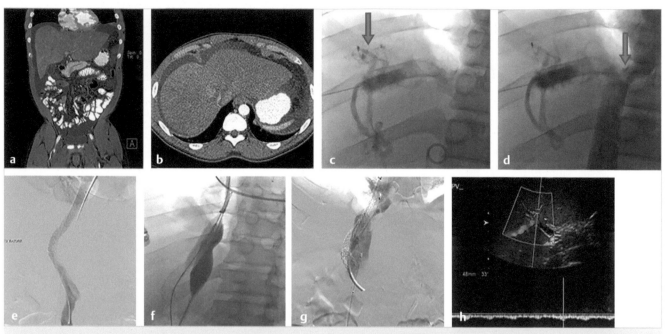

Fig. 11.25 Patient with hypereosinophilic syndrome who presents with acute abdominal pain associated with distension and lower extremity edema, consistent with Budd–Chiari syndrome. **(a, b)** Coronal and axial abdominal CT images demonstrate enlarged, edematous-appearing liver with heterogeneous, patchy enhancement and moderate ascites. The hepatic veins are not clearly identified. **(c)** Percutaneous transhepatic attempt to recanalize the hepatic vein demonstrated complete occlusion of the confluence in the IVC with spider web venous pattern representing multiple venous collaterals in the liver parenchyma (*blue arrow*). **(d)** Simultaneous hepatic venous and inferior vena cavogram demonstrates a high-degree stenosis of the IVC at the hepatic veins confluence (*blue arrow*). **(e)** Portogram after transcaval TIPS creation. **(f)** Angioplasty of the IVC. **(g)** An inferior vena cavogram postangioplasty shows significant improvement of the preexisting stenosis. **(h)** Follow-up hepatic duplex ultrasound with patent portal circulation toward the TIPS. The patient had clinical improvement of symptoms.

References

[1] Buob S, Johnston AN, Webster CR. Portal hypertension: pathophysiology, diagnosis, and treatment. J Vet Intern Med. 2011; 25(2):169–186

[2] La Mura V, Nicolini A, Tosetti G, Primignani M. Cirrhosis and portal hypertension: the importance of risk stratification, the role of hepatic venous pressure gradient measurement. World J Hepatol. 2015; 7(4):688–695

[3] Casadaban LC, Gaba RC. Percutaneous portosystemic shunts: TIPS and beyond. Semin Intervent Radiol. 2014; 31(3):227–234

[4] Parker R. Role of transjugular intrahepatic portosystemic shunt in the management of portal hypertension. Clin Liver Dis. 2014; 18(2):319–334

[5] Patidar KR, Sydnor M, Sanyal AJ. Transjugular intrahepatic portosystemic shunt. Clin Liver Dis. 2014; 18(4):853–876

[6] Copelan A, Remer EM, Sands M, Nghiem H, Kapoor B. Diagnosis and management of Budd Chiari syndrome: an update. Cardiovasc Intervent Radiol. 2015; 38(1):1–12

[7] Chen B, Wang W, Tam MD, Quintini C, Fung JJ, Li X. Transjugular intrahepatic portosystemic shunt in liver transplant recipients: indications, feasibility, and outcomes. Hepatol Int. 2015; 9(3):391–398

[8] Ferral H. The evaluation of the patient undergoing an elective transjugular intrahepatic portosystemic shunt procedure. Semin Intervent Radiol. 2005; 22(4):266–270

[9] Parvinian A, Gaba RC. Outcomes of TIPS for treatment of gastroesophageal variceal hemorrhage. Semin Intervent Radiol. 2014; 31(3):252–257

[10] Møller S, Dümcke CW, Krag A. The heart and the liver. Expert Rev Gastroenterol Hepatol. 2009; 3(1):51–64

[11] Helton WS, Belshaw A, Althaus S, Park S, Coldwell D, Johansen K. Critical appraisal of the angiographic portacaval shunt (TIPS). Am J Surg. 1993; 165 (5):566–571

[12] Casadaban LC, Gabra MG, Parvinian A, et al. Impact of transjugular intrahepatic portosystemic shunt creation on intermediate-term model for end-stage liver disease score progression. Transplant Proc. 2014; 46(5):1384–1388

[13] Gaba RC, Couture PM, Bui JT, et al. Prognostic capability of different liver disease scoring systems for prediction of early mortality after transjugular intrahepatic portosystemic shunt creation. J Vasc Interv Radiol. 2013; 24(3):411–420, 420.e1–420.e4, quiz 421

[14] Venkatesan AM, Kundu S, Sacks D, et al. Society of Interventional Radiology Standards of Practice Committee. Practice guidelines for adult antibiotic prophylaxis during vascular and interventional radiology procedures. Written by the Standards of Practice Committee for the Society of Interventional Radiology and Endorsed by the Cardiovascular Interventional Radiological Society of Europe and Canadian Interventional Radiology Association [corrected]. J Vasc Interv Radiol. 2010; 21(11):1611–1630, quiz 1631

[15] Chung H-H, Razavi MK, Sze DY, et al. Portosystemic pressure gradient during transjugular intrahepatic portosystemic shunt with Viatorr stent graft: what is the critical low threshold to avoid medically uncontrolled low pressure gradient related complications? J Gastroenterol Hepatol. 2008; 23(1):95–101

[16] Ferral H, Bilbao JI. The difficult transjugular intrahepatic portosystemic shunt: alternative techniques and "tips" to successful shunt creation. Semin Intervent Radiol. 2005; 22(4):300–308

[17] Yang Z, Han G, Wu Q, et al. Patency and clinical outcomes of transjugular intrahepatic portosystemic shunt with polytetrafluoroethylene-covered stents versus bare stents: a meta-analysis. J Gastroenterol Hepatol. 2010; 25(11):1718–1725

[18] Qi X, Liu L, Bai M, et al. Transjugular intrahepatic portosystemic shunt in combination with or without variceal embolization for the prevention of variceal rebleeding: a meta-analysis. J Gastroenterol Hepatol. 2014; 29(4):688–696

[19] Shi Y, Tian X, Hu J, et al. Efficacy of transjugular intrahepatic portosystemic shunt with adjunctive embolotherapy with cyanoacrylate for esophageal variceal bleeding. Dig Dis Sci. 2014; 59(9):2325–2332

[20] Kovács A, Schepke M, Heller J, Schild HH, Flacke S. Short-term effects of transjugular intrahepatic shunt on cardiac function assessed by cardiac MRI: preliminary results. Cardiovasc Intervent Radiol. 2010; 33(2):290–296

[21] Fili D, Falletta C, Luca A, et al. Circulatory response to volume expansion and transjugular intrahepatic portosystemic shunt in refractory ascites: Relationship with diastolic dysfunction. Dig Liver Dis. 2015; 47(12):1052–1058

[22] Colombato L, Spahr L, Martinet JP, et al. et al. Haemodynamic adaption two months later after transjugular intrahepatic portosystemic shunt (TIPS) in cirrhotic patients. Gut. 2016; 1996(39):600–604

[23] Chen S, Li X, Wei B, et al. Recurrent variceal bleeding and shunt patency: prospective randomized controlled trial of transjugular intrahepatic portosystemic shunt alone or combined with coronary vein embolization. Radiology. 2013; 268(3):900–906

[24] Xiao T, Chen L, Chen W, et al. Comparison of transjugular intrahepatic portosystemic shunt (TIPS) alone versus TIPS combined with embolotherapy in advanced cirrhosis: a retrospective study. J Clin Gastroenterol. 2011; 45(7): 643–650

[25] Ma J, Yan Z, Luo J, Liu Q, Wang J, Qiu S. Rational classification of portal vein thrombosis and its clinical significance. PLoS One. 2014; 9(11):e112501

[26] Bilbao JI, Elorz M, Vivas I, Martínez-Cuesta A, Bastarrika G, Benito A. Transjugular intrahepatic portosystemic shunt (TIPS) in the treatment of venous symptomatic chronic portal thrombosis in non-cirrhotic patients. Cardiovasc Intervent Radiol. 2004; 27(5):474–480

[27] Haskal ZJ, Rees CR, Ring EJ, Saxon R, Sacks D, Society of Interventional Radiology Technology Assessment Committee. Reporting standards for transjugular intrahepatic portosystemic shunts. J Vasc Interv Radiol. 2003; 14(9 Pt 2): S419–S426

[28] Qi X, Han G, Yin Z, et al. Transjugular intrahepatic portosystemic shunt for portal cavernoma with symptomatic portal hypertension in non-cirrhotic patients. Dig Dis Sci. 2012; 57(4):1072–1082

[29] Jourabchi N, McWilliams JP, Lee EW, Sauk S, Kee ST. TIPS placement via combined transjugular and transhepatic approach for cavernous portal vein occlusion: targeted approach. Case Rep Radiol. 2013; 2013:635391

[30] Habib A, Desai K, Hickey R, et al. Portal vein recanalization-transjugular intrahepatic portosystemic shunt using the transsplenic approach to achieve transplant candidacy in patients with chronic portal vein thrombosis. J Vasc Interv Radiol. 2015; 26(4):499–506

[31] Fanelli F, Angeloni S, Salvatori FM, et al. Transjugular intrahepatic portosystemic shunt with expanded-polytetrafluoroethylene-covered stents in non-cirrhotic patients with portal cavernoma. Dig Liver Dis. 2011; 43(1):78–84

[32] Ripamonti R, Ferral H, Alonzo M, Patel NH. Transjugular intrahepatic portosystemic shunt-related complications and practical solutions. Semin Intervent Radiol. 2006; 23(2):165–176

[33] Braillon A, Revert R, Rémond A, Auderbert M, Capron JP. Transcatheter embolization of liver capsule perforation during transvenous liver biopsy. Gastrointest Radiol. 1986; 11(3):277–279

[34] Casadaban LC, Parvinian A, Minocha J, et al. Clearing the confusion over hepatic encephalopathy after TIPS creation: incidence, prognostic factors, and clinical outcomes. Dig Dis Sci. 2015; 60(4):1059–1066

[35] Ahuja NK, Ally WA, Caldwell SH. Direct acting inhibitors of ammoniagenesis: a role in post-TIPS encephalopathy? Ann Hepatol. 2014; 13(2):179–186

[36] Zheng G, Zhang LJ, Zhong J, et al. Cerebral blood flow measured by arterial-spin labeling MRI: a useful biomarker for characterization of minimal hepatic encephalopathy in patients with cirrhosis. Eur J Radiol. 2013; 82(11):1981–1988

[37] Gaba RC, Parvinian A, Minocha J, et al. Should transjugular intrahepatic portosystemic shunt stent grafts be underdilated? J Vasc Interv Radiol. 2015; 26 (3):382–387

[38] Farsad K, Kolbeck KJ, Keller FS, Barton RE, Kaufman JA. Primary creation of an externally constrained TIPS: a technique to control reduction of the portosystemic gradient. AJR Am J Roentgenol. 2015; 204(4):868–871

[39] Boyer TD, Haskal ZJ, American Association for the Study of Liver Diseases. The role of transjugular intrahepatic portosystemic shunt (TIPS) in the management of portal hypertension: update 2009. Hepatology. 2010; 51(1):306

[40] Petersen BD, Clark TWI. Direct intrahepatic portocaval shunt. Tech Vasc Interv Radiol. 2008; 11(4):230–234

[41] Tsauo J, Yu Y, Luo X, Wang Z, Liu L, Li X. Direct intrahepatic portocaval shunt creation via the inter-strut space of the inferior vena cava stent. Clin Radiol. 2014; 69(9):896–899

[42] Hoppe H, Wang SL, Petersen BD. Intravascular US-guided direct intrahepatic portocaval shunt with an expanded polytetrafluoroethylene-covered stent-graft. Radiology. 2008; 246(1):306–314

[43] Saad WEA, Kitanosono T, Koizumi J. Balloon-occluded antegrade transvenous obliteration with or without balloon-occluded retrograde transvenous obliteration for the management of gastric varices: concept and technical applications. Tech Vasc Interv Radiol. 2012; 15(3):203–225

[44] Saad WEA, Al-Osaimi AMS, Caldwell SH. Pre- and post-balloon-occluded retrograde transvenous obliteration clinical evaluation, management, and imaging: indications, management protocols, and follow-up. Tech Vasc Interv Radiol. 2012; 15(3):165–202

[45] Saad WEA. Combining transjugular intrahepatic portosystemic shunt with balloon-occluded retrograde transvenous obliteration or augmenting TIPS with variceal embolization for the management of gastric varices: an evolving middle ground? Semin Intervent Radiol. 2014; 31(3):266–268

[46] Kirby JM, Cho KJ, Midia M. Image-guided intervention in management of complications of portal hypertension: more than TIPS for success. Radiographics. 2013; 33(5):1473–1496

[47] Saad WEA, Wagner CC, Lippert A, et al. Protective value of TIPS against the development of hydrothorax/ascites and upper gastrointestinal bleeding after balloon-occluded retrograde transvenous obliteration (BRTO). Am J Gastroenterol. 2013; 108(10):1612–1619

[48] Saad WEA, Kitanosono T, Koizumi J, Hirota S. The conventional balloon-occluded retrograde transvenous obliteration procedure: indications, contraindications, and technical applications. Tech Vasc Interv Radiol. 2013; 16(2): 101–151

[49] Saad WEA, Saad NE, Koizumi J. Stomal varices: management with decompression tips and transvenous obliteration or sclerosis. Tech Vasc Interv Radiol. 2013; 16(2):176–184

[50] Madsen MS, Petersen TH, Sommer H. Segmental portal hypertension. Ann Surg. 1986; 204(1):72–77

[51] Voros D, Mallas E, Antoniou A, et al. Splenomegaly and left sided portal hypertension. Ann Gastroenterol. 2005; 18(3):341–345

[52] Patrono D, Benvenga R, Moro F, Rossato D, Romagnoli R, Salizzoni M. Left-sided portal hypertension: successful management by laparoscopic splenectomy following splenic artery embolization. Int J Surg Case Rep. 2014; 5(10): 652–655

[53] Wang L, Liu GJ, Chen YX, Dong HP, Wang LX. Sinistral portal hypertension: clinical features and surgical treatment of chronic splenic vein occlusion. Med Princ Pract. 2012; 21(1):20–23

[54] Ferro C, Rossi UG, Bovio G, Dahamane M, Centanaro M. Transjugular intrahepatic portosystemic shunt, mechanical aspiration thrombectomy, and direct thrombolysis in the treatment of acute portal and superior mesenteric vein thrombosis. Cardiovasc Intervent Radiol. 2007; 30(5):1070–1074

[55] Henao EA, Bohannon WT, Silva MB, Jr. Treatment of portal venous thrombosis with selective superior mesenteric artery infusion of recombinant tissue plasminogen activator. J Vasc Surg. 2003; 38(6):1411–1415

[56] Sze DY, O'Sullivan GJ, Johnson DL, Dake MD. Mesenteric and portal venous thrombosis treated by transjugular mechanical thrombolysis. AJR Am J Roentgenol. 2000; 175(3):732–734

[57] Skeik N, Gits CC, Ehrenwald E, Cragg AH. Fibrinogen level as a surrogate for the outcome of thrombolytic therapy using tissue plasminogen activator for acute lower extremity intravascular thrombosis. Vasc Endovascular Surg. 2013; 47(7):519–523

[58] Jun KW, Kim MH, Park KM, et al. Mechanical thrombectomy-assisted thrombolysis for acute symptomatic portal and superior mesenteric venous thrombosis. Ann Surg Treat Res. 2014; 86(6):334–341

[59] Abdel-Aal AK, Ezzeldin IB, Hamed MF, et al. Endovascular treatment of acute portal vein thrombosis using ultrasound-accelerated catheter-directed thrombolysis. Vasc Endovascular Surg. 2014; 48(7–8):460–465

[60] De Santis A, Moscatelli R, Catalano C, et al. Systemic thrombolysis of portal vein thrombosis in cirrhotic patients: a pilot study. Dig Liver Dis. 2010; 42(6): 451–455

[61] Hoffer EK, Krohmer S, Gemery J, Zaki B, Pipas JM. Endovascular recanalization of symptomatic portomesenteric venous obstruction after pancreaticoduodenectomy and radiation. J Vasc Interv Radiol. 2009; 20(12):1633–1637

[62] Gaba RC, Garcia-Roca R, Oberholzer J. Pancreatic islet cell transplantation: an update for interventional radiologists. J Vasc Interv Radiol. 2012; 23(5):583–594, quiz 594

[63] Malinowski M, Geisel D, Stary V, et al. Portal vein embolization with plug/coils improves hepatectomy outcome. J Surg Res. 2015; 194(1):202–211

[64] Fischman AM, Ward TJ, Horn JC, et al. Portal vein embolization before right hepatectomy or extended right hepatectomy using sodium tetradecyl sulfate foam: technique and initial results. J Vasc Interv Radiol. 2014; 25(7):1045–1053

[65] van Lienden KP, van den Esschert JW, de Graaf W, et al. Portal vein embolization before liver resection: a systematic review. Cardiovasc Intervent Radiol. 2013; 36(1):25–34

[66] Malinowski M, Stary V, Lock JF, et al. Factors influencing hypertrophy of the left lateral liver lobe after portal vein embolization. Langenbecks Arch Surg. 2015; 400(2):237–246

[67] May BJ, Talenfeld AD, Madoff DC. Update on portal vein embolization: evidence-based outcomes, controversies, and novel strategies. J Vasc Interv Radiol. 2013; 24(2):241–254

[68] Patil P, Deshmukh H, Popat B, Rathod K. Spectrum of imaging in Budd Chiari syndrome. J Med Imaging Radiat Oncol. 2012; 56(1):75–83

[69] Garcia-Pagán JC, Heydtmann M, Raffa S, et al. Budd-Chiari Syndrome-Transjugular Intrahepatic Portosystemic Shunt Group. TIPS for Budd-Chiari syndrome: long-term results and prognostics factors in 124 patients. Gastroenterology. 2008; 135(3):808–815

[70] Rosenqvist K, Sheikhi R, Eriksson LG, et al. Endovascular treatment of symptomatic Budd-Chiari syndrome - in favour of early transjugular intrahepatic portosystemic shunt. Eur J Gastroenterol Hepatol. 2016; 28(6):656–660

[71] Ferral H, Behrens G, Lopera J. Budd-Chiari syndrome. AJR Am J Roentgenol. 2012; 199(4):737–745

12 Venous Anomalies and Syndromes: Classifications, Evaluation, and Treatment

Christopher R. Bailey, Scott R. Shuldiner, and Clifford R. Weiss

Summary

Venous malformations and their classification, evaluation, and treatment tend to remain poorly understood by the medical community at large. They represent a small niche in interventional radiology practice, but patients with venous anomalies will often ultimately present to interventional radiologists after evaluation and sometimes treatment by other specialists. An understanding of venous anomalies and their management is beneficial to interventional radiologists, both for purposes of managing these patients when appropriate and for understanding when to refer to a specialist with greater experience in management of these sometimes-complex patients. This chapter will review patient presentations, radiographic and clinical evaluation, and procedural details, introducing concepts related to potential outcomes and complications of treatment.

Keywords: venous malformation, venous syndromes, vascular anomalies, ISSVA classification, SEMVAFC, venous malformation imaging, sclerotherapy, sclerosants

12.1 Introduction

Venous malformations (VMs) are dilated venous channels or sacs filled with venous blood that may or may not communicate with the systemic venous system. A dysfunctional smooth muscle component leads to gradual expansion of VMs over time.[1] VMs are the most common type of vascular anomaly and can be found in isolation or in the setting of a genetic syndrome.[2] When superficial, VMs are often soft, compressible, bluish lesions. VMs can involve multiple body parts and can cross tissue and anatomic planes extending into adjacent muscles and bones, as well as along vasculature and nerves. The proper management of VMs begins with accurate diagnosis and evaluation for the extent of disease prior to selecting a targeted interventional therapy or surgical approach.[1,3,4] Pediatricians, interventionalists, dermatologists, and surgeons who diagnose and treat VMs should be well versed in the classification, imaging evaluation, and treatment options available for venous anomalies. In this chapter, we outline the currently accepted classification schemas, radiographic workup, and treatment options for a variety of VMs and venous syndromes.

12.2 Case Vignette

12.2.1 Patient Presentation

An 8-year-old boy presented with a palpable mass of his right forearm reported as intermittently painful. His mother stated that he was born with the lesion but it had grown in size over time. The lesion had first become symptomatic at age 5. He reported pain after applying pressure to the area and also with prolonged activity. The lesion did not change in size when dependent.

12.2.2 Physical Exam

Vital signs were normal. Focused exam of the right upper extremity revealed a 4×5 cm area of soft tissue swelling without discoloration over the proximal volar forearm. The lesion was painful to palpation but did not increase in size when placed in a dependent position. There was no palpable pulsation or bruit. Sensory and motor exam of the right lower extremity were unremarkable.

12.2.3 Laboratory Workup

Notable values included:
- D-dimer 2.07 mg/L (less than five times elevated from normal limits).
- Fibrinogen: 323 mg/dL (normal).

12.2.4 Imaging

Multiphase and multiplanar MRI with and without contrast was obtained. MRI revealed a lobulated and multiseptated lesion with tubular foci within the medial belly of the brachioradialis muscle. The lesion was T2 hyperintense with T2 hypointensities scattered throughout, likely representing phleboliths. There were also several fluid–fluid levels, representative of "hematocrit layering," hemorrhage, or proteinaceous material. After administration of intravenous contrast, the lesion demonstrated uniform enhancement similar in timing and appearance to the surrounding venous structures. There was no evidence of osseous invasion. Findings were compatible with solitary VM (▶ Fig. 12.1a,b).

12.2.5 Specifics of Consent

Treatment alternatives, including compression and surgical excision, were discussed, reviewing the limitations and risks of these alternatives. Risks of sclerotherapy discussed with the patient and parents included the following: thrombosis, which may be localized with associated postprocedural pain, may extend to the deep venous system with outflow occlusion or embolize with resultant, possibly significant pulmonary embolism, and, more rarely, disseminated intravascular coagulation (DIC); extravasation of sclerosant with soft tissue damage; entry of sclerosant into the deep venous system with resultant endothelial damage; allergic reaction to sclerosant; swelling of treated area with risk for compartment syndrome in the extremity; development of extremity contracture due to immobilization postprocedure; nerve damage with loss of sensory or motor function; and failure of procedure. Expectations were also set relative to the likelihood of repeat procedures for control of the chronic disorder.

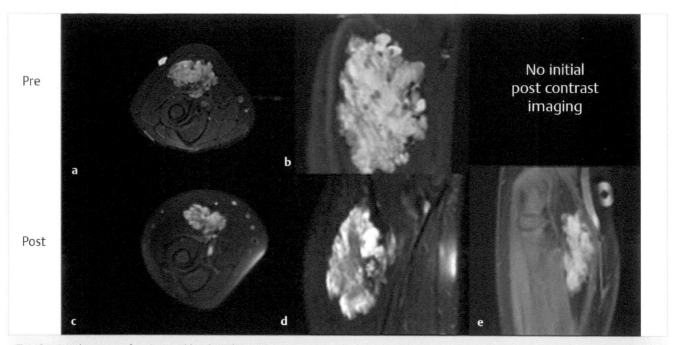

Fig. 12.1 Initial imaging of an 8-year-old male with a tender mass in his right forearm (*top row*). Axial (**a**) and sagittal (**b**) T2-weighted MR images of the right upper extremity reveals a T2-hyperintense lobulated mass with T2 hypointensities scattered throughout, likely representing phleboliths. Findings are compatible with a venous malformation. Postsclerotherapy MR imaging (*bottom row*). (**c**) T2-weighted MR postsclerotherapy reveals overall reduction in size of VM. Axial (**d**) and sagittal (**e**) postcontrast imaging also reveal a reduction in the size of the VM with areas of contrast enhancement representing residual VM.

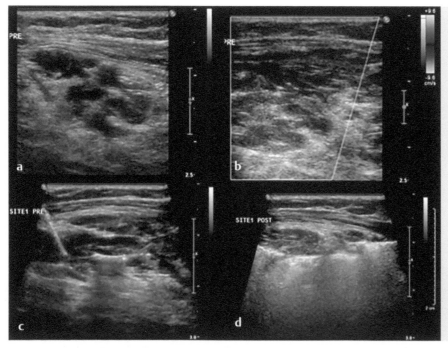

Fig. 12.2 Intraprocedural ultrasound imaging of the same 8-year-old male with a tender mass in his right forearm. (**a**) Preprocedural ultrasound revealed multiple hypoechoic tubular structures in the right forearm. (**b**) Color Doppler ultrasound demonstrated no flow appreciable flow, compatible with a venous malformation. (**c**) Ultrasound-guided percutaneous access into the lesion. (**d**) Postsclerotherapy ultrasound demonstrates increased echogenicity and acoustic shadowing at the site of sclerosant injection.

Details of Procedure

1. Informed consent was obtained and all patient questions answered.
2. Preprocedural ultrasound revealed multiple hypoechoic tubular structures in the region of the previously identified VM without appreciable flow (▶ Fig. 12.2a,b).
3. The right forearm was prepped and draped in usual sterile fashion at the location of the VM.
4. Ultrasound guidance was used to percutaneously access the VM in the right forearm/brachioradialis muscle at two sites with 21-gauge needles (▶ Fig. 12.2c).
5. Presclerotherapy venograms were performed at each access site to characterize the VM, assess size, and evaluate for presence and size of draining veins (▶ Fig. 12.3a).

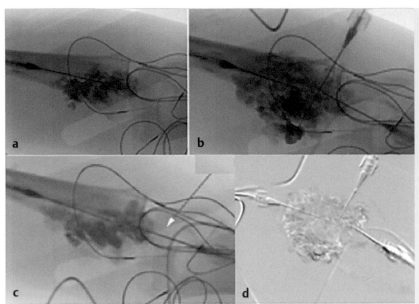

Fig. 12.3 Intraprocedural fluoroscopic images of the same 8-year-old male with a tender mass in his right forearm. **(a)** Access into the first site of the VM with preprocedural venogram defining the extent of the first site. **(b)** Access into the second site of VM with preprocedural venogram defining the extent of the second site. **(c)** Placement of a decompression needle within the second site. **(d)** Postsclerotherapy image.

6. An additional 21-gauge needle was placed into the cephalad aspect of the VM for decompression during sclerotherapy (▶ Fig. 12.3b).

7. Sotradecol foam mixture was prepared using a ratio of 1-mL 3% Sotradecol, 0.5-mL Lipiodol, 4-mL air.

8. Sotradecol foam was injected into each site under fluoroscopic guidance using negative contrast/contrast displacement technique (▶ Fig. 12.3c,d).

9. After allowing 15 minutes for the Sotradecol to act, the needles were tested for further blood return, and finding none they were removed and manual pressure applied until hemostasis was achieved. Postprocedural ultrasound revealed increased echogenicity and acoustic shadowing at the site of treatment (▶ Fig. 12.2d).

10. The patient was admitted overnight for pain control, management of postprocedure swelling, and neurovascular checks.

11. The patient was discharged the next morning without complication.

Follow-up

The patient underwent a right upper extremity duplex ultrasound in the immediate postprocedural period, which revealed a patent deep venous system without evidence of thrombosis. The patient presented for follow-up 3 days after sclerotherapy and reported slightly increased pain at the site of sclerotherapy, compatible with normal postsclerotherapy discomfort. Pain was well controlled with ibuprofen. The patient was referred for physical therapy to maintain range of motion and to prevent contractures. The patient underwent follow-up MRI approximately 2 months postsclerotherapy, which revealed greater than 50% decrease in the size of the lesion (▶ Fig. 12.1c–e). The patient was also seen in clinic at approximately 2 months post-sclerotherapy. At this time, the patient reported that he was now asymptomatic with marked improvement in soft tissue swelling of the right forearm. The patient and his family were instructed to follow-up in 1 year with an MRI or sooner if he became symptomatic again.

12.3 Epidemiology and Scope of the Problem

VMs are the most common type of vascular malformation. The estimated incidence of venous anomalies is 2%. Ninety percent of VMs are solitary, which usually indicates that the VM is sporadic. Multiple VMs account for the remaining 10% of lesions and are often related to heritable conditions or syndromes.[1,3]

12.3.1 Classification

The management of VMs often warrants a multidisciplinary approach; thus, it is important to use a common language between multiple subspecialties in order to properly define and classify these lesions with a high degree of accuracy and precision.[3] Several classification schemas have been developed, dating back to the 1970s. The most widely recognized classification system was developed and refined by the International Society for the Study of Vascular Anomalies (ISSVA).[2,4,5] Since the society's founding in 1976 by Mulliken and Young, the ISSVA has been refining its classification system on a biannual basis. The ISSVA classifies vascular anomalies based on cellular features, flow characteristics, associated clinical features and behavior, and genetics. The most recent iteration of this system was adopted in 2014.[5]

At the highest level, vascular anomalies are classified as either vascular tumors or vascular malformations (▶ Table 12.1). A vascular tumor results from aberrant cellular proliferation, whereas a vascular malformation is a regional defect in vascular morphogenesis. Vascular tumors are further subdivided into benign, malignant, and aggressive. Similarly, vascular malformations are subdivided into low-flow and high-flow lesions

Table 12.1 Adapted 2014 ISSVA classification of vascular malformations[5]

Vascular malformations	
Simple	Combined
Capillary malformation	CVM, CLM
Lymphatic malformation	LVM, CLVM
Venous malformation	CAVM
Arteriovenous malformation	CLAVM
Arteriovenous fistula	CLAVM

Abbreviations: CAVM, capillary arteriovenous malformation; CLAVM, capillary lymphatic arteriovenous malformation; CLM, capillary lymphatic malformation; CLVM, capillary lymphatic venous malformation; CVM, capillary venous malformation; LVM, lymphatic venous malformation.

Table 12.3 Adapted 2014 ISSVA combined venous malformations[5]

Combined venous malformations	
Capillary–venous malformation	CM + VM
Lymphatic–venous malformation	LM + VM
Capillary–lymphatic–venous malformation	CM + LM + VM
Capillary–venous–arteriovenous malformation	CM + VM + AVM
Capillary–lymphatic–venous–arteriovenous malformation	CM + LM + VM + AVM

Abbreviations: AVM, arteriovenous malformation; CM, capillary malformation; LM, lymphatic malformation; VM, venous malformation.

Table 12.2 Adapted 2014 ISSVA simple venous malformations[5]

Simple venous malformations
Common VM
Familial VM cutaneomucosal
Blue rubber bleb nevus (Bean) syndrome VM
Glomuvenous malformation
Cerebral cavernous malformation
Others

Abbreviation: VM, venous malformation.

Table 12.4 Adapted 2014 ISSVA genes associated with venous malformations[5]

Venous malformation	Gene
Common VM	TIE2 somatic
Familial VM cutaneomucosal	TIE2
Glomuvenous malformation	Glomulin
Cerebral cavernous malformation	KRIT1/Malcavernin/PDCD10

Abbreviation: VM, venous malformation.

Table 12.5 Adapted 2014 ISSVA venous malformations associated with other anomalies[5]

Syndrome	Malformation type and anomalies
Klippel–Trénaunay syndrome	CM + VM + /– LM + limb overgrowth
Servelle–Martorell syndrome	Limb VM + bone undergrowth
Maffucci's syndrome	VM + /– spindle-cell hemangioma + endochondroma
CLOVES syndrome	LM + VM + CM + /– AVM + lipomatous overgrowth
Proteus Syndrome	CM, VM and/or LM + asymmetric somatic overgrowth
Bannayan–Riley–Ruvalcaba	AVM + VM + macrocephaly, lipomatous overgrowth

Abbreviations: AVM, arteriovenous malformation; CM, capillary malformation; LM, lymphatic malformation; VM, venous malformation.

(e.g., venous, lymphatic vs. arterial and arteriovenous malformation), and also whether it is simple (one vascular malformation in one lesion) or combined (two or more vascular malformations in one lesion) (▶ Table 12.1).[5] With respect to VMs, the ISSVA classification schema for simple and combined VMs is shown in ▶ Table 12.2 and ▶ Table 12.3, respectively. The ISSVA also provides a table of associated genes (▶ Table 12.4) and additional anomalies associated with VMs (▶ Table 12.5).[5]

Another tool that aids in the classification of vascular anomalies is the S.E. Mitchell Vascular Anomalies Flow Chart (SEMVAFC) (▶ Fig. 12.4).[3] The SEMVAFC uses clinical symptoms, physical exam findings, and imaging to provide a clear pathway for physicians to accurately diagnose a vascular abnormality. In order to preserve a common language among the multidisciplinary team of physicians who manage these lesions, SEMFAFC is broken up into similar categories to the ISSVA classification schema. For instance, VMs are classified as slow-flow malformations under SEMVAFC.[3] Of note, the term cavernous hemangioma has previously been used to refer to VMs; in fact, this term should only be used to refer to deep hemangiomas, and cavernous hemangioma should no longer be associated with VMs.

Puig and colleagues developed a classification system specific to VMs using phlebography to help guide interventional therapy.[6] This classification is based off venous drainage of the VM and was meant to estimate the risk of central embolization, or the risk of the sclerosant agent reaching the central vasculature and causing a complication such as pulmonary vasospasm or

direct cardiotoxicity. Type 1 malformations are isolated without any peripheral drainage. Type II malformations drain into "normal" veins. Type III malformations drain into dysplastic veins. Finally, type IV malformations are venous ectasia. The authors found that patients with type I and II VMs had almost no risk of central embolization. However, patients with type III and IV VMs had a much higher risk of central embolization due to their large draining venous channels.[6]

12.3.2 Patient Presentation and Evaluation

Sporadic VMs

Superficial VMs can manifest as small varicosities or bluish mass lesions. Deeper VMs often present as soft tissue masses. Both superficial and deep VMs are typically soft and easily compressible. The lesions can sometimes enlarge with Valsalva's

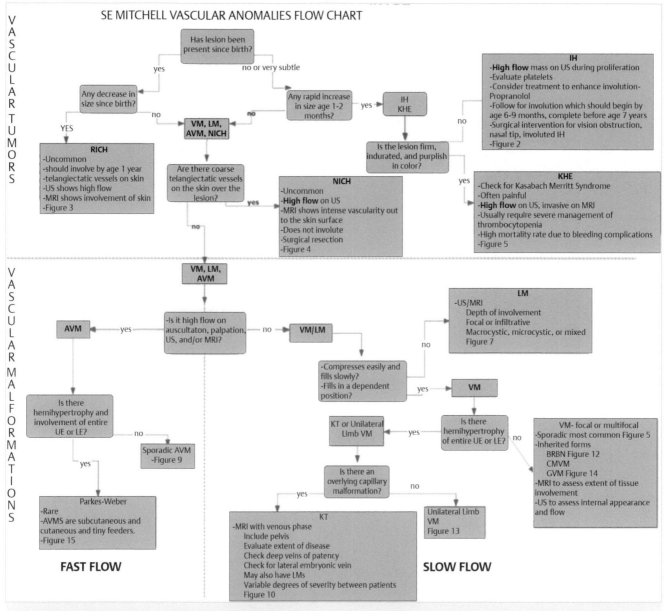

Fig. 12.4 S.E. Mitchell Vascular Anomalies Flow Chart (SEMVAFC).[3]

maneuver or when the affected area is in a dependent position due to blood pooling.[1,3,7] While VMs most commonly present during mid-to-late childhood and grow in size as time progresses, they are often present at birth. VMs typically grow as the patient grows; however, rapid growth occurs during peak hormonal levels (i.e., puberty, pregnancy, and menstrual cycles). VMs most commonly are found on the head and neck (47%), extremities (30%), and trunk (13%), but can occur anywhere on the body. As discussed above, the majority of VMs are solitary; however, when multiple VMs are present, there should be a high index of suspicion for an underlying syndrome.[1,2]

Most VMs remain asymptomatic over a patient's lifetime. When symptomatic, however, they often present with pain secondary to focal thrombosis or due to mass effect. Commonly, pain can be worse in the morning due to pooling and stasis of blood within the VM during sleep or worse after physical

activity due to pooling from increased venous pressure.[1,3,8,9] VMs can also impair function when they invade or impinge upon muscle groups, joints, and nerves. Both superficial and deep VMs can cause varying degrees of cosmetic deformity. Head and neck VMs can also cause problems with respiration, speech, swallowing, and vision.[7,10,11,12]

Venous Syndromes

Klippel–Trénaunay (KT) Syndrome

KT syndrome is characterized by VMs/varicosities, capillary–lymphatic–VMs, and bony/soft tissue hypertrophy of the limbs, which is often unilateral.[13,14,15] Though KT syndrome is thought to be a genetically sporadic syndrome, genetic associations are still being explored. With regard to the venous component of this disorder, patients present with superficial and deeper varicosities and malformations that may benefit from sclerotherapy. It is important to note that the deep venous system must be evaluated prior to intervention, since patients with KT syndrome can have absent or hypoplastic deep venous systems.[1,2,13]

Blue Rubber Bleb Nevus Syndrome (BRBNS)

BRBNS, also called Bean's syndrome, is a sporadic syndrome characterized by multiple superficial skin VMs as well as small and large bowel VMs. Due to the presence of multiple gastrointestinal VMs, these patients are at risk for gastrointestinal bleeding.[16]

Glomuvenous Malformation

Glomuvenous malformation is an autosomal dominant syndrome characterized by multiple blue nodules throughout the skin representing VMs in the presence of glomus cells (glomangiomas).[1,17]

12.4 Radiographic Evaluation

12.4.1 Ultrasound

Ultrasonographic imaging of VMs is limited. VMs usually appear as sponge-like networks of tubular structures with heterogeneous echogenicity.[18] They demonstrate either low, pure monophasic, or more typically no-flow on color Doppler ultrasound. Phleboliths may be seen as focal echogenicities within the lesion.[5,9,19,20] VMs also tend to be easily compressible with an ultrasound probe. Postsclerotherapy ultrasonographic imaging of VMs often demonstrates heterogeneous echogenicity with acoustic shadowing.[1]

12.4.2 MRI

MRI is the most sensitive imaging modality for evaluating VMs. Due to its high soft tissue resolution, MRI is particularly useful to determine the extent of a VM, confirm the diagnosis, and assess treatment response.[3,8,9] A standard multiplanar, multisequence protocol for imaging vascular abnormalities includes precontrast T1-weighted imaging, multiplanar T2-weighted imaging with fat saturation, and postcontrast multiplanar T1-weighted with fat saturation (▶ Fig. 12.5a–e). In addition to these sequences, dynamic contrast-enhanced magnetic resonance angiography (MRA),[21,22] specifically time-resolved angiography with interleaved stochastic trajectories or TWIST (Siemens, Munich, Germany),[23] is useful. TWIST provides valuable information about the timing of contrast enhancement, specifically whether the vascular lesion enhances in the venous or arterial phase, or neither. This technique also provides information about arterial or venous connections to the systemic vasculature (▶ Fig. 12.6). Additionally, delineation of specific enhancement patterns helps classify difficult-to-characterize vascular anomalies, providing interventionists and surgeons with an anatomic map for treatment planning. Indeed, the addition of TWIST to our protocol has been fruitful.[23] A recent study demonstrated that TWIST using gadofosveset accurately

classified various vascular abnormalities in the head and neck region while also providing important hemodynamic information, using one-third the dose of gadofosveset compared to other MRI contrast agents.[23] Unfortunately gadofosveset is no longer available; however, TWIST can be performed with most conventional MR contrast agents.

As VMs can infiltrate multiple soft tissue types and bone, the high soft tissue resolution provided by MRI is advantageous when assessing the extent of the lesion.[24] VMs also tend to hemorrhage internally and are prone to thrombosis, eventually leading to phlebolith formation.[1] Due to these characteristics, VMs display variable signal intensities on both T1- and T2-weighted imaging. However, VMs generally display isointense to hypointense signal intensity on T1-weighted images and hyperintense signal on T2-weighted images.[3,7,8] VMs are often lobulated lesions with tubular structures throughout. Phleboliths appear as T2 dark regions, signal voids, within the lesion. Phleboliths are a pathognomonic finding for VMs. After contrast administration, VMs enhance avidly in the late venous/delayed phase. Of note, liver hemangiomas similarly display delayed phase peripheral enhancement suggesting that liver hemangiomas are in fact VMs of the liver. Postsclerotherapy changes include a decrease in size of the lesion, with T2 dark regions representing areas of thrombosis and fibrosis[25](▶ Fig. 12.5f–j). Additionally, regions of T2 hyperintensity representing residual portions of the lesion may be present.[1,3,7,8]

12.4.3 CT

Like ultrasound, CT is not a preferred modality for imaging VMs as it provides limited information. VMs appear as an irregular mass with hyperattenuating phleboliths on CT. Contrast-enhanced CT may reveal peripheral enhancement on delayed phase imaging.[1,7]

12.5 Angiography

Angiography is rarely required for diagnosis. Prior to interventional therapy, direct contrast injection (percutaneous into the VM) is used preprocedurally to define venous outflow.

12.6 Preparation for Procedure

In addition to preprocedural imaging for diagnosis and characterization of the VM, it is advised that patients with VMs undergo hematologic testing.[1,26] Specifically, a complete blood count, coagulation panel, D-dimer, and fibrinogen must be obtained. Patients with VMs are at risk for localized intravascular coagulopathy (LIC) due to the slow venous blood flow within the VM, which promotes coagulation cascade activation.[20,26] LIC results in elevated D-dimer levels with a decrease in fibrinogen and platelets. Additionally, LIC can lead to localized thrombotic events within the VM causing pain. LIC can also lead to DIC in the setting of trauma or procedural interventions. Patients with elevated D-dimer (usually greater than five times the upper limit of normal) and low fibrinogen undergo hematology consultation and typically are placed on low-molecular-weight heparin (LMWH) for 10 days pre- and postprocedure.[1,26]

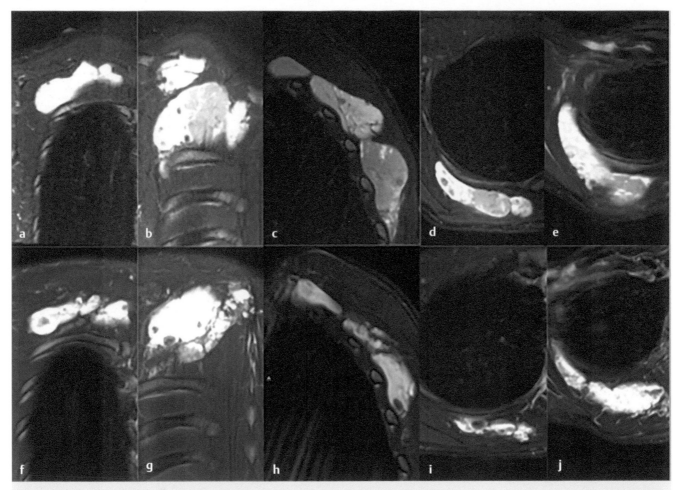

Fig. 12.5 Pre- and posttreatment MR imaging of a back and right upper extremity VM. Pretreatment coronal **(a, b)**, sagittal **(c)**, and axial **(d, e)** T2-weighted MR reveals a large, lobulated hyperintense lesion with scattered T2 hypointense regions representing phleboliths (*top row*). Posttreatment coronal **(f, g)**, sagittal **(h)**, and axial **(i, j)** T2-weighted MR reveals an overall decrease in size and T2 intensity after multiple sclerotherapy sessions.

12.6.1 Technical Tips and Tricks and Procedural Details

Sclerotherapy

Sclerotherapy is considered to be the first-line therapy in the treatment of VMs.[27] Sclerotherapy is the direct injection of sclerosants into VMs resulting in an inflammatory response that leads to thrombosis and fibrosis of the treated area.[28] The most commonly used sclerosant is ethanol, as it has the lowest rate of recurrence.[1] Ethanol must be administered carefully in order to avoid life-threatening complications such as arrhythmias, cardiovascular collapse, and hemolysis-related renal failure. Currently accepted guidelines stipulate that the dose of absolute ethanol should not exceed a total of 1 mL/kg in a single session. In addition, absolute ethanol should not be administered in aliquots greater than 0.1 mg/kg/5 min.[1] During administration, adequate hydration is necessary. Another currently accepted administration guideline pertains to sodium tetradecyl sulfate (STS). STS 3% should not be administered in aliquots greater than 0.5 mL/kg (liquid). Typically, STS is delivered as a foam, to maximize contact with vascular endothelium while limiting

dose. STS is often delivered as a foam that consists of 1-mL STS 3%, 0.5-mL lipiodol, and 4-mL air. Other sclerosant agents include sodium morrhuate, polidocanol, ethiodized oil, alcoholic solution of zein, and ethanolamine oleate.[5,28,29]

Bleomycin is a relatively newly utilized sclerosant agent that has been successfully used to treat VMs. It is a chemotherapeutic agent that causes DNA damage leading to endothelial cell death/damage and nonspecific inflammation. Bleomycin foam has been shown to be efficacious in the treatment of VMs, demonstrating improvement in symptoms after one session with few complications.[12,30] Recently, Ul Haq and colleagues demonstrated the efficacy and safety of foamed bleomycin for the treatment of a variety of VMs. The authors found that 100% of their patients reported improved symptoms after one treatment.[12] Postprocedural imaging revealed decreased VM volume (93%), decreased contrast enhancement (79%), and decreased T2 signal intensity (86%) after a single session. There were no intraprocedural complications. Twenty-two percent of patients experienced minor complications (blistering, rash, minor swelling) and 7% of patients experienced major complications (severe swelling of the treatment area). Bleomycin has a currently recommended lifetime dose limit of 400 mg or 5 mg/kg

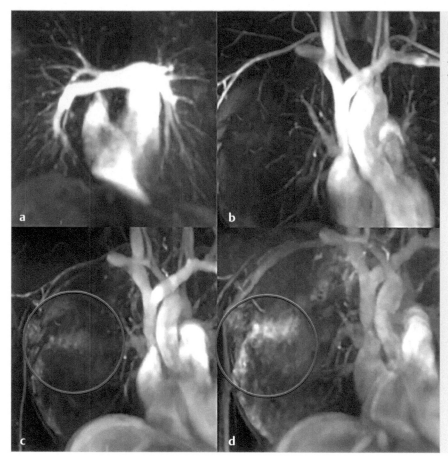

Fig. 12.6 Coronal TWIST images of the same back and right upper extremity VM. **(a)** Early arterial phase; note the VM is not visualized at this time point. **(b)** Arterial phase. **(c)** Early venous phase; the VM begins to fill (*red circle*). **(d)** Late venous phase; the VM is more densely opacified (*red circle*).

to reduce the risk of pulmonary fibrosis; using bleomycin foam instead of liquid formulations drastically reduced the amount of bleomycin required for successful treatment.[12,30]

A typical sclerotherapy procedure protocol is described below (▶ Fig. 12.7).

1. Informed consent is obtained.
2. Anesthesia is induced once the patient is in the interventional radiology suite.
3. A preprocedural ultrasound is performed to visualize the VM immediately prior to the procedure.
4. Intraprocedural nerve monitoring may be performed if the VM is in close proximity to a nerve.
5. The treatment area is prepped and draped in usual sterile fashion.
6. Ultrasound guidance is used to percutaneously access the VM, typically with a 4 or 7 cm 21-gauge needle connected to flexible tubing and a 3 mL syringe with contrast (▶ Fig. 12.7a,b).
7. Blood return confirms successful access.
8. A pneumatic cuff may be used to distend veins to allow for easier access. After access is obtained, the cuff is deflated.
9. Presclerotherapy digital subtraction angiography (DSA) venograms are performed at the access site to characterize the VM, assess size, and evaluate for presence and size of draining veins (▶ Fig. 12.7c–e):
   - If a large draining vein is identified, manual compression or a tourniquet can be used to prevent sclerosant from traveling to the systemic vasculature.

- Glue or coils may be used to occlude very large draining veins in some cases.
- A double-needle technique can also be used to reduce the risk of rupturing a type I or II VM. Double-needle technique requires the placement of two needles within the VM: one to inject sclerosant and the other to decompress the malformation as sclerosant is added.
- If there is contrast extravasation, the needle needs to be repositioned within the VM before injection of the sclerosant. Often, treatment of that section of the malformation is postponed to another date.

10. Sclerosant agent is injected into each accessed site of the VM under fluoroscopic guidance using negative contrast technique (▶ Fig. 12.7e).
11. The sclerosant should be left to dwell within the VM for 15 to 20 minutes (▶ Fig. 12.7f).
12. After the dwell time, the administration syringe is disconnected and the needle is observed for venous return (▶ Fig. 12.7g).
    - When administering bleomycin, there is no thrombosis expected, and reassessment and retreatment is not necessary.
13. If venous return is observed, another DSA venogram should be performed and steps 6 to 8 should be repeated until there is no venous return from the needle.
14. Once complete, the needles are removed and pressure is applied to the access site until hemostasis is achieved.

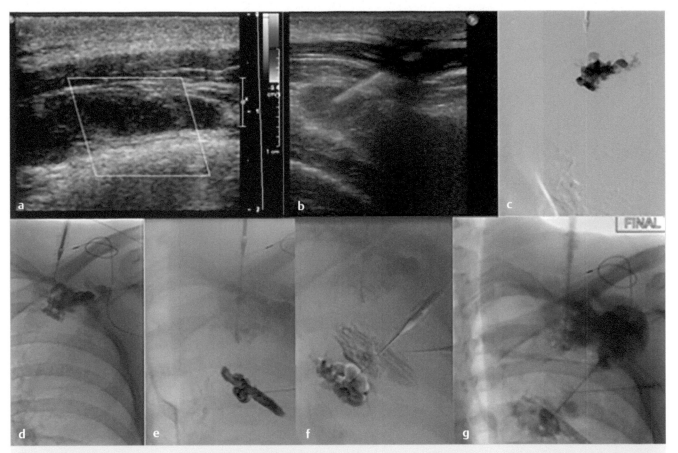

Fig. 12.7 Sclerotherapy treatment of the same back and right forearm VM. (**a, b**) Preprocedural ultrasound is performed identifying the VM with no appreciable flow, and percutaneous access is obtained. (**c**) A preprocedural venogram is then performed defining the extent of the first site. (**d**) Access into a second (**e**) and third site is obtained with venograms to define the extent of these sites. (**f**) An additional, fourth site, is accessed. Sclerosant is then injected into each site. (**g**) After letting the sclerosant dwell for 15 minutes, a postsclerotherapy image is obtained demonstrating the four treated sites.

The patient may be admitted for overnight observation and pain control. If a VM within an extremity is treated, a postprocedural ultrasound is usually obtained before discharge to confirm patency of the deep venous system.

Though ultrasound and fluoroscopy are the current gold standard imaging modalities used to performed sclerotherapy, interventional MRI has also been investigated for image guidance. MR-guided sclerotherapy has the added benefit of providing more precise imaging data at the time of intervention, allowing for the treatment of portions of VMs that cannot be seen on ultrasound such as lesions that are deep in the abdomen. Though many institutions regularly perform this next iteration of sclerotherapy, it is presently a complex and costly approach and will require further refinement before it is widely accepted and used outside of a few large centers.[1,31,32,33]

12.7 Potential Complications or Pitfalls

The overall complication rate after sclerotherapy is approximately 20%.[34] Complications after sclerotherapy can be localized or systemic. The most common localized complications are skin ulceration and blistering, especially in patients with superficial VMs. Some authors have suggested using STS, which is a less toxic sclerosant compared to absolute ethanol, to reduce the risk of skin ulceration and blistering.[1] On occasion, more serious, deeper ulcerations can occur. The treatment of ulcerations involves topical antibiotics and wound care, while deeper wounds may require more aggressive management. Nerve injury can also result when VMs extend to adjacent nerves. The use of intraprocedural nerve monitoring helps prevent nerve damage.[1] Though uncommon, acute compartment syndrome can also occur when a VM is within a fascia-bound compartment. Swelling secondary to sclerotherapy may result in increased compartment pressures leading to compression of the blood supply to structures within the treated compartment. Compartment syndrome can be managed conservatively with ice packs or with intravenous steroids in more severe cases. Systemic complications are more likely to occur after treatment of a large/extensive VM. Complications may include cardiac arrhythmias, renal failure, and hemolysis. As described above, using lower doses of sclerosant agents and splitting treatments into multiple sessions can limit systemic complications. Similarly, adequate hydration and sodium bicarbonate in the postprocedural period have been used to prevent renal injuries.[6,12,29]

12.8 Postprocedural Management and Follow-up

After discharge from the hospital, short-term follow-up is recommended, preferably at approximately 1-week postsclerotherapy. The patient should then return between 6 and 8 weeks for follow-up MRI and clinic to assess treatment response and to discuss further treatments if necessary. Sclerotherapy has been shown to decrease pain and size of the lesion in approximately 75 to 90% of cases; however, multiple sessions may be required to achieve the desired result.[1,12,29] The treatment endpoint is variable and is largely based on the patient's reported improvement (i.e., improved pain, desired cosmetic result, improved function). Once the treatment endpoint has been reached, patients should have MRI and clinical follow-up at 1-year intervals, and sooner if symptoms worsen or complications arise.

12.8.1 Noninvasive and Pharmacologic Treatments

Compression garments can be used to decrease the pooling of blood within extensive VMs of the extremities. This intervention limits stasis and expansion, resulting in decreased pain. Pharmacologic treatments have also been used to treat symptomatic VMs. As discussed above, LIC can result in recurrent, localized thrombosis that results in pain. LMWH can be administered to reduce the occurrence of thrombosis and improve the patient's coagulation profile. Aspirin can be similarly employed to reduce localized thrombotic events.[1,20,26]

12.8.2 Surgical Approaches

Prior to the advent of sclerotherapy, surgical excision of VMs was the preferred approach. While there is still a role for surgical excision, it usually occurs in combination with sclerotherapy. Sclerotherapy or coil and glue embolization prior to resection reduces the size of the lesion, allowing for an easier excisional approach.[35] Combined sclerotherapy/embolization and surgical resection/reconstruction can be particularly useful when dealing with head and neck VMs where aesthetic and functional outcomes are particularly important.[1]

12.9 Pearls of Wisdom

- The management of VMs often warrants a multidisciplinary approach; thus, it is important to use a common language between multiple subspecialties in order to properly define and classify these lesions with a high degree of accuracy and precision.
- VMs can often be diagnosed by history and physical exam alone; however, the use of MRI can aid in diagnosis and provide important anatomical information for procedural planning, and it can be used serially to monitor treatment response.
- Multisequence and multiplanar imaging as described above is a requirement for the appropriate evaluation of VMs.

- Sclerotherapy is considered to be the first-line therapy in the treatment of VMs and is indicated for symptomatic VMs (e.g., pain, functional impairments, and deformities).
- Sclerotherapy has been shown to decrease pain and size of the lesion in approximately 75 to 90% of cases; however, multiple sessions may be required to achieve the desired result.
- Careful preprocedural planning, intraprocedural monitoring, and use of low-dose sclerosant agents can limit and prevent localized and systemic postprocedural complications.

12.10 Conclusion

VMs are the most common type of vascular anomaly. Accurate diagnosis and characterization is paramount to proper management. Fortunately, current classifications schemas such as the ISSVA and SEMVAFC can help clinicians from different subspecialties to diagnosis, classify, and treat these lesions using a common language and treatment paradigms across multidisciplinary care teams. The increased standardization of MRI protocols across imaging centers and institutions will also aid in appropriate diagnosis, preprocedural planning, and postprocedure follow-up. Image-guided sclerotherapy is currently the first-line treatment for VMs. However, this may change as the development of new classes of therapies continues to evolve.

References

[1] Geschwind J, Dake M. Abrams' Angiography: Interventional Radiology. 3rd ed. Philadelphia, PA: Lippincott, Williams, & Wilkens; 2013

[2] Nozaki T, Nosaka S, Miyazaki O, et al. Syndromes associated with vascular tumors and malformations: a pictorial review. Radiographics. 2013; 33(1): 175–195

[3] Tekes A, Koshy J, Kalayci TO, et al. S.E. Mitchell Vascular Anomalies Flow Chart (SEMVAFC): a visual pathway combining clinical and imaging findings for classification of soft-tissue vascular anomalies. Clin Radiol. 2014; 69(5):443–457

[4] Miller DD, Gupta A. Histopathology of vascular anomalies: update based on the revised 2014 ISSVA classification. Semin Cutan Med Surg. 2016; 35(3): 137–146

[5] International Society for the Study of Vascular Anomalies Classification of Vascular Anomalies. Classification. Available at: issva.org/classification. Published 2014. Accessed December 1, 2016

[6] Puig S, Aref H, Chigot V, Bonin B, Brunelle F. Classification of venous malformations in children and implications for sclerotherapy. Pediatr Radiol. 2003; 33(2):99–103

[7] Flis CM, Connor SE. Imaging of head and neck venous malformations. Eur Radiol. 2005; 15(10):2185–2193

[8] Dubois J, Alison M. Vascular anomalies: what a radiologist needs to know. Pediatr Radiol. 2010; 40(6):895–905

[9] Behravesh S, Yakes W, Gupta N, et al. Venous malformations: clinical diagnosis and treatment. Cardiovasc Diagn Ther. 2016; 6(6):557–569

[10] Puttgen KB, Pearl M, Tekes A, Mitchell SE. Update on pediatric extracranial vascular anomalies of the head and neck. Childs Nerv Syst. 2010; 26(10): 1417–1433

[11] Choi DJ, Alomari AI, Chaudry G, Orbach DB. Neurointerventional management of low-flow vascular malformations of the head and neck. Neuroimaging Clin N Am. 2009; 19(2):199–218

[12] Ul Haq F, Mitchell SE, Tekes A, Weiss CR. Bleomycin foam treatment of venous malformations: a promising agent for effective treatment with minimal swelling. J Vasc Interv Radiol. 2015; 26(10):1484–1493

[13] Jacob AG, Driscoll DJ, Shaughnessy WJ, Stanson AW, Clay RP, Gloviczki P. Klippel-Trénaunay syndrome: spectrum and management. Mayo Clin Proc. 1998; 73(1):28–36

[14] Gloviczki P, Driscoll DJ. Klippel-Trenaunay syndrome: current management. Phlebology. 2007; 22(6):291–298

[15] Lindenauer SM. The Klippel-Trenaunay syndrome: varicosity, hypertrophy and hemangioma with no arteriovenous fistula. Ann Surg. 1965; 162:303–314

[16] Akutko K, Krzesiek E, Iwańczak B. Blue rubber bleb naevus syndrome [in Polish]. Pol Merkur Lekarski. 2012; 33(196):226–228

[17] Boon LM, Mulliken JB, Enjolras O, Vikkula M. Glomuvenous malformation (glomangioma) and venous malformation: distinct clinicopathologic and genetic entities. Arch Dermatol. 2004; 140(8):971–976

[18] Paltiel HJ, Burrows PE, Kozakewich HP, Zurakowski D, Mulliken JB. Soft-tissue vascular anomalies: utility of US for diagnosis. Radiology. 2000; 214(3):747–754

[19] Enjolras O, Chapot R, Merland JJ. Vascular anomalies and the growth of limbs: a review. J Pediatr Orthop B. 2004; 13(6):349–357

[20] Martin LK, Russell S, Wargon O. Chronic localized intravascular coagulation complicating multifocal venous malformations. Australas J Dermatol. 2009; 50(4):276–280

[21] van Rijswijk CSP, van der Linden E, van der Woude H-J, van Baalen JM, Bloem JL. Value of dynamic contrast-enhanced MR imaging in diagnosing and classifying peripheral vascular malformations. AJR Am J Roentgenol. 2002; 178(5): 1181–1187

[22] Ohgiya Y, Hashimoto T, Gokan T, et al. Dynamic MRI for distinguishing high-flow from low-flow peripheral vascular malformations. AJR Am J Roentgenol. 2005; 185(5):1131–1137

[23] Higgins LJ, Koshy J, Mitchell SE, et al. Time-resolved contrast-enhanced MRA (TWIST) with gadofosveset trisodium in the classification of soft-tissue vascular anomalies in the head and neck in children following updated 2014 ISSVA classification: first report on systematic evaluation of MRI and TWIST in a cohort of 47 children. Clin Radiol. 2016; 71(1):32–39

[24] Thawait SK, Puttgen K, Carrino JA, et al. MR imaging characteristics of soft tissue vascular anomalies in children. Eur J Pediatr. 2013; 172(5):591–600

[25] Flors L, Leiva-Salinas C, Maged IM, et al. MR imaging of soft-tissue vascular malformations: diagnosis, classification, and therapy follow-up. Radiographics. 2011; 31(5):1321–1340, discussion 1340–1341

[26] Dompmartin A, Acher A, Thibon P, et al. Association of localized intravascular coagulopathy with venous malformations. Arch Dermatol. 2008; 144(7):873–877

[27] Legiehn GM, Heran MKS. Venous malformations: classification, development, diagnosis, and interventional radiologic management. Radiol Clin North Am. 2008; 46(3):545–597, vi

[28] Veräjänkorva E, Rautio R, Giordano S, Koskivuo I, Savolainen O. The efficiency of sclerotherapy in the treatment of vascular malformations: a retrospective study of 63 patients. Plast Surg Int. 2016; 2016:2809152

[29] Burrows PE, Mason KP. Percutaneous treatment of low flow vascular malformations. J Vasc Interv Radiol. 2004; 15(5):431–445

[30] Azene E, Mitchell S, Radvany M, Agrawal N, Eisele D, Weiss C. Foamed bleomycin sclerosis of airway venous malformations: the role of interspecialty collaboration. Laryngoscope. 2016; 126(12):2726–2732

[31] O'Mara DM, DiCamillo PA, Gilson WD, et al. MR-guided percutaneous sclerotherapy of low-flow vascular malformations: clinical experience using a 1.5 tesla MR system. J Magn Reson Imaging. 2017; 45(4):1154–1162

[32] Boll DT, Merkle EM, Lewin JS. Low-flow vascular malformations: MR-guided percutaneous sclerotherapy in qualitative and quantitative assessment of therapy and outcome. Radiology. 2004; 233(2):376–384

[33] Lewin JS, Merkle EM, Duerk JL, Tarr RW. Low-flow vascular malformations in the head and neck: safety and feasibility of MR imaging-guided percutaneous sclerotherapy–preliminary experience with 14 procedures in three patients. Radiology. 1999; 211(2):566–570

[34] Ali S, Weiss CR, Sinha A, Eng J, Mitchell SE. The treatment of venous malformations with percutaneous sclerotherapy at a single academic medical center. Phlebology. 2016; 31(9):603–609

[35] Idle MR, Monaghan AM, Lamin SM, Grant SWJ. N-butyl-2-cyanoacrylate (NBCA) tissue adhesive as a haemostatic agent in a venous malformation of the mandible. Br J Oral Maxillofac Surg. 2013; 51(6):565–567

Index

Note: Page numbers set **bold** or *italic* indicate headings or figures, respectively.